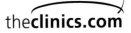

CARDIOLOGY CLINICS

Advanced 12-Lead Electrocardiography

GUEST EDITOR
S. Serge Barold, MD

CONSULTING EDITOR
Michael H. Crawford, MD

August 2006 • Volume 24 • Number 3

SAUNDERS

An Imprint of Elsevier, Inc.
PHILADELPHIA   LONDON   TORONTO   MONTREAL   SYDNEY   TOKYO

W.B. SAUNDERS COMPANY
A Division of Elsevier Inc.

Elsevier Inc. • 1600 John F. Kennedy Blvd., Suite 1800 • Philadelphia, Pennsylvania 19103-2899

http://www.theclinics.com

CARDIOLOGY CLINICS
August 2006
Editor: Karen Sorensen

Volume 24, Number 3
ISSN 0733-8651
ISBN 1-4160-3876-0

Reprints. For copies of 100 or more, of articles in this publication, please contact the Commercial Reprints Department, Elsevier Inc., 360 Park Avenue South, New York, New York 10010-1710. Tel. (212) 633-3813 Fax: (212) 462-1935 email: reprints@elsevier.com.

The ideas and opinions expressed in *Cardiology Clinics* do not necessarily reflect those of the Publisher. The Publisher does not assume any responsibility for any injury and/or damage to persons or property arising out of or related to any use of the material contained in this periodical. The reader is advised to check the appropriate medical literature and the product information currently provided by the manufacturer of each drug to be administered to verify the dosage, the method and duration of administration, or contraindications. It is the responsibility of the treating physician or other health care professional, relying on independent experience and knowledge of the patient, to determine drug dosages and the best treatment for the patient. Mention of any product in this issue should not be construed as endorsement by the contributors, editors, or the Publisher of the product or manufacturers' claims.

Cardiology Clinics (ISSN 0733-8651) is published quarterly by Elsevier Inc., 360 Park Avenue South, New York, NY 10010-1710. Months of issue are February, May, August, and November. Business and editorial Offices: 1600 John F. Kennedy Blvd., Suite 1800, Philadelphia, PA 19103-2899. Customer Service Office: 6277 Sea Harbor Drive, Orlando, FL 32887-4800. Periodicals postage paid at New York, NY, and additional mailing offices. Subscription prices are $170.00 per year for US individuals, $266.00 per year for US institutions, $85.00 per year for US students and residents, $210.00 per year for Canadian individuals, $323.00 per year for Canadian institutions, $230.00 per year for international individuals, $323.00 per year for international institutions and $115.00 per year for Canadian and foreign students/residents. To receive student/resident rate, orders must be accompanied by name of affiliated institution, data of term, and the *signature* of program/residency coordinator on institution letterhead. Orders will be billed at individual rate until proof of status is received. Foreign air speed delivery is included in all *Clinics* subscription prices. All prices are subject to change without notice. POSTMASTER: Send address changes to *Cardiology Clinics*, Elsevier Periodicals Customer Service, 6277 Sea Harbor Drive, Orlando, FL 32887-4800. **Customer Service: 1-800-654-2452 (US). From outside of the US, call 1-407-345-1000.**

Cardiology Clinics is also published in Spanish by McGraw-Hill Interamericana Editores S. A., P.O. Box 5-237, 06500, Mexico D. F., Mexico; in Portuguese by Reichmann and Alfonso Editores Rio de Janeiro, Brazil; and in Greek by Dimitrios P. Lagos, 8 Pondon Street, GR115-28 Ilissia, Greece.

Cardiology Clinics is covered in *Index Medicus, Excerpta Medica, The Cumulative Index to Nursing and Allied Health Literature* (INAHL).

Printed in the United States of America.

CONSULTING EDITOR

MICHAEL H. CRAWFORD, MD, Professor of Medicine, Lucie Stern Chair in Cardiology, University of California, San Francisco; Chief of Clinical Cardiology, University of California, San Francisco Medical Center, San Francisco, California

GUEST EDITOR

S. SERGE BAROLD, MD, Clinical Professor of Medicine, University of South Florida College of Medicine, Tampa; Cardiologist, Tampa General Hospital, Tampa, Florida

CONTRIBUTORS

CESAR ALBERTE, MD, Assistant Professor of Medicine, Indiana University School of Medicine, Krannert Institute of Cardiology, Indianapolis, Indiana

STANLEY ANDERSON, MB, BS, FRACP, Cabrini Hospital, Victoria, Australia

SHAUL ATAR, MD, Associate Professor of Medicine, Division of Cardiology, University of Texas Medical Branch, Galveston, Texas

ALEJANDRO BARBAGELATA, MD, Associate Professor of Medicine, Division of Cardiology, University of Texas Medical Branch, Galveston, Texas

S. SERGE BAROLD, MD, Clinical Professor of Medicine, University of South Florida College of Medicine, Tampa; and Cardiologist, Tampa General Hospital, Tampa, Florida

DEEPAK BHAKTA, MD, Assistant Professor of Clinical Medicine, Indiana University School of Medicine, Krannert Institute of Cardiology, Indianapolis, Indiana

YOCHAI BIRNBAUM, MD, Professor of Medicine, Director of the Intensive Cardiac Care Unit and the Heart Station, Division of Cardiology, University of Texas Medical Branch, Galveston, Texas

RORY CHILDERS, MD, Professor, Department of Medicine, Section of Cardiology, University of Chicago Medical Center, Chicago, IL

PETER CLEMMENSEN, MD, PhD, Rigs Hospital, The Heart Center, University of Copenhagen, Copenhagen, Denmark

ANNE B. CURTIS, MD, Division of Cardiology, University of South Florida College of Medicine and Tampa General Hospital, Tampa, Florida

MITHILESH K. DAS, MD, Assistant Professor of Clinical Medicine, Indiana University School of Medicine, Krannert Institute of Cardiology, Indianapolis, Indiana

BARBARA J. DREW, RN, PhD, Professor of Nursing and Clinical Professor of Medicine, Department of Physiological Nursing, University of California, San Francisco, San Francisco, California

HENRIK ENGBLOM, MD, PhD CANDIDATE, Department of Clinical Physiology, Lund University Hospital, Sweden

LEONARD GETTES, MD, Division of Cardiology, The University of North Carolina at Chapel Hill, Chapel Hill, North Carolina

MICHAEL C. GIUDICI, MD, Division of Cardiology, Genesis Heart Institute, Davenport, Iowa

NORA GOLDSCHLAGER, MD, Professor of Clinical Medicine; Associate Chief, Division of Cardiology; and Director, Coronary Care Unit, ECG Laboratory and Pacemaker Clinic, San Francisco General Hospital, San Francisco, California

ANTON GORGELS, MD, Professor, Department of Cardiology, Cardiovascular Research Institute Maastricht, Maastricht, The Netherlands

BENGT HERWEG, MD, Division of Cardiology, University of South Florida College of Medicine and Tampa General Hospital, Tampa, Florida

VINZENZ HOMBACH, MD, Professor of Medicine/Cardiology, Department of Internal Medicine II, Cardiology/Angiology/Pneumology/Sports and Rehabilitation Medicine, University Hospital of Ulm, Ulm, Germany

RICHARD H. HONGO, MD, Staff Electrophysiologist, Division of Cardiology, California Pacific Medical Center, San Francisco, California

J. WILLIS HURST, MD, MACP, Active Consultant to the Division of Cardiology, Candler Professor and Chairman, Department of Medicine Emeritus, Emory University School of Medicine, Atlanta, Georgia

MARK JOSEPHSON, MD, Director, Harvard-Thorndike Electrophysiology Institute and Arrhythmia Service, Harvard Medical School, Beth Israel Deaconess Medical Center, Boston, Massachusetts

PAUL KLIGFIELD, MD, Professor, Department of Medicine, Cornell University Medical College, New York; Director, Cardiac Graphics Laboratory; and Medical Director, Cardiac Health Center, The New York-Presbyterian Hospital, Cornell Campus, New York, New York

UDAY N. KUMAR, MD, Cardiac Electrophysiology Fellow, Division of Cardiology, Department of Medicine, University of California, San Francisco, San Francisco, California

TOBIN LIM, MD, Research Assistant, Department of Medicine, Duke University Medical Center, Durham, North Carolina

PETER W. MACFARLANE, DSc, FESC, FRCP, Professor of Electrocardiology, Division of Cardiovascular and Medical Sciences, Faculty of Medicine, University of Glasgow, Glasgow, Scotland; and Royal Infirmary, Glasgow, Scotland, United Kingdom

FRANK I. MARCUS, MD, Professor of Medicine, Department of Medicine, University of Arizona Health Sciences Center, Tucson, Arizona

JOHN M. MILLER, MD, Professor of Medicine; and Director Clinical Cardiac Electrophysiology, Indiana University School of Medicine, Krannert Institute of Cardiology, Indianapolis, Indiana

GIRISH NAIR, MD, Senior Fellow in Cardiac Electrophysiology, Indiana University School of Medicine, Krannert Institute of Cardiology, Indianapolis, Indiana

PETER OTT, MD, Assistant Professor of Clinical Medicine, Director of Arrhythmia Services, Department of Medicine, University of Arizona Health Sciences Center, Tucson, Arizona

OLLE PAHLM, MD, PhD, Associate Professor, Department of Clinical Physiology, Lund University Hospital, Sweden

RAJNI K. RAO, MD, Chief Cardiology Fellow, Division of Cardiology, Department of Medicine, University of California, San Francisco, San Francisco, California

CONTRIBUTORS

MELVIN M. SCHEINMAN, MD, Professor of Medicine, Walter H. Shorenstein Endowed Chair in Cardiology, Cardiac Electrophysiology, Division of Cardiology, Department of Medicine, University of California, San Francisco, San Francisco, California

RONALD SELVESTER, MD, Long Beach Memorial Hospital, Long Beach, California

ELIN TRÄGÅRDH, MD, PhD CANDIDATE, Department of Clinical Physiology, Lund University Hospital, Sweden

GALEN WAGNER, MD, Associate Professor of Medicine, Division of Cardiology, Duke University Medical Center, Durham, North Carolina

HEIN WELLENS, MD, Professor, Department of Cardiology, University of Maastricht; and Chairman, Department of Cardiology, University Hospital Maastricht, Maastricht, The Netherlands

ANIL V. YADAV, MD, Assistant Professor of Clinical Medicine, Indiana University School of Medicine, Krannert Institute of Cardiology, Indianapolis, Indiana

CONTENTS

> *There must be no pretense in medicine.* When a physician orders an electrocardiogram on a patient he or she must be able to interpret it. Not only that, he or she must understand the mechanism responsible for the abnormality and how the abnormality fits, or does not fit, with the other data collected from the patient.

> The standard 12-lead ECG is a common diagnostic test that provides a wealth of diagnostic information of value for clinical decision making. Its value, however, depends upon the accuracy of its recording. This article presents common errors in clinical electrocardiography including inaccurate lead placement, inappropriate serial comparisons using different lead sets, lead wire reversals, inappropriate filter settings, and excessively noisy signals. Practical information is provided to prevent errors and to improve the quality and utility of ECGs.

> The number of leads needed in clinical electrocardiography depends on the clinical problem to be solved. The standard 12-lead ECG is so well established that alternative lead systems must prove their advantage through well-conducted clinical studies to achieve clinical acceptance. Certain additional leads seem to add valuable information in specific patient groups. The use of a large number of leads (eg, in body surface potential mapping) may add clinically relevant information, but it is cumbersome and its clinical advantage is yet to be proven. Reduced lead sets emulate the 12-lead ECG reasonably well and are especially advantageous in emergency situations.

the abundance of good criteria for determining the diagnosis in cases of WQRST, they are of no use if they cannot be readily applied in an urgent clinical situation because they cannot be easily recalled or are too complex and cumbersome to use. It may be that refresher courses in the differential diagnosis of WQRST, especially for emergency physicians who are often the "first responders" to patients with WQRST, can improve physicians' diagnostic accuracy in this important disorder.

FORTHCOMING ISSUES

RECENT ISSUES

ELSEVIER
SAUNDERS

Cardiol Clin 24 (2006) xiii

CARDIOLOGY
CLINICS

Foreword

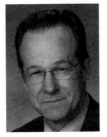

Michael H. Crawford, MD
Consulting Editor

The traditional 12-lead ECG continues to be the first-line test in the evaluation of chest pain syndromes. Characteristic ECG changes help define myocardial infarction and ischemia. Quality assurance algorithms usually require an ECG within 10 minutes of hospital arrival for the complaint of chest discomfort. It is also the mainstay in the assessment of chest pain after percutaneous coronary interventions and in the assessment of the adequacy of reperfusion after thrombolytic therapy. Thus, the ECG is the stalwart of ischemic heart disease management.

An ECG is often the first step in evaluating patients who have palpitations, syncope, or suspected cardiac arrhythmias. It may detect frequent or persistent arrhythmias, and it may reveal the substrate for arrhythmias such as left atrial enlargement, hypokalemia, long QT interval, and pre-excitation. In addition, certain ECG abnormalities may indicate a higher risk of sudden cardiac death. Finally, the ECG is useful for detecting cardiac chamber enlargement or hypertrophy.

Dr. Barold has assembled a world-class group of physicians to write the articles that appear in this issue. They are all ECG experts who keep the flame alive in a field that is mature yet not static. In addition to discussing the clinical issues mentioned above, important technical issues, pitfalls, and artifacts are covered. Computerized ECG interpretation is also discussed. Anyone who cares for patients will benefit from reading this issue.

Michael H. Crawford, MD
Division of Cardiology
Department of Medicine
University of California
San Francisco Medical Center
505 Parnassus Ave., Box 0124
San Francisco, CA 94143-0124, USA

E-mail address: crawfordm@medicine.ucsf.edu

ELSEVIER
SAUNDERS

Cardiol Clin 24 (2006) xv–xvi

CARDIOLOGY
CLINICS

Preface

Advanced 12-Lead Electrocardiography

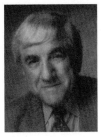

S. Serge Barold, MD
Guest Editor

The electrocardiogram (ECG) is the oldest and the most commonly used cardiology procedure. The year 2002 marked the centennial of Willem Einthoven's first recording of the ECG in a clinically applicable fashion with a string galvanometer of his design. The ECG is noninvasive, simple to record, and its cost is minimal. Possibly no other medical invention has had greater impact or is so universally used all over the world. Despite competition from many new procedures, it has remained in continuous use for 104 years. Electrocardiography obviously has strengths and weaknesses, but it remains a well-established, indispensable diagnostic tool. The clinical applicability and importance of the 12-lead ECG continue to grow in patients with all kinds of heart disease, as outlined in this issue of *Cardiology Clinics*. In this context it is important to know what the ECG can do better than other diagnostic methods.

Many relatively recent advances in electrocardiography have increased its complexity, creating a shortage of properly trained electrocardiographers.

Charles Fisch, a renowned electrocardiographer, has repeatedly emphasized this problem, and has reminded us that this issue dates back to the early days of electrocardiography as indicated by Carl Wiggers in the preface of *Principles and Practice of Electrocardiography* in 1929. Wiggers stated that "unfortunately, the training of medical manpower in the use of such apparatus and the intelligent interpretation of the electrocardiogram has not kept pace with the increased demand. Few courses in electrocardiography are included in undergraduate and postgraduate curricula in medical schools, so that opportunity for systematic instruction is decidedly restricted." Fisch was correct in stating that the issue of manpower addressed by Wiggers 87 years ago is still with us today. At the beginning of the twenty-first century there is also a loss of interest in "low-tech" electrocardiography by younger physicians and scientists. For this reason, in the United States, specialty board certification in cardiology (American Board of Internal Medicine) requires passing a separate portion of the certification examination

0733-8651/06/$ - see front matter © 2006 Elsevier Inc. All rights reserved.
doi:10.1016/j.ccl.2006.04.014

cardiology.theclinics.com

in cardiology that deals only with ECG interpretation.

The contributions to this issue of *Cardiology Clinics* are reminiscent of Fisch's 1980 statement that "He who maintains new knowledge in electrocardiography is no longer possible or contributive ignores history." The new information in this volume confirms that knowledge related to the "simple" 12-lead ECG continues to grow and assume more and more importance in daily clinical practice.

S. Serge Barold, MD
University of South Florida College of Medicine
Tampa General Hospital
5806 Mariner's Watch Drive
Tampa, FL 33615, USA

E-mail address: ssbarold@aol.com

Cardiol Clin 24 (2006) 305–307

The Interpretation of Electrocardiograms: Pretense or a Well-Developed Skill?

J. Willis Hurst, MD, MACP

Department of Medicine, Division of Cardiology, Emory University School of Medicine,
1462 Clifton Road NE, Suite 301, Atlanta, GA 30322, USA

Graduating medical students can be forgiven for being unskilled because even our most highly ranked medical schools only *introduce* students to medical skills such as history taking, physical examination, electrocardiography, and radiography. Stated another way—clinical skills are not perfected in medical school. Because this is true, such skills must be mastered during house staff training. However, it is patently apparent that house officers are not mastering the skills, and teachers are not reaching them. This is tragic, because house officer training programs were created so that trainees could become competent in the use of clinical skills. Because clinical skills are still used in the practice of medicine, it is indeed proper to be concerned about the obvious deterioration of house officer training.

This essay deals exclusively with the decline in interest and clinical competence in electrocardiography—the most commonly performed procedure by internists and family practitioners. The decline is also true for the subspecialties of internal medicine including cardiology. A few suggestions for improving the interpretive process are also discussed [1].

To perform a procedure and not be able to interpret the information yielded by the procedure is *pretense*. The patient believes the physician knows how to interpret the tracings. It is not a willful act of pretense on the part of the physician. As the author sees it—many physicians do not know that they don't know, and believe they can interpret electrocardiograms. After all, they have memorized a few patterns and a little of the language and seem

to get by. Unfortunately, their memory is limited, and they do not identify all the abnormalities in the electrocardiogram. This, of course, leads to numerous errors of omission and commission.

Why has the interpretations of electrocardiograms deteriorated and what is responsible for the mistaken view that electrocardiography is no longer needed

There are those who believe that the information yielded by an electrocardiogram has not changed in the last few decades. They argue that little new has been discovered, and that an electrocardiogram is no longer needed in the examination of the heart. They naively believe that other technology has replaced electrocardiography. I ask such skeptics if they believe we are no longer dependent on the electrocardiogram for the recognition of cardiac arrhythmia. They then admit that the electrocardiogram is needed to identify certain cardiac arrhythmias. I then point out that the treatment of acute coronary syndromes is based entirely on the abnormalities in the electrocardiogram. Therefore, the correct interpretation of the electrocardiogram is needed more now than anytime in the history of medicine.

I ask the skeptic when did he or she discover an epsilon [2] wave, a Brugada wave, [3] or an Osborn wave [4] in a tracing? I ask how do you identify primary and secondary T waves or primary and secondary S-T segments? I may also ask them to discuss the ventricular gradient and when do they use it.

It usually becomes apparent that those who downgrade the use of the electrocardiogram, but keep recording tracings, are arguing from a poorly

E-mail address: jhurst@emory.edu

thought out, but obviously defensive position. The fact is, they have lost touch with the skill.

Dependence on the computer interpretation

Many of us hailed the new computer interpretation as a great advance. Therefore, it is sad to report that it has failed us [1]. We hoped it would be accurate and would serve as a teacher to trainees. Regrettably, it is not accurate and has failed as a teacher, leaving those who wish to learn actually learning very little. Then, too, the computer software in many hospitals is 2 or more decades old, so the new information created during the last 2 decades is not recognized by the computer.

In addition, although most computers calculate the frontal plane direction of the P, QRS, and T vectors, they do not compute the spatial orientation of the vectors.

Finally, and most important, the computer readout rarely gives the physician a differential diagnosis, indicating the probability that certain types of heart disease are present. After all, that is what the clinician needs.

Poor teaching

It is clear that the deterioration of the teaching of electrocardiography is the major cause of the poor performance of graduates of house staff programs. Trainees do not rotate through a 2-month period of intensive study under the supervision of a true teacher as they did formerly. Simultaneously, teaching ward rounds have changed considerably. It is uncommon for a teaching attending to discuss and demonstrate the subtleties of the history, physical abnormalities, radiologic abnormalities, and electrocardiographic abnormalities that are germane to the diagnosis and treatment of the patient. The teaching attending often simply states what high-tech procedure is needed rather than teach electrocardiography or any other skill. Therefore, the trainee is left with the view that the electrocardiogram is no longer used in any obvious way. This actually teaches the trainee to become a subcontractor. Knowing that the teaching attending will order an echocardiogram, a nuclear test, and cardiac catherization, the trainee simply orders several procedures, including an electrocardiogram, and lets someone else make decisions based on the results of these procedures.

Now there is less teaching time than ever. The Residency Review Committee has decreased the number of hours a trainee can remain in the hospital, and this has decreased the time a true teacher can discuss the basis of electrocardiography, leaving the trainee to memorize a few patterns. Not knowing what they mean, the trainee quickly forgets them.

The method used in teaching

Here this author admits a strong bias. I have tried having trainees memorize patterns of electrocardiographic abnormalities, and have been miserably disappointed. I strongly recommend the Grant method of interpretation [5,6]. His basic work has been updated, and those who master it have a tool that can be used to interpret tracings they have never seen before [7]. The use of vector concepts leads the user to understand the cause of abnormalities found in the tracing and permits one to measure in degrees the magnitude of the abnormality. Also, the pattern worshippers should realize that the best way to learn patterns is to become proficient in the Grant method of interpretation of electrocardiograms.

How can skilled interpreters be identified?

The answer to this question is obvious—an interpreter is skilled when, after viewing an electrocardiogram, he or she can answer the following question. What heart disease, or diseases, can produce this tracing? A skilled interpreter can either identify the cardiac diagnosis or give a carefully thought out differential diagnosis.

Suggestions for improvement

Improvement will not come unless house staff training programs are restructured so that trainees can learn skills, including cognitive skills, from a true teacher of medicine. Protected time for teaching is necessary, just as protected time for research is needed by research-oriented faculty. The updated Grant methods should be taught in specially designed seminars and implemented by teaching attendings when they see patients with trainees. Trainees should become knowledgeable of the Grant method of interpretation by mid-year of their internship, and use it on every patient they see in whom an electrocardiogram has been performed. They should apply the method to each tracing they see and correlate their perception of the abnormalities with the other data collected from the patient.

The wise men and women who determine the content of board examinations should consider making the current interpretation of 12 carefully chosen electrocardiograms mandatory to pass the examination. This is justified, because many physicians other that cardiologists order electrocardiograms.

Summary

There must be no pretense in medicine. When a physician orders an electrocardiogram on a patient he or she must be able to interpret it. Not only that, he or she must understand the mechanism responsible for the abnormality and how the abnormality fits, or does not fit, with the other data collected from the patient.

Some of the reasons the teaching of electro-cardiography has declined have been discussed, and a few suggestions have been offered to improve a rather serious educational problem.

References

[1] Hurst JW. Current status of clinical electrocardiography with suggestions for the improvement of the interpretive process. Am J Cardiol 2003;92:1072–9.

[2] Hurst JW. Naming of the waves in the ECG, with a brief account of their genesis. Circulation 1998;98: 1937–42.

[3] Brugada P, Brugada J. Right bundle ranch block, persistent ST segment elevation and sudden cardiac death: a distinct clinical and electrocardiography syndrome. A multimember report. J Am Coll Cardiol 1992;20:1391–6.

[4] Osborn JJ. Experimental hypothermia; respiratory and blood pH changes in relation to cardiac function. Am J Physiol 1953;175:389–98.

[5] Grant RP. Spatial vector electrocardiography: a method for calculating the spatial electrical vectors of the heart from conventional leads. Circulation 1950;2:676–95.

[6] Grant RP. Clinical electrocardiography: the spatial vector approach. New York: McGraw-Hill Book Company; 1957. p. 1–218.

[7] Hurst JW. Interpreting electrocardiograms: using basic principles and vector concepts. New York: Marcel Dekker; 2001. p. 119–20.

Pitfalls and Artifacts in Electrocardiography

Barbara J. Drew, RN, PhD

*Department of Physiological Nursing, University of California, University of California, San Francisco,
2 Koret Way, San Francisco, CA 94143*

The ECG is a noninvasive technique that is inexpensive, simple, and reproducible. It is one of the most commonly used diagnostic tests that can be recorded rapidly with extremely portable equipment and generally is always obtainable. The ECG contains a wealth of diagnostic information routinely used to guide clinical decision making. For some conditions, such as transient myocardial ischemia, the ECG remains the reference standard for diagnosis despite the advance of many other diagnostic techniques.

ECG diagnoses are valid, however, only if electrodes are placed in correct anatomic locations, lead wires are attached to the appropriate electrode, and the recording is of good technical quality (eg, proper filtering, absence of extraneous electrical noise). In addition, if comparisons of serial ECGs are required to determine trends over time (eg, to determine whether ST-segment changes of ischemia are resolving after early reperfusion therapy), all recordings must be made using a consistent technique. For example, each ECG should be recorded with electrodes in the same location, with the patient's body in the same (supine) position, and using the same lead configuration.

This article reviews commonly encountered errors in clinical electrocardiography. Errors related to inaccurate lead placement, lead wire reversals, noisy ECG signals, inappropriate filter settings, and serial comparisons between inconsistent lead sets are reviewed. In addition, recommendations are made for preventing these pitfalls and artifacts that may lead to inappropriate therapy and adverse patient outcomes in clinical electrocardiography.

Inaccurate lead placement

Limb leads

When Einthoven [1] introduced the standard limb leads nearly 100 years ago, he measured electrical potentials from the lower left leg and right and left wrists. When the arms are extended, these three electrode sites form a triangle with points remote and nearly equidistant from the heart. This equilateral triangle is the basis for Einthoven's formula, which states that, at any given instant, the amplitude of any wave in lead II is equal to the sum of the amplitudes of the corresponding wave in leads I and III. To this day, ECG machines record leads I and II and then mathematically derive lead III using Einthoven's formula.

Wilson [2] later pointed out that because all points on a given extremity have the same potential, it does not matter whether the electrode is connected to the limb end or the trunk end of the extremity. In fact, Wilson referred to the limbs as simply extension cords of the lead wires. Wilson went on to warn, however, that if limb electrodes were placed off the limbs on to the body torso, particularly if placed within 10 to 15 inches of the heart, ECG waveforms would be altered significantly [2].

These principles are important to appreciate today in recording a standard ECG. In general, placement of the electrodes for the limb leads (right arm, left arm, left leg) can be anywhere on the limb without substantially affecting ECG waveforms and diagnostic interpretation. When limb electrodes are placed on the torso, however,

E-mail address: barbara.drew@nursing.ucsf.edu

particularly if they are moved closer to the heart (eg, arm electrodes placed closer to the sternum than the shoulders), the result may be clinically important misdiagnoses in computerized and physician interpretations [3,4].

In most cases, the change in diagnosis between a torso-positioned versus a standard ECG is either loss or appearance of Q waves of infarction in the inferior leads. Changes in ST-T waves (ST depression, T-wave inversion or flattening) also may occur and could be interpreted as acute myocardial ischemia when serial comparisons are made between standard and torso-positioned ECGs. Finally, P-, R-, and S-wave voltages may be different between standard and torso-positioned ECGs, resulting in differences regarding presence or absence of atrial overload or left ventricular hypertrophy.

The practical application of these principles is that a consistent method for placing limb electrodes should be used throughout a hospital system, especially if 12-lead ECGs are stored in a computer system for subsequent serial comparison. In some critical care and emergency hospital units, a torso-positioned 12-lead ECG is recorded continuously. Some manufacturers tout the advantage of 12-lead cardiac monitors as a substantial financial savings because cardiac monitor tracings can be substituted for ECGs previously recorded with standard ECG machines by specially trained ECG technicians. Serial comparisons should not be made between limb-positioned and torso-positioned ECGs, however, because observed differences may be caused entirely by the different lead methods.

Another potential difference in 12-lead ECGs printed at a central nurses' station in a monitored hospital unit is that the patient may not be in a supine position during the tracing. Body position changes have been reported to be the most common cause of false ST-segment monitor alarms [5] and have resulted in inappropriate therapy and adverse patient outcome [6].

Precordial leads

According to the principles laid out by Wilson [2], slight misplacement of leads that are located near the heart can produce substantial alterations in ECG waveforms. Fig. 1 shows how valuable QRS morphologic criteria to distinguish ventricular tachycardia from supraventricular tachycardia with aberrant conduction disappear when the lead V_1 electrode is moved just one intercostal space from its correct anatomic location.

Correct placement of the lead V_1 electrode is especially important because it is the first precordial lead to be positioned, and the remaining five precordial leads are placed in relation to it. Therefore, if the V_1 electrode is placed superior to its correct location, leads V_{2-6} also may be misplaced superiorly. Wenger and Kligfield [7] reported clinically important differences in precordial lead placement when serial ECGs were recorded in different hospital units by different personnel. These investigators found that leads V_1 and V_2 were misplaced superiorly in 50% of the recordings, occasionally reaching the second intercostal space. Zema and colleagues [8] reported that high and low placement of precordial electrodes produced a change in R-wave amplitude of about 1 mm per interspace, with smaller R waves when V_1 and V_2 were placed superior to the correct fourth intercostal space. Thus, the misdiagnosis of poor R-wave progression or anterior myocardial

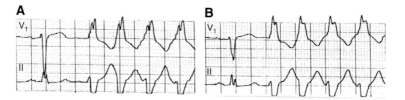

Fig. 1. (*A*) Onset of wide QRS complex tachycardia shows an rR′ pattern in lead V_1, which is unhelpful in distinguishing between ventricular tachycardia and supraventricular tachycardia with aberrant conduction. Examination of the patient revealed that the V_1 electrode was misplaced to the fifth rather than the fourth intercostal space. (*B*) After lead placement was corrected, another episode of wide QRS complex tachycardia showed an Rr′ pattern, which is strongly suggestive of ventricular tachycardia. Subsequent invasive cardiac electrophysiologic study confirmed the patient had recurrent monomorphic ventricular tachycardia. (*From* Drew BJ, Califf RM, Funk M, et al. Practice standards for electrocardiographic monitoring in hospital settings. Circulation 2004;110:2721–46; with permission.)

infarction may result from superiorly displaced precordial leads.

An important factor that complicates placement of precordial leads in women is large, pendulous breasts, particularly in obese and older women. In young women, the V_4 location in the fifth intercostal space at the midclavicular line often falls at the inferior margin of the breast where the fleshy part of the breast joins the chest wall. Thus, in young women, leads V_4 and V_5 can be placed accurately on the chest wall below the breast. In older women, however, the nipple end of the breast sags below the breast attachment to the chest wall such that visualization of the V_4 site requires lifting up the breast. In such instances, electrodes could be placed accurately in the correct intercostal space either by placing electrodes over the top of breast tissue or by lifting up the breast and placing them under the breast against the chest wall.

Research reports about which of these two options are best are conflicting. Rautaharju and colleagues [9] recommend that precordial leads be placed over the top of the breast, because in so doing they found only negligible attenuation of R-wave voltage. Colaco and colleagues [10], however, found that women who had large breasts (bra size D or greater) had clinically significant attenuation of R waves in the anterior precordial leads V_{1-4}. They also reported that if precordial leads were misplaced inferiorly (ie, below pendulous breasts), R-wave voltage in leads V_{5-6} were attenuated. These investigators also reported the prevalence of poor R-wave progression was 19% in women compared with 11% in men. They concluded that this 8% gender difference might have been caused in part by electrodes being placed on top of breast tissue because there was no evidence of prior anterior infarction in most of the women who had poor R-wave progression.

Because of these conflicting research findings, it seems reasonable to place electrodes under the breast, especially in large-breasted or obese women, to minimize the likelihood of altering R-wave voltage. If technicians are uncomfortable lifting up breast tissue in women, placement over the breast in the correct anatomic location is acceptable, however. An unacceptable method is to place precordial leads superior or inferior to the breast, because R-wave voltage and progression will be altered.

Occasionally, inaccurate precordial lead placement is necessary in hospitalized patients because of chest wounds, placement of defibrillator pads, or for other reasons. In such circumstances, the alternative electrode sites should be clearly identified on the final ECG.

Inappropriate serial comparisons using different lead sets

A phenomenon occurring in current hospital settings that may make serial ECG comparisons misleading is that patients may have cardiac monitors that provide 12-lead ECG tracings that are mathematically derived from a reduced number of leads [11,12]. Such derived 12-lead ECGs are comparable to the standard ECG for diagnoses important in the immediate care setting, such as distinguishing ventricular tachycardia from supraventricular tachycardia with aberrant conduction, detection of new bundle-branch block, and ST-segment changes of acute myocardial ischemia [13–16]. For serial comparisons that require measurement of precise amplitudes (eg, to determine whether voltages indicative of left ventricular hypertrophy have decreased or whether ST-segment elevations have resolved following reperfusion therapy), however, derived and standard ECG comparisons should not be made. Fig. 2 illustrates ST-segment amplitude differences between simultaneously recorded derived and standard leads in a patient who had acute myocardial infarction enrolled in a prospective clinical trial to compare the two lead methods in patients presenting to the emergency department with chest pain [15].

Therefore, as in the case for torso-positioned ECGs, 12-lead ECGs recorded from reduced lead sets should not be compared serially with 12-lead ECGs recorded in the standard way [17].

Limb lead wire reversals

There are five limb lead wire reversals that produce abnormal ECG findings. A sixth error in connecting the ECG cable, reversal of the right leg (RL) and left leg (LL) electrodes, does not alter the ECG because potentials recorded from the right and left legs are practically the same.

Right arm–left arm reversal

The most common error when attaching an ECG cable to a patient is right arm (RA)–left arm (LA) lead wire reversal, which means that lead I looks upside down (inverted P, QRS, and T waves). If the P wave is upright and only the

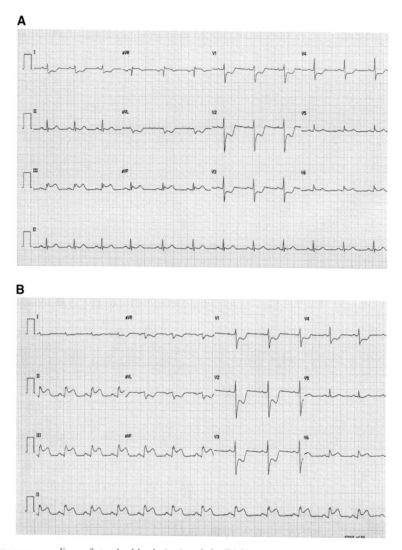

Fig. 2. Simultaneous recordings of standard leads (*top*) and the EASI system that derives a 12-lead ECG using just 5 electrodes (Philips Co., Andover, MA) (*bottom*). Although both ECGs indicate acute inferior myocardial infarction, ST-segment amplitudes differ considerably between the two methods. Thus, if the top tracing had been recorded in the emergency department with a standard ECG machine before fibrinolytic therapy, and the bottom tracing had been recorded minutes later in the coronary care unit with a bedside cardiac monitor, serial comparison between the two lead methods would have suggested erroneously that ST-segment deviation was getting worse. (*From* Philips Company, Andover, MA; with permission [EASI recording].)

QRS is negative, the problem is not lead wire reversal but an abnormal QRS axis, most likely resulting from some pathology causing extreme right axis deviation. If, however, the P wave is inverted also, there are two possible causes: (1) RA-LA lead wire reversal, or (2) dextrocardia. It is a simple matter to distinguish between these two conditions by examining a set of leads that do not depend upon proper placement of arm electrodes (ie, the precordial leads). In RA-LA lead wire reversal, the precordial leads will look normal with a small R wave in V_1 that progressively increases in consecutive V leads until it is maximally positive in V_5 or V_6. In contrast, an individual born with the heart positioned on the right side in mirror-image fashion (sinus inversus) will have no R-wave progression, with a negative QRS complex in lead V_6 (Fig. 3).

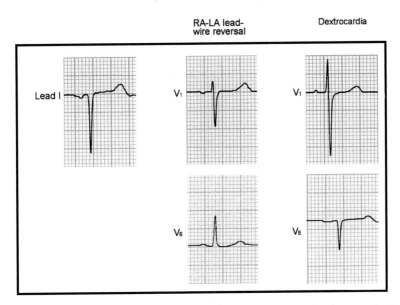

Fig. 3. Method to distinguish RA-LA lead wire reversal from dextrocardia. When there is a negative P and QRS complex in lead I, examine the precordial leads to determine whether they have normal R-wave progression (RA-LA reversal does not affect precordial leads) or abnormal R-wave progression with a negative QRS in V_6 (dextrocardia affects the precordial leads because the heart is not on the left side).

Left arm–left leg reversal

LA-LL reversal means that lead I on the ECG is actually lead II, lead II is actually lead I, and lead III is upside down because the positive and negative poles are reversed. In addition, leads aVL and aVF are reversed. This type of reversal may be difficult to identify because it may not appear out of the ordinary except for left axis deviation, which is common in hospitalized patients. One clue is the appearance of a P wave in "lead I" that is larger in amplitude than in "lead II." The "lead I" P wave actually represents the P wave of the true lead II, which typically has the largest P-wave amplitude of any limb lead.

Right arm–left leg reversal

RA-LL reversal causes lead I to be the inverse of lead II, lead II to be the inverse of lead I, and lead II is upside down because the positive and negative poles are reversed. In addition, aVR and aVF are reversed. This situation produces highly abnormal-looking limb leads, with leads I, II, III, and aVF being negative and aVR being upright. During sinus rhythm, it is highly unlikely to have a QRS axis in the bizarre quadrant of $-90°$ to $\pm 180°$, which is typical of this type of lead reversal.

Reversals involving the right leg and right or left arm

In reversals involving one of the arm lead wires switched with the RL lead wire, one lead (either lead II in the case of RA-RL reversal or lead III in the case of LA-RL reversal) records a zero potential difference between the legs, resulting in a flat line (termed a "far-field" signal).

Technically unacceptable ECG recordings

Excessively noisy signals

Hospitals are filled with equipment that can be a source of electrical artifact during the recording of an ECG. Moreover, ECGs recorded in the emergency department or other immediate care setting where patients may be restless or confused may be plagued with a noisy signal. Fig. 4 shows an example of a noisy signal that simulates ventricular tachycardia. Knight and colleagues [18] reported on the clinical implications of the misdiagnosis of artifact as ventricular tachycardia in 12 patients. Clinical consequences of the misdiagnoses in these patients included unnecessary cardiac catheterization in three patients, unnecessary medical therapies including intravenous antiarrhythmic agents in nine patients,

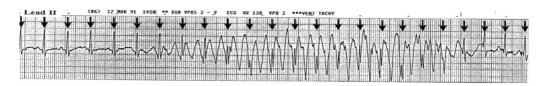

Fig. 4. False cardiac monitor alarm showing a noisy signal simulating ventricular tachycardia. Arrows point out the normal QRS complexes that can be discerned if one looks carefully and uses calipers to confirm their timing.

precordial thumps in two patients, implantation of a permanent pacemaker in one patient, and insertion of an implantable cardioverter-defibrillator in one patient. Moreover, hospital costs were high because of unnecessary testing, and patients were transferred to a higher level of intensive care or treated longer than necessary in the hospital.

Inappropriate filter settings

The problem of unacceptably noisy ECG recordings makes it tempting for clinicians to reprogram high-frequency filter settings to a lower number on ECG machines, especially in emergency departments and other immediate care settings. Clinical guidelines for recording a standard 12-lead ECG specify a high-frequency filter setting of no lower than 100 Hz [19]. Lowering the high-frequency filter from 100 to 40 Hz will eliminate noise caused by 60-cycle interference and other artifact. Clinically important high-frequency signals (eg, pacemaker stimuli or notches in the QRS complex) will be eliminated also, however.

The low-frequency filter should be set no higher than 0.05 Hz to avoid distortion of the ST segment [19]. Clinicians may violate this rule to minimize baseline wander and other artifacts, however.

In patients who have severe pain, tremor, or some other cause of an unacceptably noisy ECG signal, the filter switch on the ECG machine can be used after all attempts to eliminate the interference have failed. The change in filter setting should be documented on the final ECG.

Summary/clinical implications

The value of the ECG depends upon the accuracy of how it is obtained. Currently, many different types of health personnel record ECGs, including physician office workers, minimally trained hospital aides, ECG technicians, nurses from a variety of hospital units, and house staff. Thus, the potential exists for inconsistent

recording methods that are especially problematic when accurate diagnosis depends on comparison of serial ECG tracings. It is important to have a hospital/clinic policy for the recording of ECGs that includes appropriate filter settings, diagrams of accurate lead placement, and most commonly encountered errors. Training of personnel should include a return demonstration to identify difficulties identifying anatomic landmarks and to clear up any other inconsistent techniques or misconceptions. Finally, a quality improvement program should monitor the incidence of common errors such as RA-LA lead wire reversal and provide retraining when indicated.

References

[1] Einthoven W. The different forms of the human electrocardiogram and their signification. Lancet 1912; 1:853.
[2] Wilson FN. The distribution of the potential differences produced by the heart beat within the body and at its surface. Am Heart J 1929–1930;5:599–616.
[3] Gamble P, McManus H, Jensen D, et al. A comparison of the standard 12-lead electrocardiogram to exercise electrode placements. Chest 1984;85(5): 616–22.
[4] Bennett FT, Bennett KR, Markov AK. Einthoven's triangle: lead errors and an algorithm for solution. Am J Med Sci 2005;329(2):71–7.
[5] Drew BJ, Wung SF, Adams MG, et al. Bedside diagnosis of myocardial ischemia with ST-segment monitoring technology: measurement issues for real-time clinical decision-making and trial designs. J Electrocardiol 1998;30:157–65.
[6] Drew BJ, Adams MG. Clinical consequences of ST-segment changes caused by body position mimicking transient myocardial ischemia: hazards of ST-segment monitoring? J Electrocardiol 2001;34:261–4.
[7] Wenger W, Kligfield P. Variability of precordial electrode placement during routine electrocardiography. J Electrocardiol 1996;29:179–84.
[8] Zema MJ, Luminais SK, Chiaramida S, et al. Electrocardiographic poor R wave progression III: the normal variant. J Electrocardiol 1980;13:135–42.
[9] Rautaharju PM, Park L, Rautaharju FS, et al. A standardized procedure for locating and

documenting ECG chest electrode positions. J Electrocardiol 1998;31(1):17–29.

[10] Colaco R, Reay P, Beckett C, et al. False positive ECG reports of anterior myocardial infarction in women. J Electrocardiol 2000;33(Suppl): 239–44.

[11] Dower GE, Yakush A, Nazzal SB, et al. Deriving the 12-lead electrocardiogram from four (EASI) electrodes. J Electrocardiol 1988;21:S182–7.

[12] Nelwan SP, Kors JA, Meij SH, et al. Reconstruction of the 12-lead electrocardiogram from reduced lead sets. J Electrocardiol 2004;37:11–8.

[13] Drew BJ, Scheinman MM, Evans GT. Comparison of a vectorcardiographically derived 12-lead electrocardiogram with the conventional electrocardiogram during wide QRS complex tachycardia, and its potential application for continuous bedside monitoring. Am J Cardiol 1992;69:612–8.

[14] Drew BJ, Adams MG, Pelter MM, et al. ST segment monitoring with a derived 12-lead electrocardiogram is superior to routine CCU monitoring. Am J Crit Care 1996;5:198–206.

[15] Drew BJ, Pelter MM, Wung SF, et al. Accuracy of the EASI 12-lead electrocardiogram compared to the standard 12-lead electrocardiogram for diagnosing multiple cardiac abnormalities. J Electrocardiol 1999;32(Suppl):38–47.

[16] Drew BJ, Pelter MM, Brodnick DE, et al. Comparison of a new reduced lead set ECG with the standard ECG for diagnosing cardiac arrhythmias and myocardial ischemia. J Electrocardiol 2002; 35(Suppl):13–21.

[17] Drew BJ, Califf RM, Funk M, et al. Practice standards for electrocardiographic monitoring in hospital settings. Circulation 2004;110:2721–46.

[18] Knight BP, Pelosi F, Michaud GF, et al. Clinical consequences of electrocardiographic artifact mimicking ventricular tachycardia. N Engl J Med 1999; 341:1270–4.

[19] Society for Cardiological Science and Technology. Clinical guidelines by consensus, number 1: recording a standard 12-lead electrocardiogram. London, England: Society for Cardiological Science and Technology; 2005.

ELSEVIER
SAUNDERS

CARDIOLOGY
CLINICS

Cardiol Clin 24 (2006) 317–330

How many ECG leads do we need?

Elin Trägårdh, MD, PhD candidate*,
Henrik Engblom, MD, PhD candidate, Olle Pahlm, MD, PhD

Department of Clinical Physiology, Lund University Hospital, SE-221 85 Lund, Sweden

The number of leads used and the electrode placement in a standard ECG have remained the same for over half a century although the technology behind the method has developed greatly (Fig. 1). It is well known that the sensitivities of current standard 12-lead ECG criteria for detecting many cardiac diseases—such as acute myocardial infarction (MI) and ventricular hypertrophy—are poor. To increase the diagnostic ability of the ECG, many alternative lead systems have been proposed, but none has yet received general acceptance in the cardiology community.

The issue of the optimal number of leads is of great interest to researchers, as becomes apparent when researching the literature on the subject. Some investigators argue that a small number of leads will suffice; others maintain that the greater the number of leads, the better. This article aims to answer the question of how many ECG leads actually are necessary by presenting some of the most widely studied lead sets. Also discussed are researchers' efforts to enhance the sensitivity and specificity of the ECG in detecting acute MI and the capability of the ECG to diagnose other cardiac conditions.

The development of the standard 12-lead ECG

The first surface ECG recorded on humans was performed in 1887 by Waller [1], but the leads that were first used for diagnostic electrocardiography were three-limb leads introduced by Einthoven [2]. In the earliest ECG recording systems, the patient's arms were inserted into jars of conducting solution, which were connected to a sensitive galvanometer. This method made it possible to measure the potential differences between the

two arms (lead I), the left leg and the right arm (lead II), and the left leg and the left arm (lead III).

In the early 1930s, Wilson [3,4] introduced a "central terminal," which he hypothesized would allow measurements of the potential variation at a single point, giving rise to the incorrect term "unipolar leads." Indeed, all leads measure the potential difference between two poles. The original Einthoven leads were "two-electrode leads," whereas other standard leads used a single electrode as one pole and averaged inputs from multiple electrodes as the second pole. When inputs from all three limb electrodes were averaged, the resulting "central terminal" served as the second pole, thus creating a "V" lead. The lead system defined six additional chest leads to be recorded, labeled V1, V2, V3, V4, V5, and V6.

In the early years of ECG recordings, there was no standardization of placement of the precordial leads, making it difficult to compare studies. In 1938, the first standardization was made by the Cardiac Society of Great Britain and Ireland in conjunction with the American Heart Association [5]. Later that same year, the electrode positions of leads V1 to V6 as known today were described [6,7]. The standardized placement of the precordial leads was a committee decision, made with the specific intent of standardizing research.

The Wilson central terminal also enabled three other limb leads: VR, VL, and VF. These leads, however, were of low voltage in general and were replaced by augmented (aV) leads by removing input from the electrode that provided the first pole from the averaged second pole. Augmented limb leads, developed in 1942, measure the potential differences between the left arm and the average of the potentials at the right arm and left leg (lead aVL). In a similar fashion, it was possible to design two other augmented limb

* Corresponding author.
E-mail address: elin.tragardh@med.lu.se (E. Trägårdh).

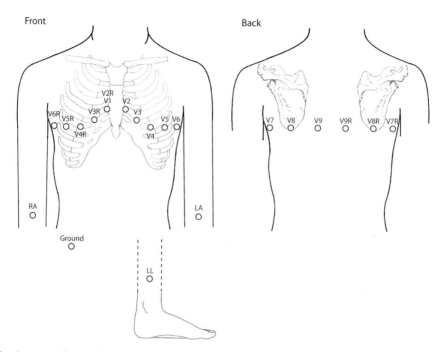

Fig. 1. The placement of precordial and limb electrodes. In the frontal view (left) the electrode placement for the standard 12-lead ECG is shown: V1 to V6. The right-sided electrodes are also shown, which are mirror images of leads V2 to V6. On the back view (right) the posterior electrodes V7 to V9 and V7R to V9R are shown. LA, left arm; LL, left leg; RA, right arm.

leads, aVR and aVF [8], creating the standard 12-lead ECG used today.

In some situations it is not feasible to use the standard electrode placement for limb leads because of noise from skeletal muscle (eg, during percutaneous transluminal coronary angioplasty and during stress tests). In 1966, Mason and Likar [9] introduced a system in which limb electrodes are instead placed on the torso (Fig. 2). In this system, the arm electrodes are placed in the left or right infraclavicular fossa, medial to the border of the deltoid muscle and 2 cm below the lower border of the clavicle. The left leg electrode is placed in the anterior axillary line, halfway between the costal margin and the crest of the ilium. Studies have shown, however, that the electrical axis may change and that ECG findings indicating inferior or posterior infarcts are lost in 69% and 31% of patients, respectively, compared with findings in ECGs recorded with standard electrode placement [10,11]. Hence, when interpreting an ECG, it is important to know if it has been recorded using Mason-Likar electrode placement.

Additional precordial leads

It is well known that the sensitivity of current 12-lead ECG criteria is poor for detecting acute MI

[12,13]. There are three principal reasons. First, the infarct may be too small to affect the cardiac electrophysiology reflected by an ECG. Second, the location of the infarction might not be "observed" by a 12-lead ECG because of its limited coverage of the precordium. It also is possible that the precordial electrodes in a standard 12-lead ECG are not optimally placed to detect acute MI and ischemia. For example, Saetre and colleagues [14] found that leads derived from electrodes placed in the left axilla and on the back could differentiate ECG changes that occurred during percutaneous coronary intervention of the first diagonal and left circumflex (LCX) arteries, respectively.

Third, the location of ischemia in acute infarction might be observed by the 12-lead ECG as ST depression when, in fact, it should be considered "ST elevation equivalent." This consideration of the inverse of a standard lead as the equivalent of an additional lead (eg, lead aVR and lead −aVR) may negate the need to create additional leads by placement of additional electrodes [15].

In addition to precordial leads V1 to V6, other precordial torso leads can be used as well. Posterior leads V7 (left posterior axillary line), V8 (left midscapular line), and V9 (left border of the spine) are all located in the same horizontal plane as lead

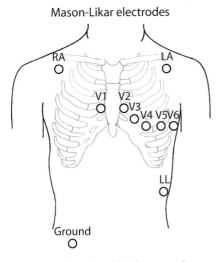

Mason-Likar electrodes

Fig. 2. Mason-Likar electrode placement. In comparison with the electrode placement for the standard 12-lead ECG, the limb leads are moved proximally when recording the 12-lead ECG according to the Mason-Likar system. The upper limb leads are placed in the infraclavicular fossa medial to the border of the deltoid muscle and 2 cm below the lower border of the clavicle. The lower limb lead is moved to the anterior axillary line, halfway between the costal margin and the crest of the ilium. LA, left arm; LL, left leg; RA, right arm.

V6. Leads V3R to V9R are located on the right side of the chest in the same location as corresponding to the location of the left-sided leads V3 to V9. V2R is therefore the same as V1 (Fig. 1).

Posterior leads

Posterior MI occurs when either the LCX or a branch of the right coronary artery (RCA) supplying blood to the posterior wall of the left ventricle is occluded. Because there are no posterior electrodes in a standard 12-lead ECG, the diagnosis of posterior MI depends on ST depression in anterior leads [16]. Currently, patients who do not have ST-segment elevation in a standard ECG are not recommended for thrombolytic therapy [17]. Moreover, there are reports of ST elevation in posterior leads in the absence of changes in anterior leads [18]. It is important to diagnose posterior MI because it often is associated with complications such as mitral valve regurgitation [19] and poor patient prognosis [20,21]. Accordingly, there has been much interest in the study of posterior chest leads in the past few years.

In one such study, ECG patterns in posterior chest leads (V7–V9) were studied in 225 normal male subjects about to undergo military training

[22]. The investigators found that none of the subjects had ST elevation at the J point exceeding 0.5 mm. The prevalence of 0.5- to 1.0-mm ST elevation at 80 milliseconds after the J point in lead V7 was 8.9%, 5.8% and 3.1% in leads V7, V8, and V9, respectively. In only two subjects did the ST elevation reach 1 mm in amplitude. The results indicate that ST elevation in leads V7 to V9 at the J point or of more than 1 mm 80 milliseconds after the J point can be considered abnormal.

In acute MI, it is important to open the occluded artery as soon as possible after the onset of symptoms. It is desirable to identify the culprit artery by surface ECG to facilitate coronary intervention. A prospective ECG analysis during angioplasty for single-vessel disease involving LCX or RCA found that the most common ECG change during RCA occlusion was ST-segment elevation in leads II, aVF, and III (95%), and that the most common change during LCX occlusion was posterior ST elevation in leads V7 to V9 (68%) [23]. Therefore, the use of posterior leads may help in distinguishing between occlusion of the RCA and occlusion of the LCX.

Many studies have demonstrated that posterior leads are useful for identifying acute posterior MI not detected by the standard ECG [19,21,24–26]. Zalenski and colleagues [26] found that the addition of V4R, V8, and V9 in patients admitted to a cardiac-monitored unit with a provisional diagnosis of MI or unstable angina increased the sensitivity of ST-segment elevation detection from 47.1% to 58.8%, with no loss of specificity. Biochemical markers were used to diagnose MI, and percutaneous coronary intervention was not performed in the study.

In another study, however, Zalenski and colleagues [27] found that the accuracy of detecting ST-segment elevation in acute MI was improved only modestly by the addition of leads V7 to V9. The sensitivity increased from 57.7% to 59.7%, whereas the specificity decreased from 91% to 89.4%.

In a study of low-risk patients presenting with chest pain suggestive of acute coronary syndromes, posterior leads were not found to increase the detection rate of ischemia [28]. Low-risk patients were identified by a normal 12-lead ECG, absence of arrhythmias or hemodynamic instability, and one negative serum cardiac troponin I assay. Different studies have used different levels of ST elevation in posterior leads as diagnostic of acute MI. Some authors have used a criterion of 1 mm, whereas studies with an angiography gold standard have considered 0.5 mm of ST elevation to be diagnostic [29].

Right-sided leads

Right ventricular infarction rarely occurs in isolation [30] but occur in more than 30% of cases of inferior left ventricular MI [31]. Patients who have right ventricular infarct involvement have a worse prognosis [32,33], a significantly higher incidence of depressed right ventricular function [34], and a high risk of developing high-degree atrioventricular nodal block compared to infarcts with no right ventricular involvement [35]. Usually, there are only inconclusive signs of right ventricular infarction in the standard 12-lead ECG. Chou and colleagues [36] concluded that ST elevation of 1 mm or more in lead V1, in the absence of other explanations for the ST elevation, should raise suspicion of right ventricular involvement. Other studies [37–39], however, do not support this criterion because of its low sensitivity. One method that can be used to observe the right ventricle better is to apply right-sided leads. Andersen and colleagues [40] described ST deviations in the right chest leads V3R to V7R during transient balloon occlusion of the coronary arteries. They found that ST elevation always evolved in leads V5R and V6R when the RCA was occluded and was 100% discriminative for RCA occlusion compared with occlusion of either of the two left coronary arteries. ST elevation within normal range or ST depression could be seen in leads V3R and V4R during RCA occlusion.

Morgera and colleagues [41] studied 82 normal subjects and found that an rS pattern was always present in V3R and was present in V4R in 91% of subjects. qR or qS patterns were seen in V6R in 26% of the subjects, in V5R in 10% of subjects, and in V4R in 2% of subjects. In a study by Andersen and colleagues [42], 109 normal subjects were studied. An rS configuration was found in V3R in 98% and in V4R in 91%. A qS configuration was found most frequently in V6R (16%). They also investigated the ST deviation 40 and 80 milliseconds after the J point. Measurements of the ST segment made 80 milliseconds after the last QRS deflection showed significantly more deviation from the isoelectric line than measurements made 40 milliseconds after the last QRS deflection. They concluded that ST-segment deviation should be measured 40 milliseconds after the last QRS deflection and should be at least 0.6 mm to be considered abnormal.

Many studies have evaluated right-sided precordial leads in acute MI and have found a high but variable sensitivity for detecting right ventricular MI [27,37–39,41,43]. Croft and colleagues [37] studied 33 patients who had enzymatically confirmed MI, using myocardial scintigraphy as the criterion gold standard. They found that ST elevation of 1 mm or greater in one or more of leads V4R to V6R is both highly sensitive (90%) and specific (91%) in identifying acute right ventricular infarction. Braat and colleagues [38] reported similar results, with a sensitivity of 93% and a specificity of 95% in lead V4R, which was found to be the best right-sided lead for detecting right ventricular MI. Later, they also performed a study using angiography as the criterion gold standard [43]. Forty-two patients who had inferior MI were included, 17 of whom had right ventricular MI. The sensitivity for detecting right ventricular MI was 100% for lead V4R, and the specificity was 87%. Lopez-Sendon and colleagues [39] found 100% sensitivity and 68% specificity in detecting right ventricular MI in lead V4R.

Another study compared the standard 12-lead ECG with 12-lead ECG plus the addition of V4R to V6R in 533 patients who had chest pain [27]. They found that the sensitivity increased from 57.7% to 64.4% with the addition of V4R to V6R. The specificity, however, decreased from 91% to 85.6%. Most of the studies used 1 mm as the cut-off value [27,37,38,41,43], but others have used 0.5 mm [39,41]. An autopsy study by Morgera and colleagues [41] compared sensitivity and specificity when using a 1-mm or 0.5-mm cut-off in lead V4R. With 0.5 mm as the cut-off, the sensitivity was 76%, and the specificity was 86%. With 1 mm as the cut-off, the sensitivity was 57%, and the specificity was 100%.

The use of right-sided precordial leads has also been investigated during exercise tests, with divergent results. Some studies have shown that the addition of right-sided leads does not increase the sensitivity of the ECG for the detection of myocardial ischemia [44,45], but another study showed that the sensitivity improved greatly [46]. Some studies indicate that the addition of right-sided chest leads could be of use in the early diagnosis of acute pulmonary embolism [47,48].

Body surface potential mapping

The standard 12-lead ECG is derived from only 10 electrodes. Hence, it offers a limited coverage of the body surface potential distribution caused by the depolarization and repolarization of the myocardium. Therefore, local electrical events in the myocardium may not be reflected in the standard 12-lead ECG. Body surface potential mapping (BSPM) is a method that provides better coverage of the body surface potential distribution by performing recordings at multiple sites (24–240) on the body surface. This approach is not novel; in fact, the first example of a potential map was published in 1889 by Waller [49], who performed 10 to 20 ECG recordings at various points on the surface of the human body. Since then, normal BSPM patterns have been established [50,51], and abnormal patterns of BSPM have been explored. In addition to this empiric use of BSPM, aimed at obtaining descriptive information of cardiac electrical behavior, BSPM has evolved from the so-called "classical forward" and "inverse" problems of electrocardiography. The former focuses on how the electrical activity from electrical sources present in the heart is propagated to the epicardium (near-field problem) or to the body surface (far-field problem) [52]. The latter focuses on how the electrical activity recorded at the body surface can be used to derive details about the electrical activity in the heart (ie, epicardial potentials) [53]. Both problems require information of high spatial resolution from the body surface, which can be obtained through BSPM. The theoretical aspects of BSPM are not discussed further in this article. Instead, the more clinical aspects of BSPM are discussed.

Clinical implications

Several studies involving BSPM in patients with MI have been published [54–74]. A study by Kornreich and colleagues [55] included 177 patients who had MI and 184 normal subjects. Criteria based on six features from three locations (mostly ST-T measurements) derived from 120-lead BSPM data yielded a specificity of 95% and sensitivity of 95% for diagnosing MI. The three locations were the right subclavian area, the left posterior axillary region, and the left leg. The 12-lead ECG had the same specificity but a sensitivity of 88% for the same number of features. The leads with the greatest discriminating power were found outside the 12-lead ECG. Furthermore, it has been shown that the sensitivity for right ventricular MI increased from 42% for right ventricular leads to 58% for BSPM [57]. In the

same study, the sensitivity increased from 1% for posterior leads to 27% for BSPM.

The 12-lead ECG has a sensitivity of about 50% for detection of acute MI. Menown and colleagues [56] studied 635 patients who had chest pain, of whom 325 had MI (according to the World Health Organization criteria for acute MI), and 125 controls. Subjects were randomly assigned to either a learning or a test set. The 64-lead anterior BSPM data showed an overall correct acute MI classification of 74%.

The standard 12-lead ECG is known to have low sensitivity for detection of acute MI in the presence of left bundle branch block. Sgarbossa and colleagues [75] showed a sensitivity of 33%, and Hands and colleagues [76] showed a sensitivity of 17% for detecting acute MI in the presence of left bundle branch block. Maynard and colleagues [58], however, have shown that the sensitivity can be increased to 67% using BSPM.

BSPM also has been shown useful in evaluating the clinical efficacy of reperfusion therapy [77,78]. In a study of 67 patients who had acute MI undergoing coronary angiography 90 minutes after fibrinolytic therapy, Menown and colleagues [77] showed that BSPM had a sensitivity of 97% and a specificity of 100% for detecting patients who had established reperfusion (Thrombolysis in Myocardial Infarction [TIMI] grade 2–3 flow). In comparison, all ST-resolution patterns on the standard 12-lead ECG showed a sensitivity of 59% and a specificity of 50%.

The 12-lead ECG is used frequently for assessing stress-induced ischemia in coronary artery disease. Using BSPM, Manninen and colleagues [79] showed that regional stress-induced ischemia can be identified at sites on the body surface not covered by the standard 12-lead ECG. Montague and colleagues [80] demonstrated that ischemic repolarization changes were detectable and quantifiable by BSPM at low levels of cardiac stress in patients who had one-vessel disease when the usual ECG criteria of myocardial ischemia frequently were absent. Furthermore, Boudik and colleagues [81] showed that BSPM during dipyridamole stress can be used to differentiate between normal subjects, patients who have syndrome X, and patients who have coronary artery disease. The sensitivity and specificity for detecting syndrome X were 71% and 78%, respectively.

BSPM also has been shown to increase the diagnostic accuracy of left ventricular hypertrophy criteria [82] as well as the ability to estimate left ventricular mass from an ECG [83,84] in comparison to a standard 12-lead ECG. In addition, BSPM has been shown to be useful in identifying accessory pathways in patients who have Wolff-Parkinson-White syndrome [85–91].

Why is body surface potential mapping not clinical routine?

It is clear that BSPM provides more information regarding the cardiac electrical field than the standard 12-lead ECG. Why then is BSPM not more clinically established? First, recording the large number of leads and displaying them appropriately is time consuming, making the procedure unsuitable for clinical settings. This obstacle has, to a large extent, been overcome by the development of electrode strips that are easier to apply and by modern computer technology. Modern BSPM systems can acquire and process maps in less than 30 seconds. Second, the great amount of information received from BSPM has been difficult to interpret and classify correctly; however, a variety of statistical methods have been devised that allow measurements of cardiac patients to be compared with those of healthy subjects of various ages, sex, and body habitus. Interpretation schemes are now available, also. Nonetheless, correct interpretation and classification of maps remain challenging tasks and require a deep understanding of body surface potential distribution. In a recent study of 389 patients presenting to an emergency department with chest pain, Carley and colleagues [92] showed that BSPM offered a relatively small increase in sensitivity (from 40% to 47.1%), and a comparable decrease in specificity (from 93.7% versus 85.6%) for detecting acute MI in comparison to a standard 12-lead ECG. In this study, the BSPM maps were interpreted by emergency physicians trained in BSPM, not by cardiologists with a special interest in BSPM. Additionally, this study was performed in an emergency setting with unselected patients, thus reflecting the clinical reality of a typical emergency department.

Although BSPM offers better coverage of the body surface potential distribution, further studies of the diagnostic capability of BSPM in different clinical settings are needed to establish it as a clinical routine examination.

Reduced lead sets

Although there are clear advantages in using additional leads in certain circumstances,
problems might occur even when using only the 10 electrodes of the standard 12-lead ECG. Multiple electrodes and wires interfere with auscultation, echocardiograms, resuscitation efforts, and chest radiographs. Noise levels created by limb movement detected by multiple leads make interpretation difficult, and the discomfort to patients caused by so many electrodes tends to be high. Additionally, rapid and accurate electrode placement can be difficult in emergency situations. Fewer electrodes placed at more easily accessed locations could facilitate ECG acquisition for both patient and staff.

Frank leads

Today, the standard 12-lead ECG is the most common method for studying the electrophysiology of the heart. Vectorcardiography is another method that was first described in the early twentieth century. A vectorcardiogram traces the sum of the heart's electrical activity in a three-dimensional space throughout the cardiac cycle. Three orthogonal leads, Vx, Vy, and Vz, are used. The most commonly used and best-studied orthogonal lead system is that of Frank [93]. In this lead system, seven electrodes are used (Fig. 3, upper panel). Five of the electrodes are positioned around the heart on the torso (on the left and right side of the thorax, on the sternum, on the back, and on the left side of the chest, at an angle of 45° with respect to the center of the thorax), one electrode is positioned on the back of the neck, and one on the left foot. From the contributing measurements of these leads, the orthogonal leads Vx, Vy, and Vz are derived. Typically, the leads are analyzed in pairs and presented as loops. The amplitudes of the two leads are measured at the same time and plotted in a diagram, with the amplitude of one lead appearing on the x-axis and the amplitude of the other lead appearing on the y-axis (Fig. 4). The leads are combined pair-wise to a frontal plane (x and y), a transversale plane (x and z), and a sagittal plane (y and z). The shape, direction of rotation, and area of the loop are then analyzed.

Continuous vectorcardiographic registration with Frank leads has been shown to have substantial potential for monitoring patients who have acute MI [94,95] and may help in identifying candidates for emergency coronary angiography [95]. It also has been shown to correlate more closely with enzymatically estimated infarct size in patients who have Q-wave infarction than

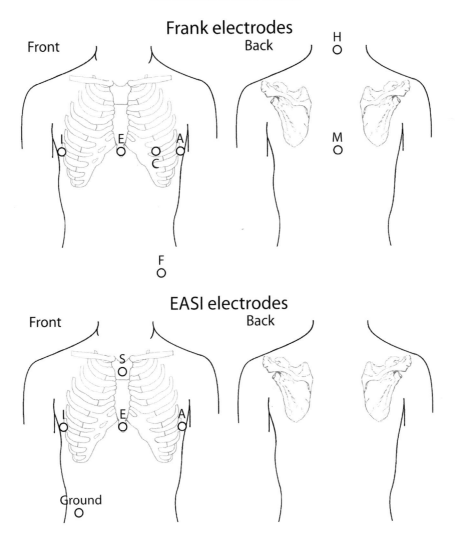

Fig. 3. Comparison between Frank and EASI electrode placement. The E, A, and I electrodes are identical for the two placements. In the EASI setting, however, no electrodes are required on the back.

does QRS scoring of the standard 12-lead ECG [96]. The Common Standards for Quantitative Electrocardiography working party, however, concludes that vectorcardiography has slightly lower specificity and although a slightly higher sensitivity than standard 12-lead ECG [97].

Derived 12-lead ECG

In 1988 Dower [98] introduced a "derived" 12-lead ECG, using five torso electrodes, four recording and one ground. Because three electrodes from the original Frank lead configuration

(E, A, and I) were used, he labeled it the "EASI 12-lead ECG" (Fig. 3, lower panel). In addition, he used a fourth electrode (S). The fifth ground electrode can be placed anywhere. The electrodes are placed on easily identified anatomic points on the torso: the E electrode on the lower sternum, the A and I electrodes on the left and right mid-axillary lines, respectively, at the same transverse level as E, and the S electrode on the sternum manubrium. The electrodes record three ECG leads: A-I (horizontal vector), E-S (vertical vector), and A-S (anterior-posterior vector). Each of the 12 standard ECG leads is derived as a weighted linear

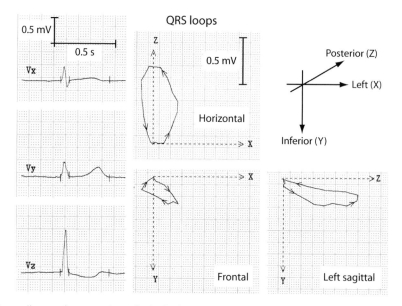

Fig. 4. A vectorcardiogram from a patient who had a large anterior myocardial infarction. To the left the three orthogonal leads Vx, Vy, and Vz are shown. From these leads the QRS loops shown to the right in the frontal, horizontal, and left sagittal planes were derived. As seen in the horizontal and left sagittal planes, the anterior electrical forces are completely absent as a result of the large anterior infarction.

sum of the signals from these three leads using the following formula:

$$L_{derived} = a(A - I) + b(E - S) + c(A - S),$$

where L represents any ECG lead and a, b, and c represent coefficients determined to optimize the fit between the standard 12-lead ECG and the derived ECG [99].

Basic comparisons between standard 12-lead ECG and EASI-derived 12-lead ECG have concluded that differences between PR, QRS, QT, and QTc intervals are small. Some differences in cardiac axes, especially in T-wave axes, have been found, but EASI still accurately detected right/left bundle branch block and fascicular blocks [100,101].

Accurate diagnosis of both myocardial arrhythmias and ischemia often requires analysis of multiple leads. Many hospital wards, however, rely on only two leads (most often leads II and V1) for ECG monitoring. Continuous monitoring of the EASI-lead ECG has been found to be superior to monitoring with leads II and V1 for diagnosing transient myocardial ischemia in patients who have unstable coronary syndromes [102]. Leads II and V1 were shown to miss 64% of ischemic ST changes detected by EASI; 75%

of the missed events were clinically silent. Moreover, EASI-derived ECG has been found to be diagnostically equivalent to standard 12-lead ECG for the detection of cardiac arrhythmias [100,101].

The diagnostic capabilities of the EASI system have been found to be equivalent to the standard 12-lead ECG for the detection of acute ischemia [101–104], acute MI [105], and prior MI [100,101,103,106]. Another application might be in the ambulance setting. Sejersten and colleagues [107] showed that the EASI lead system can provide an alternative to the standard 12-lead ECG to facilitate data acquisition and possibly save time in emergency situations. So far, few studies have been performed in children, where it also is important to simplify ECG recordings. A basic study by Pahlm and colleagues [108] concluded that EASI leads in children have the same high levels of "goodness-of-fit" to replicate conventional 12-lead ECG waveforms as reported in adults. The EASI lead system has been approved by the US Food and Drug Administration for assessing normal, abnormal, and paced cardiac rhythms and for detecting myocardial ischemia in patients with chest pain or silent ischemia by monitoring ST-segment elevation or depression.

Because there is individual variation between standard 12-lead ECG and EASI ECG it is advised that clinicians only use one method when making serial ECG comparisons.

Derived precordial leads

Another approach to a reduced number of leads is to exclude certain leads from the ECG recording and instead reconstruct the excluded leads from the existing leads, using either general or patient-specific reconstruction. Nelwan and colleagues [109] studied how well the 12-lead ECG can be reconstructed from different lead subsets, always including limb leads I and II and at least one precordial lead. Patients who had unstable angina were monitored with extremity electrodes at the Mason-Likar locations and precordial leads at the standard positions. They concluded that general construction allows reconstruction of one or two precordial leads, whereas patient-specific construction allows up to four leads to be reconstructed. The best lead subset with four removed precordial leads was I, II, V2, and V5. The patient-specific reconstruction, however, presupposes a previously recorded ECG and is affected over time, probably by postural changes. In a comparison of general construction, patient-specific construction (using leads I, II, V2, and V5), and EASI leads, it was found that, when comparing ST60, patient-specific construction showed a more accurate reconstruction of the standard ECG than did the other two methods [110].

One advantage to using this system is that all limb leads and two precordial leads are known to be true leads, although the system uses more electrodes than the EASI lead system.

24-view ECG

Some investigators propose that there is no need for additional leads if the standard 12-lead ECG system could be used more effectively [15]. It is widely considered that ST elevation occurs when an injury current develops between normal and transmurally ischemic myocardium [111]. The flow of this current creates a vector toward leads with positive poles facing that area of the myocardium, seen as ST elevation. Any electrode on the other side of the heart will instead record an ST depression. For example, to see ST elevation in patients who have posterior infarcts, one would have to apply posterior thoracic electrodes (as discussed previously) or to produce a 24-view ECG in which displays of negative views of all standard leads are regarded as well (Fig. 5).

The classical standard 12-lead display includes two subsets of limb leads (I, II, III, and aVL, aVR, aVF) and the chest leads V1 to V6. It is, however, equally possible to regroup the limb leads into an orderly sequence [112]. This sequence displays the cardiac electrical activity in the frontal plane in a logical order: aVL, I, −aVR, II, and aVF, III, with each separated by

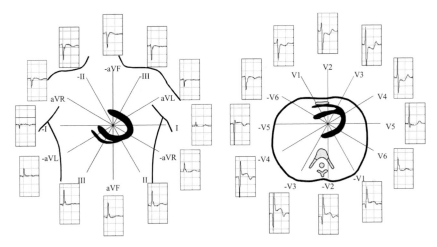

Fig. 5. The 24 views of the standard 12-lead ECG are shown as recorded from a patient receiving angioplasty balloon occlusion in a nondominant left circumflex coronary artery. QRS complexes and T waves from single cardiac cycles recorded simultaneously in the six frontal plane leads viewed from the front (*left*) and the six transverse plane leads viewed from below (*right*) are arranged like numbers around a clock face. (*From:* Pahlm-Webb U, Pahlm O, Sadanandan S, et al. A new method for using the direction of ST-segment deviation to localize the site of acute coronary occlusion: the 24-view standard electrocardiogram. Am J Med 2002;113(1):75–8; with permission.)

30°. This sequence could be enlarged further to include all inverted leads in the frontal plane, just as −aVR has been inverted in the orderly sequence. In the same manner, an inversion of the precordial leads V1 to V6 could also be used. Thus, an ST depression in lead V1 would present as an ST elevation in lead −V1, just as an ST depression in lead aVR would present as an ST elevation in lead −aVR. The 24-view ECG does not require the placement of additional electrodes, because all information is available in the 12-lead ECG. An alternative of the 24-view ECG is simply to allow ST deviation (elevation or depression) in the standard 12-lead ECG to be diagnostic of acute MI. Further studies are needed, however, before any ECG diagnostic guidelines can be changed.

Summary

There is no single right answer to the question of how many leads are needed in clinical electrocardiography. This question must be answered in the context of the clinical problem to be solved. The standard 12-lead ECG is so well established that alternative lead systems must prove their advantage through well-conducted clinical studies to achieve clinical acceptance. Certain additional leads seem to add valuable information in specific patient groups. The use of a large number of leads (such as in body surface potential mapping) may add clinically relevant information; however, it is still cumbersome, and its clinical advantage is yet to be proven. Reduced lead sets emulate the 12-lead ECG reasonably well and are especially advantageous in the emergency situation.

References

[1] Waller A. A demonstration on man of electromotive changes accompanying the hearts beat. J Physiol 1887;8:229–34.

[2] Einthoven W. The different forms of the human electrocardiogram and their signification. Lancet 1912;1:853–61 [reprinted in Am Heart J 1950;40: 195–211].

[3] Wilson F, MacLeod A, Barker P. The potential variations produced by the heart beat at the apices of Einthovens triangle. Am Heart J 1931;7:207–11.

[4] Wilson F, MacLeod A, Barker P, et al. The electrocardiogram in myocardial infarction with particular reference to the initial deflections of the ventricular complex. Heart 1933;16:155–99.

[5] Committee of the Cardiac Society of Great Britain and Ireland and Committee of the American Heart Association. Standardisation of precordial leads. Lancet 1938; 221.

[6] Barnes A, Pardee H, White P, et al. Standardization of precordial leads. Am Heart J 1938;15:107–8.

[7] Barnes A, Pardee H, White P, et al. Standardization of precordial leads: supplementary report. Am Heart J 1938;15:235–9.

[8] Goldberger E. A simple, indifferent, electrocardiographic electrode of zero potential and a technique of obtaining augmented, unipolar, extremity leads. Am Heart J 1942;23:483–92.

[9] Mason RE, Likar I. A new system of multiple-lead exercise electrocardiography. Am Heart J 1966; 71(2):196–205.

[10] Papouchado M, Walker PR, James MA, et al. Fundamental differences between the standard 12-lead electrocardiography and the modified (Mason-Likar) exercise lead system. Eur Heart J 1987; 8(7):725–33.

[11] Sevilla DC, Dohrmann ML, Somelofski CA, et al. Invalidation of the resting electrocardiogram obtained via exercise electrode sites as a standard 12-lead recording. Am J Cardiol 1989;63(1):35–9.

[12] Speake D, Terry P. Towards evidence based emergency medicine: best BETs from the Manchester Royal Infirmary. First ECG in chest pain. Emerg Med J 2001;18(1):61–2.

[13] Blanke H, Cohen M, Schlueter GU, et al. Electrocardiographic and coronary arteriographic correlations during acute myocardial infarction. Am J Cardiol 1984;54(3):249–55.

[14] Saetre HA, Selvester RH, Solomon JC, et al. 16-lead ECG changes with coronary angioplasty. Location of ST-T changes with balloon occlusion of five arterial perfusion beds. J Electrocardiol 1992;24(Suppl):153–62.

[15] Pahlm-Webb U, Pahlm O, Sadanandan S, et al. A new method for using the direction of ST-segment deviation to localize the site of acute coronary occlusion: the 24-view standard electrocardiogram. Am J Med 2002;113(1):75–8.

[16] Brady WJ. Acute posterior wall myocardial infarction: electrocardiographic manifestations. Am J Emerg Med 1998;16(4):409–13.

[17] The Joint European Society of Cardiology/ American College of Cardiology Committee. Myocardial infarction redefined – A consensus document of The Joint European Society of Cardiology/American College of Cardiology Committee for the Redefinition of Myocardial Infarction. Eur Heart J 2000;21:1502–13.

[18] Khaw K, Moreyra AE, Tannenbaum AK, et al. Improved detection of posterior myocardial wall ischemia with the 15-lead electrocardiogram. Am Heart J 1999;138(5 Pt 1):934–40.

[19] Matetzky S, Freimark D, Feinberg MS, et al. Acute myocardial infarction with isolated ST-segment elevation in posterior chest leads V7–9: "hidden" ST-segment elevations revealing acute posterior infarction. J Am Coll Cardiol 1999; 34(3):748–53.

[20] Oraii S, Maleki M, Tavakolian AA, et al. Prevalence and outcome of ST-segment elevation in posterior electrocardiographic leads during acute myocardial infarction. J Electrocardiol 1999; 32(3):275–8.

[21] Matetzky S, Freimark D, Chouraqui P, et al. Significance of ST segment elevations in posterior chest leads (V7 to V9) in patients with acute inferior myocardial infarction: application for thrombolytic therapy. J Am Coll Cardiol 1998;31(3):506–11.

[22] Chia BL, Tan HC, Yip JW, et al. Electrocardiographic patterns in posterior chest leads (V7, V8, V9) in normal subjects. Am J Cardiol 2000;85(7): 911–2.

[23] Kulkarni AU, Brown R, Ayoubi M, et al. Clinical use of posterior electrocardiographic leads: a prospective electrocardiographic analysis during coronary occlusion. Am Heart J 1996;131(4):736–41.

[24] Agarwal JB. Routine use of a 15-lead electrocardiogram for patients presenting to the emergency department with chest pain. J Electrocardiol 1998; 31(Suppl):172–7.

[25] Agarwal JB, Khaw K, Aurignac F, et al. Importance of posterior chest leads in patients with suspected myocardial infarction, but nondiagnostic, routine 12-lead electrocardiogram. Am J Cardiol 1999;83(3):323–6.

[26] Zalenski RJ, Cooke D, Rydman R, et al. Assessing the diagnostic value of an ECG containing leads V4R, V8, and V9: the 15-lead ECG. Ann Emerg Med 1993;22(5):786–93.

[27] Zalenski RJ, Rydman RJ, Sloan EP, et al. Value of posterior and right ventricular leads in comparison to the standard 12-lead electrocardiogram in evaluation of ST-segment elevation in suspected acute myocardial infarction. Am J Cardiol 1997;79(12): 1579–85.

[28] Ganim RP, Lewis WR, Diercks DB, et al. Right precordial and posterior electrocardiographic leads do not increase detection of ischemia in low-risk patients presenting with chest pain. Cardiology 2004;102(2):100–3.

[29] Wung SF, Drew BJ. New electrocardiographic criteria for posterior wall acute myocardial ischemia validated by a percutaneous transluminal coronary angioplasty model of acute myocardial infarction. Am J Cardiol 2001;87(8):970–4.

[30] Andersen HR, Falk E, Nielsen D. Right ventricular infarction: frequency, size and topography in coronary heart disease: a prospective study comprising 107 consecutive autopsies from a coronary care unit. J Am Coll Cardiol 1987;10(6):1223–32.

[31] Haji SA, Movahed A. Right ventricular infarction–diagnosis and treatment. Clin Cardiol 2000;23(7): 473–82.

[32] Correale E, Battista R, Martone A, et al. Electrocardiographic patterns in acute inferior myocardial infarction with and without right ventricle involvement: classification, diagnostic and prognostic value, masking effect. Clin Cardiol 1999;22(1): 37–44.

[33] Andersen HR, Nielsen D, Lund O, et al. Prognostic significance of right ventricular infarction diagnosed by ST elevation in right chest leads V3R to V7R. Int J Cardiol 1989;23(3):349–56.

[34] Braat SH, Brugada P, De Zwaan C, et al. Right and left ventricular ejection fraction in acute inferior wall infarction with or without ST segment elevation in lead V4R. J Am Coll Cardiol 1984;4(5): 940–4.

[35] Braat SH, de Zwaan C, Brugada P, et al. Right ventricular involvement with acute inferior wall myocardial infarction identifies high risk of developing atrioventricular nodal conduction disturbances. Am Heart J 1984;107(6):1183–7.

[36] Chou TC, Van der Bel-Kahn J, Allen J, et al. Electrocardiographic diagnosis of right ventricular infarction. Am J Med 1981;70(6):1175–80.

[37] Croft CH, Nicod P, Corbett JR, et al. Detection of acute right ventricular infarction by right precordial electrocardiography. Am J Cardiol 1982;50(3): 421–7.

[38] Braat SH, Brugada P, de Zwaan C, et al. Value of electrocardiogram in diagnosing right ventricular involvement in patients with an acute inferior wall myocardial infarction. Br Heart J 1983;49(4): 368–72.

[39] Lopez-Sendon J, Coma-Canella I, Alcasena S, et al. Electrocardiographic findings in acute right ventricular infarction: sensitivity and specificity of electrocardiographic alterations in right precordial leads V4R, V3R, V1, V2, and V3. J Am Coll Cardiol 1985;6(6):1273–9.

[40] Andersen HR, Thomsen PE, Nielsen TT, et al. ST deviation in right chest leads V3R to V7R during percutaneous transluminal coronary angioplasty. Am Heart J 1990;119(3 Pt 1):490–3.

[41] Morgera T, Alberti E, Silvestri F, et al. Right precordial ST and QRS changes in the diagnosis of right ventricular infarction. Am Heart J 1984; 108(1):13–8.

[42] Andersen HR, Nielsen D, Hansen LG. The normal right chest electrocardiogram. J Electrocardiol 1987;20(1):27–32.

[43] Braat SH, Brugada P, den Dulk K, et al. Value of lead V4R for recognition of the infarct coronary artery in acute inferior myocardial infarction. Am J Cardiol 1984;53(11):1538–41.

[44] Ueshima K, Kobayashi N, Kamata J, et al. Do the right precordial leads during exercise testing contribute to detection of coronary artery disease? Clin Cardiol 2004;27(2):101–5.

[45] Shry EA, Eckart RE, Furgerson JL, et al. Addition of right-sided and posterior precordial leads during stress testing. Am Heart J 2003;146(6):1090–4.

[46] Michaelides AP, Psomadaki ZD, Dilaveris PE, et al. Improved detection of coronary artery disease by exercise electrocardiography with the use of

right precordial leads. N Engl J Med 1999;340(5): 340–5.

[47] Akula R, Hasan SP, Alhassen M, et al. Right-sided EKG in pulmonary embolism. J Natl Med Assoc 2003;95(8):714–7.

[48] Chia BL, Tan HC, Lim YT. Right sided chest lead electrocardiographic abnormalities in acute pulmonary embolism. Int J Cardiol 1997;61(1):43–6.

[49] Waller AD. On the electromotive changes connected with the beat of the mammalian heart, and of the human heart in particular. Philos Trans R Soc 1889;180:169–94.

[50] Taccardi B. Distribution of heart potentials on the thoracic surface of normal human subjects. Circ Res 1963;12:341–52.

[51] Nahum LH, Mauro A, Chernoff HM, et al. Instantaneous equipotential distribution on surface of the human body for various instants in the cardiac cycle. J Appl Physiol 1951;3(8):454–64.

[52] Gulrajani RM, Roberge FA, Mailloux GE. The forward problem of electrocardiography. In: Macfarlane P, Lawrie T, editors. Comprehensive electrocardiology: theory and practice in health and disease. New York: Pergamon Press; 1989. p. 197–236.

[53] Gulrajani RM, Roberge FA, Savard P. The inverse problem of electrocardiography. In: Macfarlane P, Lawrie T, editors. Comprehensive electrocardiology: theory and practice in health and disease. New York: Pergamon Press; 1989. p. 237–88.

[54] Montague TJ, Smith ER, Spencer CA, et al. Body surface electrocardiographic mapping in inferior myocardial infarction. Manifestation of left and right ventricular involvement. Circulation 1983; 67(3):665–73.

[55] Kornreich F, Rautaharju PM, Warren J, et al. Identification of best electrocardiographic leads for diagnosing myocardial infarction by statistical analysis of body surface potential maps. Am J Cardiol 1985;56(13):852–6.

[56] Menown IB, Patterson RS, MacKenzie G, et al. Body-surface map models for early diagnosis of acute myocardial infarction. J Electrocardiol 1998;31(Suppl):180–8.

[57] Menown IB, Allen J, Anderson JM, et al. Early diagnosis of right ventricular or posterior infarction associated with inferior wall left ventricular acute myocardial infarction. Am J Cardiol 2000;85(8): 934–8.

[58] Maynard SJ, Menown IB, Manoharan G, et al. Body surface mapping improves early diagnosis of acute myocardial infarction in patients with chest pain and left bundle branch block. Heart 2003;89(9):998–1002.

[59] Yamada K, Toyama J, Sugenoya J, et al. Body surface isopotential maps. Clinical application to the diagnosis of myocardial infarction. Jpn Heart J 1978;19(1):28–45.

[60] Vincent GM, Abildskov JA, Burgess MJ, et al. Diagnosis of old inferior myocardial infarction by body surface isopotential mapping. Am J Cardiol 1977;39(4):510–5.

[61] Vesterinen P, Hanninen H, Karvonen M, et al. Temporal analysis of the depolarization wave of healed myocardial infarction in body surface potential mapping. Ann Noninvasive Electrocardiol 2004;9(3):234–42.

[62] Toyama S, Suzuki K, Koyama M, et al. The body surface isopotential mapping of the QRS wave in myocardial infarction. a comparative study of the scintigram with thallium-201. J Electrocardiol 1982;15(3):241–8.

[63] Toyama S, Suzuki K, Koyama M. The isopotential mapping of the T wave in myocardial infarction. J Electrocardiol 1980;13(4):323–30.

[64] Pham-Huy H, Gulrajani RM, Roberge FA, et al. A comparative evaluation of three different approaches for detecting body surface isopotential map abnormalities in patients with myocardial infarction. J Electrocardiol 1981;14(1):43–55.

[65] Osugi J, Ohta T, Toyama J, et al. Body surface isopotential maps in old inferior myocardial infarction undetectable by 12 lead electrocardiogram. J Electrocardiol 1984;17(1):55–62.

[66] Ohta T, Toyama J, Ohsugi J, et al. Correlation between body surface isopotential maps and left ventriculograms in patients with old anterior myocardial infarction. Jpn Heart J 1981;22(5):747–61.

[67] Ohta T, Kinoshita A, Ohsugi J, et al. Correlation between body surface isopotential maps and left ventriculograms in patients with old inferoposterior myocardial infarction. Am Heart J 1982; 104(6):1262–70.

[68] Medvegy M, Preda I, Savard P, et al. New body surface isopotential map evaluation method to detect minor potential losses in non-Q-wave myocardial infarction. Circulation 2000;101(10):1115–21.

[69] Kornreich F, Montague TJ, Rautaharju PM. Identification of first acute Q wave and non-Q wave myocardial infarction by multivariate analysis of body surface potential maps. Circulation 1991; 84(6):2442–53.

[70] Hirai M, Ohta T, Kinoshita A, et al. Body surface isopotential maps in old anterior myocardial infarction undetectable by 12-lead electrocardiograms. Am Heart J 1984;108(4 Pt 1):975–82.

[71] Flowers NC, Horan LG, Sohi GS, et al. New evidence for inferoposterior myocardial infarction on surface potential maps. Am J Cardiol 1976; 38(5):576–81.

[72] Flowers NC, Horan LG, Johnson JC. Anterior infarctional changes occurring during mid and late ventricular activation detectable by surface mapping techniques. Circulation 1976;54(6):906–13.

[73] De Ambroggi L, Bertoni T, Rabbia C, et al. Body surface potential maps in old inferior myocardial

infarction. Assessment of diagnostic criteria. J Electrocardiol 1986;19(3):225–34.

[74] Ackaoui A, Nadeau R, Sestier F, et al. Myocardial infarction diagnosis with body surface potential mapping, electrocardiography, vectorcardiography and thallium-201 scintigraphy: a correlative study with left ventriculography. Clin Invest Med 1985;8(1):68–77.

[75] Sgarbossa EB, Pinski SL, Barbagelata A, et al. Electrocardiographic diagnosis of evolving acute myocardial infarction in the presence of left bundle-branch block. GUSTO-1 (Global Utilization of Streptokinase and Tissue Plasminogen Activator for Occluded Coronary Arteries) Investigators. N Engl J Med 1996;334(8):481–7.

[76] Hands ME, Cook EF, Stone PH, et al. Electrocardiographic diagnosis of myocardial infarction in the presence of complete left bundle branch block. Am Heart J 1988;116(1 Pt 1):23–31.

[77] Menown IB, Allen J, Anderson JM, et al. Noninvasive assessment of reperfusion after fibrinolytic therapy for acute myocardial infarction. Am J Cardiol 2000;86(7):736–41.

[78] Cahyadi YH, Takekoshi N, Matsui S. Clinical efficacy of PTCA and identification of restenosis: evaluation by serial body surface potential mapping. Am Heart J 1991;121(4 Pt 1):1080–7.

[79] Manninen H, Takala P, Makijarvi M, et al. Recording locations in multichannel magnetocardiography and body surface potential mapping sensitive for regional exercise-induced myocardial ischemia. Basic Res Cardiol 2001;96(4):405–14.

[80] Montague TJ, Johnstone DE, Spencer CA, et al. Body surface potential maps with low-level exercise in isolated left anterior descending coronary artery disease. Am J Cardiol 1988;61(4):273–82.

[81] Boudik F, Anger Z, Aschermann M, et al. Dipyridamole body surface potential mapping: noninvasive differentiation of syndrome X from coronary artery disease. J Electrocardiol 2002;35(3):181–91.

[82] Kornreich F, Montague TJ, Rautaharju PM, et al. Identification of best electrocardiographic leads for diagnosing left ventricular hypertrophy by statistical analysis of body surface potential maps. Am J Cardiol 1988;62(17):1285–91.

[83] Kornreich F, Montague TJ, van Herpen G, et al. Improved prediction of left ventricular mass by regression analysis of body surface potential maps. Am J Cardiol 1990;66(4):485–92.

[84] Holt JH Jr, Barnard AC, Kramer JO Jr. Multiple dipole electrocardiography: a comparison of electrically and angiographically determined left ventricular masses. Circulation 1978;57(6):1129–33.

[85] Yamada K, Toyama J, Wada M, et al. Body surface isopotential mapping in Wolff-Parkinson-White syndrome: noninvasive method to determine the localization of the accessory atrioventricular pathway. Am Heart J 1975;90(6):721–34.

[86] Tseng YZ, Hsu KL, Chiang FT, et al. The use of body surface potential map for identifying sites of accessory pathway in patients with Wolff-Parkinson-White syndrome. Jpn Heart J 1998;39(4):445–55.

[87] Liebman J, Zeno JA, Olshansky B, et al. Electrocardiographic body surface potential mapping in the Wolff-Parkinson-White syndrome. Noninvasive determination of the ventricular insertion sites of accessory atrioventricular connections. Circulation 1991;83(3):886–901.

[88] Iwa T, Magara T. Correlation between localization of accessory conduction pathway and body surface maps in the Wolff-Parkinson-White syndrome. Jpn Circ J 1981;45(10):1192–8.

[89] Dubuc M, Nadeau R, Tremblay G, et al. Pace mapping using body surface potential maps to guide catheter ablation of accessory pathways in patients with Wolff-Parkinson-White syndrome. Circulation 1993;87(1):135–43.

[90] De Ambroggi L, Taccardi B, Macchi E. Body-surface maps of heart potentials: tentative localization of pre-excited areas in forty-two Wolff-Parkinson-White patients. Circulation 1976;54(2):251–63.

[91] Benson DW Jr, Sterba R, Gallagher JJ, et al. Localization of the site of ventricular preexcitation with body surface maps in patients with Wolff-Parkinson-White syndrome. Circulation 1982;65(6):1259–68.

[92] Carley SD, Jenkins M, Jones KM. Body surface mapping versus the standard 12 lead ECG in the detection of myocardial infarction amongst emergency department patients: a Bayesian approach. Resuscitation 2005;64(3):309–14.

[93] Frank E. An accurate, clinically practical system for spatial vectorcardiography. Circulation 1954;13(4):737–49.

[94] Dellborg M, Topol EJ, Swedberg K. Dynamic QRS complex and ST segment vectorcardiographic monitoring can identify vessel patency in patients with acute myocardial infarction treated with reperfusion therapy. Am Heart J 1991;122(4 Pt 1):943–8.

[95] Dellborg M, Steg P, Simoons M, et al. Vectorcardiographic monitoring to assess early vessel patency after reperfusion therapy for acute myocardial infarction. Eur Heart J 1995;16(1):21–9.

[96] Dellborg M, Herlitz J, Risenfors M, et al. Electrocardiographic assessment of infarct size: comparison between QRS scoring of 12-lead electrocardiography and dynamic vectorcardiography. Int J Cardiol 1993;40(2):167–72.

[97] Willems JL, Abreu-Lima C, Arnaud P, et al. Assessment of the diagnostic performance of ECG computer programs and cardiologists. In: Common standards for quantitative electrocardiography.

CSE 10th progress report. Leuven (Belgium): Acco; 1990. p. 197–236.

[98] Dower GE, Yakush A, Nazzal SB, et al. Deriving the 12-lead electrocardiogram from four (EASI) electrodes. J Electrocardiol 1988;21(Suppl): S182–7.

[99] Feild DQ, Feldman CL, Horacek BM. Improved EASI coefficients: their derivation, values, and performance. J Electrocardiol 2002;35(Suppl):23–33.

[100] Klein M, Key-Brothers I, Feldman C. Can the vectorcardiographically derived EASI ECG be a suitable surrogate for the standard ECG in selected circumstances? Proc Comput Cardiol 1997;5(3): 721–4.

[101] Drew BJ, Pelter MM, Wung SF, et al. Accuracy of the EASI 12-lead electrocardiogram compared to the standard 12-lead electrocardiogram for diagnosing multiple cardiac abnormalities. J Electrocardiol 1999;32(Suppl):38–47.

[102] Drew BJ, Adams MG, Pelter MM, et al. ST segment monitoring with a derived 12-lead electrocardiogram is superior to routine cardiac care unit monitoring. Am J Crit Care 1996;5(3): 198–206.

[103] Rautaharju PM, Zhou SH, Hancock EW, et al. Comparability of 12-lead ECGs derived from EASI leads with standard 12-lead ECGS in the classification of acute myocardial ischemia and old myocardial infarction. J Electrocardiol 2002; 35(Suppl):35–9.

[104] Feldman CL, MacCallum G, Hartley LH. Comparison of the standard ECG with the EASIcardiogram for ischemia detection during exercise

monitoring. Proc Comput Cardiol 1997;24: 343–5.

[105] Wehr G, Peters R, Khalife K, et al. A vector-based 5 electrode 12-lead ECG (EASI) is equivalent to the conventional 12-lead ECG for diagnosis of myocardial ischemia. J Am Coll Cardiol 2002; 39(Suppl):122A.

[106] Horacek BM, Warren JW, et al. Diagnostic accuracy of derived versus standard 12-lead electrocardiograms. J Electrocardiol 2000;33(Suppl):155–60.

[107] Sejersten M, Pahlm O, Pettersson J, et al. The relative accuracies of ECG precordial lead waveforms derived from EASI leads and those acquired from paramedic applied standard leads. J Electrocardiol 2003;36(3):179–85.

[108] Pahlm O, Pettersson J, Thulin A, et al. Comparison of waveforms in conventional 12-lead ECGs and those derived from EASI leads in children. J Electrocardiol 2003;36(1):25–31.

[109] Nelwan SP, Kors JA, Meij SH, et al. Reconstruction of the 12-lead electrocardiogram from reduced lead sets. J Electrocardiol 2004;37(1):11–8.

[110] Nelwan SP, Crater SW, Meij SH, et al. Simultaneous comparison of three derived 12-lead ECGs with standard ECG at rest and during percutaneous coronary occlusion. J Electrocardiol 2004; 37(Suppl):171–2.

[111] Wagner GS. Marriott's practical electrocardiography. 10th edition. Philadelphia: Lippincott Williams & Wilkins; 2001.

[112] Anderson ST, Pahlm O, Selvester RH, et al. Panoramic display of the orderly sequenced 12-lead ECG. J Electrocardiol 1994;27(4):347–52.

CARDIOLOGY CLINICS

Cardiol Clin 24 (2006) 331–342

Consideration of Pitfalls in and Omissions from the Current ECG Standards for Diagnosis of Myocardial Ischemia/Infarction in Patients Who Have Acute Coronary Syndromes

Galen Wagner, MD[a],*, Tobin Lim, MD[a], Leonard Gettes, MD[d],
Anton Gorgels, MD[e], Mark Josephson, MD[f], Hein Wellens, MD[e],
Stanley Anderson, MB, BS, FRACP[g], Rory Childers, MD[h],
Peter Clemmensen, MD, PhD[i], Paul Kligfield, MD[k],
Peter Macfarlane, PhD[b], Olle Pahlm, MD, PhD[c],
Ronald Selvester, MD[j]

[a]Division of Cardiology, Department of Medicine, Duke University Medical Center,
2400 Pratt Street, RM 0306, Durham, NC 27705, USA
[b]Division of Cardiovascular and Medical Sciences, Section of Cardiology, Royal Infirmary,
Glasgow G31 2ER, Scotland, UK
[c]Department of Clinical Physiology, Lund University Hospital, LunSE-221 85 Lund, Sweden
[d]Division of Cardiology, The University of North Carolina at Chapel Hill, CB #7075, Bioinformatics Building,
130 Mason Farm Road, 4th Floor, Chapel Hill, NC 27599-7075, USA
[e]Department of Cardiology, Cardiovascular Research Institute Maastricht,
PO Box 5800, 6202 Maastricht, The Netherlands
[f]Harvard-Thorndike Electrophysiology Institute and Arrhythmia Service, Cardiology,
Harvard Medical School, Beth Israel Deaconess Medical Center,
185 Pilgrim Road, Baker 4, Boston, MA 02215, USA
[g]Cabrini Hospital, 18 Bay Street, Victoria 3186, Australia
[h]Section of Cardiology, University of Chicago Medical Center,
5841 S. Maryland Avenue, Chicago, IL 60637, USA
[i]Rigs Hospital, The Heart Center, University of Copenhagen, Blegdamsvej 9, 2100 Copenhagen, East Denmark
[j]Long Beach Memorial Hospital, 6298 East Ocean Boulevard, Long Beach, CA 90803, USA
[k]Department of Medicine, Cardiac Health Center, New York-Presbyterian Hospital,
525 East 68th Street, New York, NY 10021, USA

The ECG is the key clinical test available for the emergency determination of the patients with acute coronary syndromes who are indeed having acute myocardial ischemia/infarction. In these individuals, the process of evolution from potentially reversible ischemia to irreversible infarction occurs during the minutes to hours following coronary artery occlusion. Because the etiology is typically thrombosis, the correct clinical decision regarding reperfusion therapy is crucial.

Reperfusion using either intravenous thrombolytic therapy or intracoronary intervention has become the standard of care for the subgroup of

* Corresponding author.
   E-mail address: Galen.wagner@duke.edu
(G. Wagner).

patients who have acute coronary syndrome who meet ECG criteria for ST elevation myocardial infarction (STEMI); but is considered contraindicated for all others characterized by the broad term "non-STEMI". It has become clear, however, that the non-STEMI subgroup with ST depression in certain ECG leads should be considered "STEMI-equivalent" and similarly considered for reperfusion therapy. The application of STEMI criteria alone results in high specificity but unacceptably low sensitivity [1].

For many years, the standards for application of the ECG for decision support for patients who have acute coronary syndrome have been unchanged [2,3]. During the past 5 years, however, groups such as the American Heart Association (AHA), European Society of Cardiology (ESC), and American College of Cardiology (ACC) have initiated working groups to evolve new diagnostic standards [4]. As data become available to produce sufficient documentation of new criteria in peer-review journals, the pitfalls in current standards are corrected. This process, however, requires the passage of time. This review emerged from the efforts of an AHA working group to develop new standards for clinical application of electrocardiology. The general document has been completed by Kligfield and colleagues [5], and specific documents regarding ischemia/infarction and other aspects of electrocardiography are in development. The pitfalls in the current diagnostic standards regarding ischemia/infarction that have been identified by sufficiently documented studies will be corrected. This article refers only to the pitfalls in and omissions from current standards for which new standards will potentially emerge in future years.

The ECG provides diagnostic information that complements that from other clinical methods during the sequential phases of the myocardial ischemia/infarction process (as identified by the AHA Working Group) [6].

- The ischemic phase persists during the initial minutes when only potentially reversible ischemia is present because the viability of the jeopardized myocardium is maintained by anaerobic metabolism.
- The infarcting phase occurs during the hours when some protection is provided by collateral vessels and ischemic preconditioning.
- The reperfusing phase occurs during the minutes following spontaneous or therapeutic restoration of coronary flow.

- The healing phase occurs during the weeks when necrosis and inflammation are replaced by scar in the infarcted portion and stunning is replaced by contraction in the salvaged portion [4].
- The chronic phase occurs during the months and years when residual scar coexists with compensating myocardium.

This article focuses on the pitfalls in the existing ECG criteria for the diagnosis of the ischemic and infarcting phases of the ischemia/infarction process. Other articles in this issue by Atar and colleagues consider the diagnosis of STEMI, and of reperfusion based on presence of resolution of ST-segment elevation. As indicated in the article on diagnosis of STEMI by Atar and colleagues, there are current strong criteria for both identification and localization, and ways to attain high specificity. The sensitivity of these criteria is only about 50%, however, and it is undetermined what portion of ECG false negatives is caused by true "ECG silence". Because at the time of initial emergency evaluation it is not possible to determine whether the ischemic or infarcting phase is present, the term "ischemia/infarcting phase" is used. The ST-segment changes of transmural ischemia may mask the Q-wave changes of infarction, and the Q-wave changes of ischemia may resolve when myocardium is salvaged by reperfusion. Indeed, recent studies have documented a 13% to 17% incidence of aborted infarction when patients receive immediate reperfusion therapy triggered by the acute ECG changes of ischemia/infarction [7,8].

Criteria for diagnosis of ischemia/infarction

Patients who have acute myocardial ischemia/infarction constitute a minority of the vast numbers of individuals with the broad range of symptoms suggestive of acute coronary syndrome who indeed require emergency diagnosis and therapy. ECG standards for detection of the presence, location, acuteness, severity, and extent of myocardium jeopardized by acute coronary occlusion provide support for the clinical decisions required to maximize salvage and minimize morbidity and mortality. High ECG diagnostic accuracy is required because

- The subsequent health of the individual is so critically influenced by infarcted myocardium.
- The typical thrombotic cause of the coronary occlusion is potentially reversible.

- Intravenous or intracoronary reperfusion therapy has both high economic cost and high risk of serious adverse consequences.

Acute coronary thrombosis typically produces potentially reversible myocardial ischemia within seconds, which then evolves to infarction within minutes in the absence of reperfusion [9]. The ECG changes associated with this process can be categorized into those affecting repolarization (ie, the ST segment and T wave) and those affecting depolarization (ie, the QRS complex). Following acute coronary occlusion, as contrasted with exercise-induced ischemia, the initial ECG change is deviation of the T waves toward the involved myocardial region [6]. These hyperacute T-wave changes typically are accompanied by or followed by similarly directed deviation of the ST segment from the TP/PR baseline. This ST-segment deviation is indicated by ST elevation in the ECG leads directed toward the involved region and by ST depression in leads directed away from the involved region. These ST deviations are produced by the flow of injury currents generated by voltage gradients across the boundary between the ischemic and non-ischemic myocardium during the resting and early repolarization phases of the ventricular action potential [10,11]. Questions remain about the exact location and configuration of this boundary and the mechanism of generation of the injury current.

The involved myocardial region is determined by identifying the ECG lead or spatially contiguous pair of leads with the maximal positive or negative ST deviation. This method is in contrast to that for ischemia of increased myocardial demand, where the direction of ST-segment deviation on the surface ECG does not accurately localize the involved region [12].

Pitfalls in the current diagnostic standards

The current criterion for the diagnosis of acute myocardial ischemia/infarction is ST-segment elevation of at least 0.1 mV in two contiguous ECG leads (an 0.2-mV threshold is required in precordial leads V1 to V3) [3].

There are pitfalls in each of the three components of this standard, however:

1. Two contiguous leads
2. ST segment elevation
3. A single diagnostic deviation threshold for both genders and all age groups

An additional pitfall is the inconsistency of the terms used for ECG designation of the regions of the left ventricle involved by acute ischemia/infarction in regard to those adopted as standards for cardiac imaging [13]. Each of these pitfalls and potential methods for their elimination are considered.

Two contiguous leads

It is difficult to determine which of the ECG leads are really contiguous (adjacent) unless they are displayed in the order of their sequential viewpoints of the cardiac electrical activity. Only the six chest leads are currently displayed in their contiguous order: V1, V2, V3, V4, V5, and V6. The limb leads usually are displayed in two separate groups of three: I, II, and III, and aVR, aVL, and aVF. This display is the existing standard despite the 30-year experience in Sweden with the orderly (Cabrera) display of aVL, I, −aVR, II, aVF, III (Fig. 1) [14]. Indeed, this change was endorsed in the 2000 ESC/ACC consensus guidelines [4]. The orderly (Cabrera) sequence of frontal plane leads is contrasted with the classic sequence in Fig. 1. It should be noted that the classic display of the frontal plane included lead aVR, but the orderly display replaces this lead with lead −aVR. This lead replacement provides six spatially contiguous leads and therefore five pairs of spatially contiguous leads in the frontal as well as in the transverse plane. Only three pairs of spatially contiguous leads are provided by the classic limb lead display: aVL and I, II and aVF, and aVF and III.

ST elevation

In any of the 12 standard ECG leads with their positive poles directed toward the region of ischemia/infarction, ST segment elevation would be recorded, and STEMI would be diagnosed. In leads with their negative poles directed toward the involved region, however, ST-segment depression would be recorded; and "non-STEMI" would be diagnosed. As illustrated in Fig. 2, neither the 150° arc in the frontal plane including the positive poles of the six orderly displayed limb leads (Fig. 2B) nor the 150° arc in the transverse plane including the positive poles of the six orderly displayed chest leads (Fig. 2C) provide views of the basal and middle segments of either the anterosuperior or posterolateral left ventricular (LV) walls.

Just as lead aVR and lead −aVR are two distinct ECG leads, each of the other 11 standard leads has

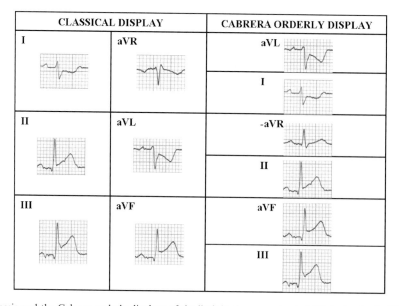

Fig. 1. The classic and the Cabrera orderly displays of the limb leads are contrasted. Note that lead aVR in the classic display is replaced by lead –aVR in the Cabrera orderly display.

a reciprocal (antipodal, inverted, mirror-lake) counterpart. Thus the 10 recording electrodes required to generate the standard 12-lead ECG potentially provide a 24-lead ECG, because all 12 leads are bipolar. Leads I, II, and III are universally accepted as bipolar because two physical electrodes are used for their generation. Alternatively, the negative poles of the augmented limb leads aVR, aVL, and aVF are provided by the average of the potentials recorded by the other two limb electrodes, and the negative poles of the chest leads V1, V2, V3, V4, V5, and V6 are provided by Wilson's central terminal that includes the potentials recorded from all three of the limb electrodes [16]. The 12 leads in each plane can be viewed around the two 360° perimeters as "clockface displays" (Fig. 3) [17,18].

The pitfall of requiring ST elevation for acute ischemia/infarction diagnosis has profound implications in this era when reperfusion therapy is considered to be indicated in the presence of STEMI but contraindicated in the presence of non-STEMI.

This "non-STEMI" group is large and heterogeneous; including four very different sub-groups based on their ECG appearance:

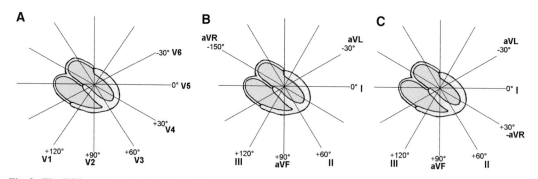

Fig. 2. The ECG leads are displayed in relation to a schematic view of the heart in its typical position in the thorax as documented by cardiac MRI [15] in the (A) transverse and (B and C) frontal planes. The chest leads are displayed in their classical orderly sequence in A, and the limb leads in the classic nonorderly sequence in B. The limb leads are then displayed in the Cabrera orderly sequence in C. Note lead aVR at −150° in B and lead –aVR at +30° in C.

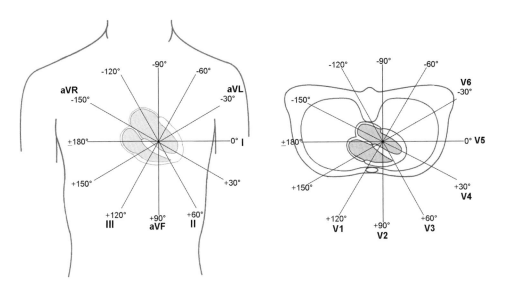

Fig. 3. The full 24-lead ECG is presented as clock-face displays of the frontal (*left*) and the transverse (*right*) planes. The schematic views of the heart are as in Fig. 2.

1. NORMAL - Those with essentially normal ECGs
2. NON-SPECIFIC ST-T - Those with minimal ST segment elevation or T wave inversion
3. CONFOUNDED - Those with ECG confounding factors such as ventricular hypertrophy or bundle branch block
4. STEMI EQUIVALENT - Those with ST depression but no ECG confounding factors

Only individuals in the STEMI EQUIVALENT sub-group should be considered candidates for reperfusion therapy. Indeed, individuals in the CONFOUNDED subgroup may have conditions such as hypertension induced LV hypertrophy that increase their potential for intracerebral bleeding complications of thrombolytic therapy.

It has been shown that sensitivity for posterolateral infarction can be increased by recording from nonstandard posterior chest leads V7 to V9 [19,20]. The placement of these additional electrodes has not been widely accepted, however. Further studies are required to determine if use of these additional electrodes increases the sensitivity for diagnosis of acute coronary occlusion beyond that achieved by consideration of either the 24-lead ECG or STEMI-equivalent ST depression in the 12-lead ECG. Indeed, patients who have even the most proximal site of thrombotic occlusion, the left main coronary, have widespread ischemia manifested primarily by ST depression, with ST elevation typically only in two noncontiguous leads (limb lead aVR and chest lead V1) [21,22].

A single diagnostic ST-deviation threshold

The pitfall of a single diagnostic ST-deviation threshold has been addressed in the 2006 *New ECG Standards* of the AHA, ESC, and ACC. Studies by Macfarlane and colleagues [23] have been used to establish age- and gender-specific thresholds for the diagnosis of STEMI in the standard 12-lead ECG. Future studies are required to establish such thresholds for ST-segment elevation in the negative leads or for STEMI-equivalent ST depression in the standard leads. Reference to the tables of normal values in Macfarlane and Lawrie [24], however, reveals that more than 0.1-mV ST elevation in leads V2 and V3 is the mean normal level in middle-aged white males. Indeed, this is the reason that higher STEMI thresholds are required for these leads than the 0.1-mV threshold required for the other standard leads. Thus, a threshold of even less than 0.1 mV of oppositely directed ST deviation will be required to achieve adequate sensitivity for diagnosis of lateral wall ischemia/infarction.

Myocardial locations of ischemia/infarction

A common diagnostic pitfall is inconsistency in the terms used to designation the locations of the ischemia/infarction process in the LV myocardium. A map of the coronary arteries and the LV regions of ischemia/infarction resulting from their occlusion is presented in Fig. 4 [25]. Like the Mercator projection of a map of the earth, these Mercator views provide a planar perspective of the spatial relationships of the anatomy and pathology to the basal, middle, and apical segments of the walls of the LV. The LV is divided into four walls: the anteroseptal and anterosuperior walls supplied by the left anterior descending (LAD) coronary artery, the posterolateral wall supplied by the left circumflex (LCX) coronary artery, and the inferior wall supplied from the posterior descending coronary artery (the terminal aspect of either the right coronary artery [RCA 90%] or LCX [10%]). Table 1 relates the sites of coronary occlusion to the involved segments of the LV walls.

The LAD supplies perforating branches into the septal wall and diagonal branches into the anterosuperior wall as it continues on its course from the left main coronary in the groove between the right ventricle (RV) and LV (see Fig. 4).

Occlusion of the mid to distal LAD produces ischemia/infarction primarily in the apical segment of the anteroseptal wall (Fig. 5A). Occlusion proximal to the first diagonal branch produces involvement extending into the middle segment of that wall and also the middle and apical segments of the anterosuperior wall and the apical segments of the posterolateral and inferior walls (Fig. 5B). When the occlusion is in the first diagonal branch, the basal and middle segments of the anterior wall are involved (Fig. 5C). Previously the term "high lateral" has been applied, but a better term would be "anterosuperior" ischemia/infarction. When the occlusion is even proximal to the first septal perforating branch, left or right bundle-branch block may occur.

The LCX supplies marginal branches into the anterosuperior wall as it continues on its course from the left main coronary in the groove between the left atrium and ventricle (see Fig. 4). In about 90% of individuals it is nondominant and

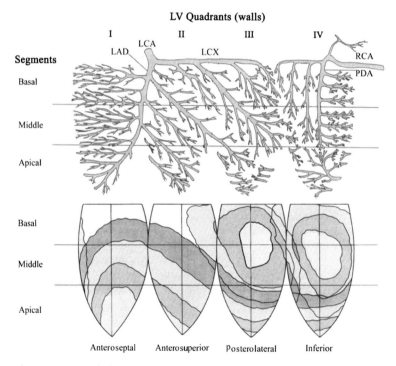

Fig. 4. Mercator views are presented of the coronary arteries (*above*) and the left ventricle (*below*). They have been divided circumferentially into quadrants to coincide with the left ventricular walls (I, anteroseptal; II, anterosuperior; III, posterolateral; IV, inferior) and longitudinally into basal, middle, and apical segments. The RV has been removed to provide a clear view of the interventricular septum in the entire anteroseptal quadrant and in the most anterior aspect of the inferior quadrant. The left ventricular myocardium has been color-coded, with light blue representing the extents of ischemia/infarction resulting from distal occlusions of each of the major coronary arteries, yellow representing the extents of involvement resulting from proximal occlusions of the LCX or RCA, and dark blue representing the extent of involvement resulting from proximal occlusion of the LAD.

Table 1
Sites of ischemia/infarction resulting from occlusion of the major coronary arteries

Ischemia/Infarct Term	LV Wall(s)	Wall Segment(s)	Coronary Artery	Level
Anteroseptal	Anteroseptal	Apical	LAD	Mid-distal
Extensive anterior	Anteroseptal	Apical/middle	LAD	Proximal
	Anterosuperior	Apical/middle		
	Posterolateral	Apical		
	Inferior	Apical		
Mid-anterior[a]	Anterosuperior	Basal/middle	Diagonal or marginal	Proximal
Posterolateral[a]	Posterolateral	Basal	LCX	Mid-distal
Extensive lateral	Posterolateral	Basal/middle	LCX	Proximal
	Anterosuperior	Basal		
Inferolateral	Inferior	Basal/middle	RCA	Mid
	Posterolateral	Basal		
Extensive inferior	Inferior (and RV)	Basal/middle	RCA	Proximal
Inferior	Inferior	Basal/middle	Posterior descending	Proximal

Abbreviations: LAD, left anterior descending coronary artery; LCX, left circumflex coronary artery; RCA, right coronary artery; RV, right ventricular.

[a] Represented on the 12 lead ECG as STEMI-equivalent ST depression.

terminates within that groove. LCX occlusion distal to its first marginal branch produces ischemia/infarction primarily in the basal segment of the posterolateral wall (Fig. 5D). This term should replace "posterior" or "postero-lateral" to coincide with the term typically used when the myocardium is visualized directly by clinical imaging techniques [26,27]. Occlusion proximal to the first marginal branch produces involvement extending into the middle segment of the posterolateral wall and also the basal and middle segments of the anterosuperior wall (Fig. 5E). Occlusion in the marginal branch involves segments of the anterosuperior wall similar to those described for the diagonal branch of the LAD (see Fig. 5C).

The RCA is dominant in about 90% of individuals because, after coursing (and supplying RV branches) in the groove between the right atrium and ventricle, it turns abruptly as the posterior descending branch in the groove between the RV and LV (see Fig. 4). Occlusion of the RCA distal to the first RV branch produces ischemia/infarction primarily in the basal and middle segments of the inferior wall with variable extension into the posterolateral wall (Fig. 5F). Occlusion proximal to the first RV branch produces involvement of that ventricle, as well as the aspects of the LV indicated previously (Fig. 5G). Occlusion of the posterior descending branch of the dominant coronary produces involvement limited to the basal and middle segments of the inferior wall (Fig. 5H).

Fig. 5C and D indicate that the acute mid anterior ischemia/infarction resulting from diagonal or marginal occlusion would be represented by ST deviation toward leads –III and –aVF and that the acute posterolateral ischemia/infarction resulting from LCX occlusion would be represented by ST deviation toward leads –V1 and –V2. An alternative to considering the full 24-lead ECG is considering ST depression in the 12-lead ECG as STEMI-equivalent. This concept may be difficult to adopt clinically, however, because ST depression typically is considered indicative of ischemia caused by increased metabolic demand rather than ischemia/infarction caused by occlusion of coronary flow.

Even occlusion in the most proximal portion (left main) of the left coronary artery produces only STEMI-equivalent ECG changes (Fig. 5I). Indeed, the direction of the ST-segment deviation is the same as typically occurs with the ischemia of increased metabolic demand during a positive stress test. As indicated in the figure, there is usually a large magnitude of ST depression, and, of course, the patient is typically hemodynamically unstable.

Omissions from the current diagnostic standards

Important additions to the ECG evaluation of patients who have acute myocardial ischemia/infarction would be provided by formal indices of the three key aspects of this pathologic process: extent, acuteness, and severity. Indeed algorithms for each of these aspects have been developed, and literature regarding their validation has been accumulating for many years. None of these indices has yet been incorporated into commercial diagnostic algorithms, however, and each is too

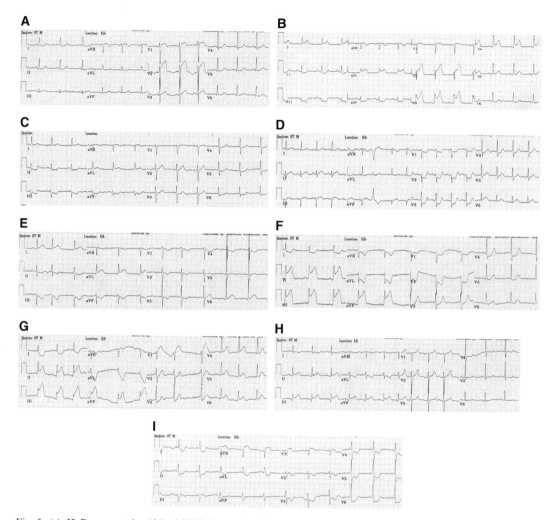

Fig. 5. (*A–H*) Representative 12-lead ECGs for each of the eight regions of ischemia/infarction included in Table 1. In the order in Table 1, the infarcts are termed (*A*) anteroseptal, (*B*) extensive anterior, (*C*) anterosuperior, (*D*) posterolateral, (*E*) anterolateral, (*F*) inferolateral, (*G*) extensive inferior, and (*H*) inferior. (*I*) More global LV involvement resulting from main left occlusion is also included.

complex for routine manual clinical application. Examples of presenting ECGs of patients who have inferior (Fig. 6) and anterior (Fig. 7) STEMI are accompanied by the calculated extent (Aldrich score), acuteness (Anderson-Wilkins score), and severity (Sclarovsky-Birnbaum grade).

Ischemia/infarction extent

The Aldrich score for application on the presenting ECG for estimation of the extent of myocardium at risk for infarction in the absence of successful reperfusion therapy was introduced in 1988 [28]. It is based on the slope of the relationship between the amount in millimeters of

ST segment elevation on the presenting ECG and the Selvester QRS score on the predischarge ECG [29] and is expressed as "% LV infarcted."

Fig. 6 presents the use of the Aldrich formula for estimation of the extent of inferior wall ischemia/infarction based on the amount of ST elevation in leads II, III, and aVF in two representative patients:

% myocardim at risk of infarction

$$= 3[0.6(\text{sum ST elevation II, III, aVF}) + 2].$$

Fig. 7 presents the use of the Aldrich formula regarding anteroseptal and anterosuperior wall involvement:

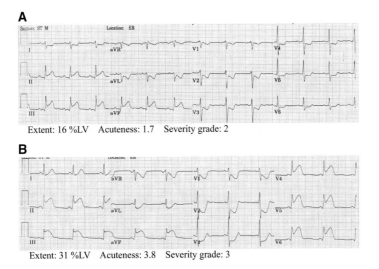

Extent: 16 %LV   Acuteness: 1.7   Severity grade: 2

Extent: 31 %LV   Acuteness: 3.8   Severity grade: 3

Fig. 6. Two presenting ECGs indicating (*A,B*) inferolateral ischemia/infarction of varying extent, acuteness, and severity. The Aldrich extent score, Anderson-Wilkins acuteness score, and Sclarovsky-Birnbaum ischemia grade are indicated beneath each ECG.

% myocardim at risk of infarction

$$= 3[1.5(\# \text{ of leads with ST elevation}) - 0.4]$$

Ischemia/infarction acuteness

The Anderson-Wilkins score for application on the presenting ECG for estimation of the acuteness of the ischemia/infarction process was introduced in 1995 [30]. It was based on the concept developed by Selvester and colleagues of the serial hyperacute, acute, and subacute phases of the acute ischemia/infarction process and is based on the relative amounts of tall T waves and abnormal Q waves in all leads with ST-segment elevation [31]. The Anderson-Wilkins score is provided as a continuous scale from 4.0 (hyperacute) to 1.0 (subacute) based on the comparative hyperacute T waves versus abnormal Q waves in each of the leads with ST-segment elevation. The

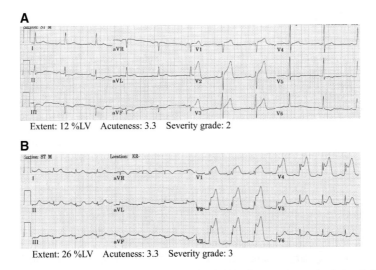

Extent: 12 %LV   Acuteness: 3.3   Severity grade: 2

Extent: 26 %LV   Acuteness: 3.3   Severity grade: 3

Fig. 7. Two presenting ECGs indicating (*A*) anteroseptal and (*B*) extensive anterosuperior ischemia/infarction of varying extent, acuteness, and severity. The format of presentation of the three indices is the same as in Fig. 6.

lead-specific thresholds for both the abnormally increased T-wave amplitudes and increased Q-wave durations are presented in the original reference [30].

The Anderson-Wilkins score has been calculated for the four representative patients in Figs. 6 and 7 using the formula:

4(# leads with tall T **yes**/abnormal Q **no**)
+3(# leads with neither **yes**)
+2(# leads with tall T **no**/abnormal Q **yes**)
+1(# leads with both **yes**)
divided by the Total # leads with
ST-segment elevation

The original acuteness score was recently modified by Heden and colleagues [32] to provide a similarly even distribution of scores in patients who have inferior and anterior ischemia/infarction by reducing the threshold for abnormal Q-wave duration.

Ischemia/infarction severity

The Sclarovsky-Birnbaum score for application on the presenting ECG for estimation of the severity of the ischemia/infarction process was introduced in 1990 [33]. It was based on the concept that the severity of the ischemia/infarction process is determined by the degree of myocardial protection provided by the combination of collateral vessels and ischemic preconditioning. The Sclarovsky-Birnbaum score is expressed as grades 1 (least severe), 2 (moderately severe), and 3 (most severe). Indeed, grade 1 of ischemia is rarely present in patients presenting with acute myocardial ischemia/infarction. Differentiation between grades 2 and 3 severity requires observation of each lead with ST elevation for the presence of "terminal QRS distortion." This distortion is characterized in leads with a terminal R wave by a large ST-segment elevation to R-wave amplitude ratio, and in leads with a terminal S wave by its total disappearance. A recent study by Billgren and colleagues [34] documents a high level of interobserver agreement in calculation of the Sclarovsky-Birnbaum score and provides an appendix with calculation rules.

The Sclarovsky-Birnbaum ischemia grade is indicated for each of the four representative patients in Figs. 6 and 7. Indeed for each figure, examples A were selected for these illustrations because they have the ST elevation without QRS

distortion typical of grade 2 ischemia; and examples B were selected because they have the tombstone-like QRS distortion typical of grade 3 ischemia.

Summary

Pitfalls have been identified in the current standards for use of the ECG in patients presenting with symptoms of acute coronary syndromes to identify those who have probable acute coronary thrombosis–induced myocardial ischemia/infarction. Indeed, there are pitfalls in every aspect of standards for the use of this common but inexpensive method for diagnosing this common but critical clinical problem. The acute ischemia/infarction diagnostic criteria require identification of two contiguous leads, even though the classic display fails to present the limb leads in the same orderly sequence as the chest leads. These criteria require the presence of ST elevation even though acute occlusion of several branches of the coronary arteries, and even of the main left coronary artery, can produce only ST depression in the 12 lead ECG. These criteria have continued to be age and gender nonspecific until corrected in new standards documents. There have been inconsistencies in the terms used to designate the involved myocardial regions, with retention of terms such as "posterior," even though myocardial imaging methods have documented more in-vivo correct alternative terms.

Algorithms for identification of key aspects of the ischemia/infarction process including extent, acuteness, and severity that are too detailed for routine manual application have not been incorporated into commercial ECGs, even though they have been well documented in the literature for 10 to 20 years. Additional studies are needed to validate these indices using non-ECG reference standards. Unfortunately historical time from symptom onset is not a sufficiently accurate estimate of the time of the acute coronary occlusion, and formerly available clinical imaging methods have lacked the precision to serve as standards for ischemia/infarction extent and severity. As additional studies of these indices emerge, future working groups of the international cardiovascular societies will have the opportunity to consider their adoption as new standards for ECG evaluation of individuals who have acute coronary syndromes and who might benefit from reperfusion before their ischemic myocardium undergoes irreversible infarction.

Acknowledgment

The authors acknowledge the key contributions to this document by the AHA Working Group for Establishing New Electrocardiographic Standards chaired by Leonard Gettes. There has been extensive input by the Subgroup on Acute Ischemia/Infarction, some of whom serve as co-authors of this article.

References

[1] Diderholm E, Andren B, Frostfeldt G, et al. ST depression in ECG at entry indicates severe coronary lesions and large benefits of an early invasive treatment strategy in unstable coronary artery disease; the FRISC II ECG sub study. The Fast Revascularization during InStability in Coronary artery disease. Eur Heart J 2002;23:41–9.

[2] Optimal electrocardiography. 10th Bethesda Conference. Am J Cardiol 1978;41:111–91.

[3] Surawicz B. Pathogenesis and clinical significance of primary T wave abnormalities. In: RC Schlant RD, Hurst W, editors. Advances in electrocardiography. New York: Grune and Stratton; 1972. p. 377–422.

[4] The Joint European Society of Cardiology/American College of Cardiology Committee. Myocardial infarction redefined—a consensus document of the Joint ESC/ACC Committee for the Redefinition of Myocardial Infarction. JACC2000:36:959–969 and EHJ2000:21:1502–1513.

[5] Kligfield P, Gettes L, Bailey JJ, et al, and the AHA writing group. Standards for Electrocardiography, Part II: The ECG and its Technology. In final AHA review.

[6] Wagner GS, Wagner NB, White R, et al. The 12 lead ECG in acute myocardial infarctionAcute coronary care. 2nd edition. : Mosby-Yearbook, Inc.; 1994.

[7] Lamfers EJP, Schut A, Hertzberger DP, et al. Prehospital versus hospital fibrinolytic therapy using automated versus cardiologist electrocardiographic diagnosis of myocardial infarction: abortion of myocardial infarction and unjustified fibrinolytic therapy. Am Heart J 2004;147:509–15.

[8] Taher T, Fu Y, Wagner GS, et al. aborted myocardial infarction in patients with ST segment elevation—insights from the ASSENT 3 ECG substudy. J Am Coll Cardiol 2004;44:38–43.

[9] Reimer KA, Lowe JE, Rasmussen MM, et al. The wavefront phenomenon of ischemic cell death. Circulation 1977;56(5):786–94.

[10] Samson WE, Scher AM. Mechanism of ST segment alteration during acute myocardial injury. Circ Res 1960;8:780–7.

[11] Downar E, Janse MJ, Durrer D. The effect of acute coronary artery occlusion on subepicardial transmembrane potentials in the intact porcine heart. Circulation 1977;56:217–24.

[12] Mark DB, Hlatky MA, Lee KI, et al. Localizing coronary artery obstruction with the exercise treadmill test. Ann Intern Med 1987;106:53–5.

[13] Bayés de Luna A, Cino JM, et al. Concordance of Electrocardiographic Patterns and Healed Myocardial Infarction Location Detected by Cardiovascular Magnetic Resonance. Am J Cardiol 2006;97:443–51.

[14] White T. Ordningsföljden för extremitets-acledningarna i EKG. Lakartidningen 1971;68:1352–6.

[15] Foster JE, Martin TN, Wagner GS, et al. Determination of Left Ventricular Long-Axis Orientation using MRI: changes during the respiratory and cardiac cycles in normal and diseased subjects. J Clinical Physiology and Functional Imaging 2005;25:286–92.

[16] Bacharova L, Selvester RH, Engblom H, et al. Where is the central terminal located? In search of understanding the use of the Wilson Central Terminal for production of 9 of the standard 12 ECG leads. JECG 2005;119–27.

[17] Pahlm-Webb U, Pahlm O, Sadanandan S, et al. A new method for using the direction of ST segment deviation to localize the site of acute coronary occlusion: the 24-view standard ECG. Am J Med 2002; 113:75–8.

[18] Sadanandan S, Hochman JS, Kolodziej A, et al. Clinical and angiographic characteristics of patients with combined anterior and inferior ST segment deviation on the initial ECG during acute MI. Am Heart J 2003;146:653–61.

[19] Matetzky S, Freimark D, Chouraqui P, et al. Significance of ST segment elevations in posterior chest leads (V7–V9) in patients with acute inferior myocardial infarction: application for thrombolytic therapy. J Am Coll Cardiol 1998;31:506–11.

[20] Menown IBA, Allen J, Anderson J, et al. Early diagnosis of right ventricular or posterior infarction associated with inferior wall left ventricular acute myocardial infarction. Am J Cardiol 2000;85:934–8.

[21] Barrabes JA, Figueras J, Moure C, et al. Prognostic significance of ST segment depression in lateral leads 1, aVL, V5 and V6 on the admission electrocardiogram in patients with a first acute myocardial infarction without ST segment elevation. J Am Coll Cardiol 1813;2000:35.

[22] Barrabes JA, Figueras J, Moure C, et al. Prognostic value of lead aVR in patients with a first non-ST-segment elevation acute myocardial infarction. Circulation 2003;108:814.

[23] MacFarlane PW. Age, sex and the ST amplitude in health and disease. J Electrocardiol 2001; 34(Suppl):235–41.

[24] Macfarlane PW, Lawrie TDV. Appendix I: normal limits. In: Comprehensive electrocardiology: theory and practice in health and disease. New York: Pergamon Press; 1989. p. 1442–525.

[25] Wagner NB, Wagner GS, White RD. The twelve lead ECG and the extent of myocardium at risk of acute infarction: cardiac anatomy and lead locations, and

the phases of serial changes during acute occlusion. In: Califf RM, Mark DB, Wagner GS, editors. Acute coronary care in the thrombolytic era. Chicago: Year Book Medical Publishers; 1988. p. 31–45.

[26] Bayes de Luna A, Cino JM, Pujadas S, et al. Concordance of electrocardiographic patterns and healed myocardial infarction location detected by cardiovascular magnetic resonance. Am J Cardiol 2006; 97:443–51.

[27] Cino JM, Pujadas S, Carreras F, et al. Utility of contrast-enhanced cardiovascular magnetic resonance (CE-CMR) to assess how likely is an infarct to produce a typical ECG pattern. J Cardiovasc Magn Reson 2006;8:335–44.

[28] Aldrich HR, Wagner NB, Boswick J, et al. Use of initial ST segment for prediction of final electrocardiographic size of acute myocardial infarcts. Am J Cardiol 1988;61:749–63.

[29] Hindman NB, Schocken DD, Widmann M, et al. Evaluation of a QRS scoring system for estimating myocardial infarct size. V. Specificity and method

of application of the complete system. Am J Cardiol 1985;55:1485–90.

[30] Wilkins ML, Pryor AD, Maynard C, et al. An electrocardiographic acuteness score for quantifying the timing of a myocardial infarction to guide decisions regarding reperfusion therapy. Am J Card 1995;75: 617–20.

[31] Anderson ST, Wilkins M, Weaver WD, et al. Electrocardiographic phasing of acute myocardial infarction. J Electrocardiol 1993;25(Suppl):3–5.

[32] Heden B, Ripa R, Persson E, et al. A modified Anderson-Wilkins ECG acuteness score for anterior or inferior myocardial infarction. Am Heart J 2003; 146:797–803.

[33] Sclarovsky S, Mager A, Kusniec J, et al. Electrocardiographic classification of acute myocardial ischemia. Isr J Med Sc 1990;26 535–533.

[34] Billgren T, Birnbaum Y, Sgarbossa EB, et al. Detailed definition and intraobserver agreement for the electrocardiographic Sclarovsky-Birnbaum ischemia grading system. JECG 2002;35(Suppl):201–2.

ELSEVIER
SAUNDERS

Cardiol Clin 24 (2006) 343–365

CARDIOLOGY
CLINICS

Electrocardiographic Diagnosis of ST-elevation Myocardial Infarction

Shaul Atar, MD, Alejandro Barbagelata, MD,
Yochai Birnbaum, MD*

*Division of Cardiology, University of Texas Medical Branch, 5.106 John Sealy Annex,
301 University Boulevard, Galveston, TX 77555, USA*

The ECG is the most useful and feasible diagnostic tool for the initial evaluation, early risk stratification, triage, and guidance of therapy in patients who have chest pain. There is currently a growing trend for 12-lead ECGs to be recorded in the field by paramedics and transmitted by cellular telephone or fax to the target emergency department. It is conceivable that emergency department physicians will be involved in triaging patients in the prehospital phase to hospitals offering primary percutaneous coronary intervention (PCI), which is now recognized to be a superior reperfusion strategy than thrombolytic therapy [1].

Patients who have ST-segment elevation or new left bundle-branch block are usually referred for immediate reperfusion therapy, whereas those who do not have ST-segment elevation are being treated initially with medications [2,3]. Patients are diagnosed as having anterior, inferior-posterior, or lateral myocardial infarction based on the patterns of ST deviation, and assessment of risk is usually based on simple crude measurements of the absolute magnitude of ST-segment deviation or the width of the QRS complexes [4]. Much more information concerning the exact site of the infarct related lesion, prediction of final infarct size, and estimation of prognosis can be obtained from the admission ECG without extra cost or time. Although some clinicians believe that with the increased use of primary PCI in

patients who have ST-elevation myocardial infarction (STEMI) this information is no longer needed, there are many instances in which, even with immediate coronary angiography, identification of the infarct-related site and estimation of the myocardial area supplied by each of the branches distal to the coronary artery occlusion is difficult. In some patients, more than one occlusive lesion may be found, and identification of the acutely thrombosed lesion may not always be apparent. In other cases, total occlusion of side branches at bifurcation of coronary arteries may be missed during coronary angiography.

It is important to appreciate that the ECG provides information about a totally different aspect of pathophysiology in STEMI than does the coronary angiogram. Coronary angiography identifies vessel lumen anatomy, whereas the ECG reflects the physiology of the myocardium during acute ischemia. For this reason, it is possible to observe severe coronary stenoses on angiography without ECG evidence of acute ischemia. On the other hand, it is possible to observe restored vessel patency while the ECG continues to show signs of ongoing "ischemia" or "injury pattern" caused by the no-reflow phenomenon, reperfusion injury, or myocardial damage that has already developed before reperfusion occurs. Thus, although coronary angiography remains the reference standard for identifying the infarct-related artery, the ECG remains the reference standard for identifying the presence, location, and extent of acute myocardial ischemia and injury. Moreover, with current imaging techniques, including contrast ventriculography, echocardiography, and radionuclide

* Corresponding author.
  E-mail address: yobirnba@utmb.edu (Y. Birnbaum).

perfusion imaging, differentiation of ischemic but still viable myocardium from necrotic myocardium during the acute phase of STEMI is not feasible, but such differentiation may be possible with a correct interpretation of the ECG.

Nevertheless, several conditions other than STEMI may present with ST elevation and need immediate recognition to avoid false treatment [5]. These conditions include left ventricular hypertrophy with secondary repolarization abnormalities, early repolarization pattern, Prinzmetal's angina, chronic left ventricular aneurysm, acute pericarditis, pulmonary embolism, and the Brugada syndrome. Moreover, studies have pointed out that in a healthy population, more than 90% of men between the ages of 16 and 58 years have ST-segment elevation of 1 to 3 mm in one or more of the precordial leads, mainly in lead V_2 [6]. The prevalence of these changes declined with age, reaching 30% in men over the age of 76 years, whereas in women the prevalence is only 20% and is constant throughout the ages [7].

Some of the patients who have acute chest pain and ST elevation may subsequently have an increase in cardiac markers without any further ECG changes (no ST resolution, no new Q-wave development, and no T-wave inversion). These patients may have non-STEMI with baseline ST elevation, or pseudo STEMI, as shown in Fig. 1.

On the other hand, there are patients who have transient ST elevation who have ST resolution without an increase in the cardiac markers. Although some of them may have acute pericarditis, Prinzmetal's angina, or aborted myocardial infarction [8], many simply have transient early repolarization or pseudo-pseudo STEMI. This last entity has not been well characterized. The clinician encountering a patient who has suggestive symptoms and ST elevation must make rapid therapeutic decisions concerning urgent revascularization without waiting for the results of cardiac markers. It is currently uncertain how many patients who had pseudo or pseudo-pseudo STEMI have been included in randomized trials of STEMI. For example, in a recent analysis of the Hirulog and Early Reperfusion or Occlusion (HERO)-2 trial, 11.3% of the patients who had ST-segment elevation who received reperfusion therapy did not have enzymatically confirmed myocardial infarction [9]. Increasing the threshold for ST elevation (ie, 2 mm in the precordial leads) may decrease the occurrence of false-positive cases but may result in reduced sensitivity and underuse of reperfusion therapy. Comparison with previous ECG recordings or repeating ECG recordings for evolution of subtle changes, along with selective use of echocardiography, may enable the clinician to increase the accuracy of diagnosing true

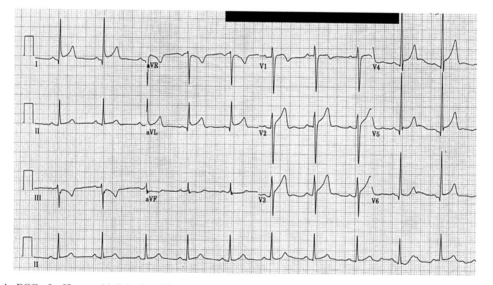

Fig. 1. ECG of a 57-year-old diabetic and hypertensive man admitted with chest pain of 3 hours' duration. ECG shows left ventricular hypertrophy and ST elevation in the anterolateral leads with reciprocal changes in the inferior leads. Subsequently his creatine kinase muscle-brain increased to 28.9 pg/mL, and his troponin I was positive. His ECG 3 years before admission showed the same pattern of ST elevation. Repeat ECGs during current admission did not show resolution of ST elevation, T-wave inversion, or development of new Q waves. The diagnosis is pseudo STEMI.

STEMI that may benefit from urgent reperfusion therapy.

This article concentrates on the information that can be obtained from the admission ECG in patients who have STEMI. In particular, it discusses the association of various ECG patterns of the acute phase of STEMI with estimation of infarct size and prognosis and the correlation of various ECG patterns with the underlying coronary anatomy.

Factors that determine prognosis in ST-elevation myocardial infarction

The immediate prognosis in patients who have STEMI is inversely related to the amount of myocardial reserves (total myocardial mass less the myocardium involved in the acute STEMI [ischemic area at risk], scarred territories caused by previous myocardial infarction or fibrosis, and remote ischemic myocardial segments supplied by critically narrowed coronary arteries). Among patients who do not have prior myocardial infarction or major pre-existing stenotic lesions in the coronary arteries, prognosis is directly related to the size of the ischemic myocardium supplied by the culprit coronary artery distal to the occlusion. In patients who have low myocardial reserves because of previous myocardial infarctions or diffuse fibrosis, however, even a relatively small infarction may be detrimental. Moreover, in patients who have diffuse severe coronary artery disease, a small myocardial infarction may interfere with the delicate balance and induce remote ischemia by obliterating collateral flow or creating a need for (compensatory) augmentation of contractility in the remote noninfarcted segments supplied by stenosed coronary arteries. Therefore, in addition to accurate diagnosis, there is a need for early estimation of the size of the ischemic myocardium at risk and myocardial reserves.

The ECG may help in assessing the size of the ischemic myocardial area at risk, may help in differentiation between subendocardial (nontransmural) and transmural ischemia, and may assist in identifying the presence of previous infarctions (abnormal Q waves in leads not involved in the present infarction; for example, abnormal Q waves in the precordial leads in a patient who has inferior ST elevation) [10]. Furthermore, some ECG patterns may indicate the presence of diffuse coronary artery disease and remote ischemia [11–13].

On admission, part of the myocardial area at risk (supplied by the culprit coronary artery) might have already undergone irreversible damage. The proportion of the ischemic area at risk that has undergone irreversible necrosis depends on the total ischemic time and on the rate of progression of the wave front of necrosis. The rate of progression of necrosis is highly variable and is dependent on the presence of residual perfusion through collateral circulation [14] or incomplete or intermittent occlusion of the infarct related artery [15], as well as on metabolic factors including ischemic preconditioning [16].

ECG changes during the acute phase of ST-elevation myocardial infarction

Shortly after occlusion of a coronary artery, serial ECG changes are detected by leads facing the ischemic zone, as shown in Fig. 2. First, the T waves become tall, symmetrical, and peaked (grade 1 ischemia); second, there is ST elevation (grade 2 ischemia) without distortion of the terminal portion of the QRS; and third, changes in the terminal portion of the QRS complex may appear (grade 3 ischemia) [17–19]. The changes in the terminal portion of the QRS are explained by prolongation of the electrical conduction in the Purkinje fibers in the ischemic region. The delayed conduction decreases the degree of cancellation,

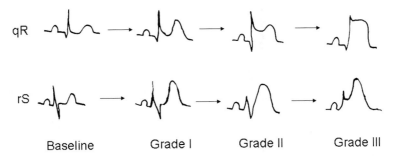

Fig. 2. The grades of ischemia in leads with baseline qR configuration (*upper row*) and leads with baseline rS configuration (*lower row*).

346 ATAR et al

resulting in an increase in R-wave amplitude in leads with terminal R wave and a decrease in the S-wave amplitude in leads with terminal S wave on the surface ECG [20,21]. The Purkinje fibers are less sensitive to ischemia than the contracting myocytes [22]. Hence, for an alteration in the terminal portion of the QRS to occur, there probably should be a severe and prolonged ischemia that would affect the Purkinje fibers [23]. In patients who have collateral circulation, no changes are detected in the QRS complex during balloon angioplasty [20]. Thus, absence of distortion of the terminal portion of the QRS, despite prolonged ischemia, may be a sign for myocardial protection (probably by persistent myocardial flow caused by subtotal occlusion or collateral circulation or by myocardial preconditioning). The disappearance of the S waves in leads with terminal S (RS configuration), mainly leads V_1 to V_3, can be recognized easily (Fig. 3). In contrast, the absolute R-wave height is influenced by many

other variables. Therefore, the absolute R-wave amplitude is not helpful in determining the severity of ischemia. Changes in the R-wave amplitude can be detected reliably only by continuous ECG monitoring; comparison of the admission ECG with previous ECG recordings often is difficult because of differences in ECG instruments and different placement of the precordial electrodes. Therefore, a second empiric criterion for leads with terminal R configuration was developed. This criterion relates the J point of the ST to the R-wave amplitude in leads with terminal R waves (qR configuration). As shown in Fig. 4, a ratio of 0.5 or greater indicates grade 3 ischemia [17,19]. Although the transition between the grades of ischemia is gradual and continuous, for practical clinical purposes it is convenient to define grade 2 ischemia as ST elevation greater than 0.1 mV without distortion of the terminal portion of the QRS and grade 3 as ST elevation with distortion of the terminal portion of the QRS (emergence

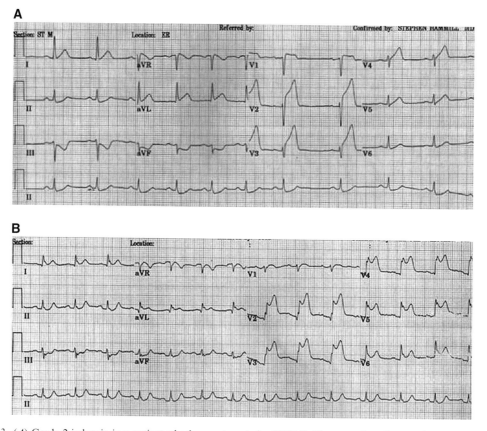

Fig. 3. (A) Grade 2 ischemia in a patient who has acute anterior STEMI. There are deep S waves in leads V_1 to V_3. (B) Grade 3 ischemia in a patient who has acute anterior STEMI. There is loss of S waves in leads V_1 to V_3, and the J point/R wave ratio is greater than 0.5 in leads V_4 and V_5.

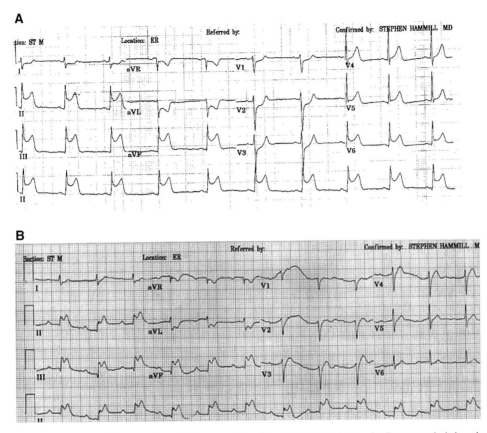

Fig. 4. (*A*) Grade 2 ischemia in a patient who has acute inferolateral STEMI. The J point:R wave ratio is less than 0.5. (*B*) Grade III ischemia in a patient who has acute inferior STEMI. There is first-degree atrioventricular block, and the J point:R wave ratio is greater than 0.5 in leads II, III, and aVF.

of the J point > 50% of the R wave in leads with qR configuration, or disappearance of the S wave in leads with an Rs configuration (see Figs. 3, 4) [17,24–28]. Only later, the T waves become negative, the amplitude of the R waves decreases, and Q waves may appear. Only a minority of patients who have STEMI presents with grade 3 ischemia upon admission. Although the underlying mechanism for this difference is still unclear, grade 3 ischemia has large implications regarding prognosis, as discussed later.

Diagnosis of acute ST-elevation myocardial infarction

In a patient who has typical symptoms, the presence of ST-segment elevation, especially when accompanied with reciprocal changes, is highly predictive of evolving STEMI. Several investigators, however, reported that the sensitivity of the ECG

for acute myocardial infarction may be as low as 50% [29–31]. In most of these studies only one admission ECG was analyzed. Hedges and colleagues [32] used the admission and a second ECG performed 3 to 4 hours after admission and found serial ECG changes in 15% of the patients. Continuous ECG monitoring or multiple ECG recordings over time or during fluctuations in the intensity of symptoms were not performed, however. Repeated ECG recordings may improve the ability to detect subtle ischemic changes. Furthermore, as determined by independent reviewers, 49% of the missed acute myocardial infarctions could have been diagnosed through improved ECG-reading skills or by comparing the current ECG with a previous one [30]. It should be remembered that acute myocardial infarction detected by elevated creatine kinase muscle-brain (MB) or troponin levels without ST elevation is not an indication for urgent reperfusion therapy. The only exception is new left bundle-branch block in a patient who has acute chest pain. Menown and colleagues [33] studied the sensitivity and specificity of the admission ECG for diagnosing acute myocardial infarction by studying patients who had (n = 1041) or did not have (n = 149) chest pain. Acute myocardial infarction was defined by the presence of chest pain of 20 minutes' duration or longer, elevation of creatine kinase two times or more the upper laboratory normal reference level (creatine kinase-MB activity $\geq 7\%$ if the etiology of the total creatine kinase was equivocal), or elevation of creatine kinase less than two times the upper laboratory normal reference level accompanied by serial ECG changes consistent with new myocardial infarction (new Q waves ≥ 0.03 seconds' duration or new persistent T-wave inversion in two or more contiguous leads). The best ECG variables for the diagnosis of acute myocardial infarction were ST elevation greater than 0.1 mV in more than one lateral or inferior lead or ST elevation greater than 0.2 mV in more than one anteroseptal precordial lead. These criteria correctly classified 83% of subjects, with a sensitivity of 56% and a specificity of 94%. Changing the degree of ST elevation significantly modified both the sensitivity (45%–69%) and the specificity (81%–98%). The addition of multiple QRST variables (Q waves, ST depression, T-wave inversion, bundle-branch block, axes deviations, and left ventricular hypertrophy) increased specificity but only marginally improved overall classification [33].

Estimation of the size of ischemic myocardium at risk

There is no currently defined reference standard to measure the ischemic area at risk in the acute setting. The extent of regional wall motion abnormalities can be appreciated easily soon after admission by two-dimensional echocardiography or left ventriculography. With both methods, however, a differentiation between old scars and the acutely ischemic but viable zones is not always possible. Because of the effect of stunning, regional wall motion may persist for long periods of time after reperfusion has occurred [34]. Moreover, differentiation of transmural from subendocardial ischemia/infarction is not always possible, because akinesis may occur when only the inner myocardial layers are ischemic [35].

Several studies have tried to estimate the ischemic area at risk or final infarct size by the admission ECG. In these studies, either the number of leads with ST deviation (elevation or depression) [36–39] or the absolute amplitude of ST deviation [4,36,39–41] was used. The results were conflicting, however. Arnold and Simoons [4] have evaluated the "expected infarct size without thrombolysis" by multivariate regression analysis in 885 patients in the rt-PA/placebo and rt-PA/PTCA trial conducted by the European Cooperative Study Group and validated the findings in 533 patients from the Intracoronary Streptokinase trial of the Interuniversity Cardiology Institute of The Netherlands and in 1741 patients from the Intravenous Streptokinase in Acute Myocardial Infarction study; both trials contained a nonthrombolyzed control group. They defined an infarct size score that included the absolute sum of the amplitude of ST deviation, the QRS width exceeding 0.12 seconds, anterior STEMI location, Killip class 3 or 4 on admission, and delay from symptom onset to treatment allocation and found that the expected infarct size correlated well with the actual enzymatic infarct size in the nonthrombolyzed patients of the latter two studies. Limitation of infarct size by thrombolytic therapy was greatest in patients who had a large expected infarct size and was absent in patients who had a small expected infarct size. Similarly, 1-year mortality reduction was greatest in patients who had a large expected infarct size without thrombolysis.

Aldrich and colleagues [36] studied 144 patients who had STEMI who did not receive thrombolytic therapy. The best correlation between the final ECG Selvester QRS scoring system (an estimation of infarct size) and the admission ECG was found using the magnitude of ST elevation in leads II, III, and aVF in inferior STEMI and the number of leads with ST elevation in anterior STEMI. Another study in patients who received reperfusion therapy showed only a weak correlation between the Aldrich score and either the ischemic area at risk or final infarct size, as measured by pretreatment and predischarge technetium-99m (Tc-99m) sestamibi scans, respectively [38]. The Aldrich formula was related more to the collateral score than to the ischemic area at risk or final infarct size [38]. Clemmensen and colleagues [37] reported a good correlation between the final Selvester score and the number of leads with ST elevation ($r = 0.70$) in anterior STEMI. Neither the magnitude of ST segment elevation in all leads nor the number of leads with ST elevation correlated with the final Selvester score in inferior STEMI. Clements and colleagues [39] also reported only a weak correlation between myocardial area at risk (as assessed by Tc-99m sestamibi scan) and the number of leads with ST deviation, total ST deviation, total ST elevation, or total ST depression. The myocardial area at risk correlated modestly ($r = 0.58$) with total ST deviation in anterior STEMI and with total ST depression normalized to the R wave ($r = 0.70$) in inferior STEMI. Because of large standard errors (9%–15% of the left ventricle), however, these formulas for estimation of the myocardial area at risk cannot be used in the clinical setting for estimation of infarct size [39]. Birnbaum and colleagues [42] showed that among patients with first anterior STEMI, the correlation between either the number of leads with ST elevation or the sum of ST elevation and the extent and severity of regional left ventricular dysfunction (both at 90 minutes after initiation of thrombolytic therapy and at predischarge) was poor.

These ECG studies were based on the assumption that each lead represents the same amount of myocardium and that a similar size of ischemic area in different locations of the left ventricle will result in similar magnitude of ST deviation in the same number of leads. The 12-lead ECG does not represent all myocardial regions equally, however. The inferior and anterior walls of the left ventricle are well represented, but the lateral, posterior, septal, and apical regions are relatively ECG silent [43,44]. Moreover, ischemia in opposed regions may attenuate or augment ST deviation. For example, in patients who have ischemia of the high anterolateral and inferior regions caused by proximal occlusion of a dominant left circumflex coronary artery (LCX), attenuation of ST deviation in leads I, aVL, and the inferior leads may occur, whereas subendocardial high anterolateral ischemia may augment ST-segment elevation in the inferior leads. Posterior myocardial infarction is commonly associated with ST depression in the precordial leads V_1 to V_3 [45], whereas right ventricular infarction may cause ST elevation in leads V_1 and V_2 [46]. In concomitant right ventricle and posterior myocardial infarction, the opposing forces may neutralize each other, and therefore, no ST deviation may occur in these leads. Because different leads represent different areas of the myocardium, a different coefficient probably should be used for each lead and even for each type of infarction. To overcome the unequal representation of the myocardium by the different leads, another technique has been suggested

[47,48]. In this technique the maximal points of the Selvester QRS score are given to each lead with ST elevation greater than 0.1 mV. The sum of these initial scores is considered to represent the percentage of the left ventricle that is ischemic. This method was compared with thallium-201 perfusion scans in 28 patients (10 patients on admission and 18 patients on day 5 after reperfusion therapy) [47]. A good correlation was found between this potential Selvester score and the extent of thallium-201 perfusion defect ($r = 0.79$; $P < .005$). Birnbaum and colleagues [42] found only a weak correlation between the maximal potential Selvester score and the extent or severity of left ventricular dysfunction among patients who had first anterior STEMI and underwent left ventriculography at 90 minutes after initiation of thrombolytic therapy and at predischarge. On the other hand, in patients receiving streptokinase for STEMI, Wong and colleagues [49] found that the initial Selvester QRS score and T-wave inversion grade were the only predictors of myocardial salvage ($P < .001$), with no difference between anterior and nonanterior STEMI [49].

Another qualitative approach for predicting final infarct size by the admission ECG based on the grades of ischemia has been reported by Birnbaum and colleagues [26,27,42,50]. In the Thrombolysis in Myocardial Infarction–4 (TIMI-4) trial, patients presenting with grade 3 ischemia (n = 85) on admission had a larger infarct as assessed by creatine kinase release over 24 hours ($P = .023$), and a larger predischarge Tc-99m sestamibi defect size ($P = .001$) [26]. In a comparison of patients with first anterior STEMI who were assigned randomly to thrombolytic therapy or conservative treatment, the final QRS Selvester score was lowered by thrombolytic therapy only in patients who had grade 2 ischemia on enrollment, but not grade 3 [27]. Overall, final QRS Selvester score was higher for patients who had grade 3 than grade 2 ischemia on enrollment, both in those who received and in those who did not receive thrombolytic therapy. Among patients with a first anterior STEMI who participated in the Global Use of Streptokinase and t-PA for Occluded Coronary Arteries (GUSTO)-I angiographic substudy and underwent angiography both at 90 minutes after initiation of thrombolytic therapy and at predischarge, patients who had grade 2 ischemia on enrollment had higher left ventricular ejection fraction at 90 minutes than patients who had grade 3 ischemia [42]. The difference in global left ventricular function was related mainly to the severity of regional dysfunction in the involved segments and less to the extent of involvement (size of the area at risk) [42]. On predischarge evaluation, the grade 3 group tended to have lower left ventricular ejection fraction and had significantly more chords with dysfunction and more severe regional dysfunction than the grade 2 group. The number of dysfunctional chords tended to decrease from 90 minutes to predischarge in the grade 2 group, whereas it tended to increase in the grade 3 group. This finding may reflect partial recovery from stunning at the predischarge ventriculography in the grade 2 group [42]. There was no difference in the time to therapy or the success of thrombolysis between the grade 2 and 3 groups. Thus, it seems that the difference in infarct size between the grade 2 and grade 3 groups is explained by more severe ischemia and not by larger ischemic area at risk, longer ischemia, or lower rates of successful reperfusion [42]. Findings from the Acute Myocardial Infarction Study of Adenosine trial confirmed this hypothesis [50]. In this study, patients who received thrombolytic therapy were assigned randomly to pretreatment with intravenous adenosine or placebo. For placebo-treated patients, the median pretreatment Tc-99m sestamibi single-photon-emission CT (SPECT) perfusion defect (ischemic area at risk) did not differ significantly between grade 2 and grade 3 patients; however, the median infarction index (infarct size/area at risk) was smaller in patients who had grade 2 ischemia (66% versus 90%; $P = .006$). Overall, infarct size was related to baseline ischemia grade ($P = .0121$) and was reduced by adenosine treatment ($P = .045$). In a recently published study, Billgren and colleagues [51] have assessed the relation of baseline ECG ischemia grades to area at risk and myocardial salvage [100(area at risk − infarct size)/area at risk] in 79 patients who underwent primary PCI for first STEMI and had technetium Tc-99m sestamibi SPECT before PCI and predischarge final infarct size. Patients were classified as having grade 2 ischemia (ST elevation without terminal QRS distortion in any of the leads; n = 48), grade 2.5 ischemia (ST elevation with terminal QRS distortion in 1 lead, n = 16), or grade 3 ischemia (ST elevation with terminal QRS distortion in ≥ two adjacent leads; n = 15). Time to treatment and area at risk were comparable among groups. Myocardial salvage, as a percentage of the area at risk, tended to be smaller for the grade 3 ischemia group than in the other two groups (65%, 65%, and 45%, for grade 2,

2.5, and 3, respectively; $P = .16$). Salvage was dependent on time only in the grade 3 group. The authors conclude that patients who have grade 3 ischemia have rapid progression of necrosis over time and less myocardial salvage, and that grade 3 ischemia is a predictor of smaller myocardial salvage by primary PCI.

Most, but not all, studies have shown that, as a group, patients who have inferior STEMI and ST depression in leads V_1–V_3 have larger infarcts than their counterparts who do not have ST depression, as evidenced by higher peak creatine kinase release; more extensive wall motion abnormalities; larger defect size by thallium-201, Tc-99m, and positron emission tomography; and higher QRS scores of infarct size [13,52–57]. In addition, ST elevation in lead V_6 in patients who have inferior STEMI also is associated with larger myocardial infarction [58]. Others have reported that ST elevation in the posterior leads (V_7–V_9) in patients who have inferior STEMI is associated with larger infarct size [59]. It is unclear whether there is additive value for ST elevation in leads V_7 to V_9 over V_6 alone.

Many variables, such as the width of the chest wall, the distance of the electrode from the ischemic zone, the myocardial mass, and the presence of ischemic preconditioning and collateral circulation, have a major influence on the absolute magnitude of ST deviation. Therefore, currently, there is no accurate method for estimating the area at risk by the admission ECG that can be used in the individual patient, although, in general, patients who have ST deviation (elevation plus depression) in large number of leads or high absolute sum of ST deviation have a larger myocardial infarction than patients who have ST deviation in a small number of leads or low sum of ST deviation [4,40]. There are patients who have a relatively large infarction who have only minor absolute ST deviation. Infarct size underestimation in these patients may lead to underuse of reperfusion therapy. The grades of ischemia predict final infarct size but not the size of the ischemic area at risk.

Differentiation between viable and necrotic myocardium at the ischemic area at risk

Although with echocardiography old myocardial scars with thinning of the ventricular wall and dense echo reflections can be identified, none of the direct imaging modalities (contrast ventriculography and echocardiography) can differentiate between ischemic but viable myocardium and myocardium that has already undergone irreversible necrosis in the acute stage of infarction. Q waves were traditionally considered as a sign of myocardial necrosis [60]. The mechanism and significance of Q waves that appear very early in the course of STEMI in leads with ST elevation are probably different, however [60–63]. Fifty-three percent of the patients who had STEMI admitted within 1 hour of onset of symptoms had abnormal Q waves on presentation, even before reperfusion therapy had been initiated [61]. It has been suggested that Q waves that appear within 6 hours from onset of symptoms do not signify irreversible damage and do not preclude myocardial salvage by thrombolytic therapy [64]. Furthermore, Q waves that appear early in the course of acute ischemia may be transient and disappear later [64,65]. Several authors have found early Q waves to be associated with larger ischemic zone and ultimate infarct size [61,66]. Such Q waves have been explained by a transient loss of electrophysiologic function caused by intense ischemia [60,64]. In contrast, some investigators found that Q waves develop rapidly only after reperfusion [62,63,67]. It has been suggested that the presence of Q waves may be masked by the injury current during ischemia [63], and they frequently can be seen only after resolution of the injury current. These changes, however, may reflect reperfusion injury, interstitial edema, or hemorrhage that later may resolve partially [67]. Ninety minutes after thrombolytic therapy, however, TIMI flow grade 3 is achieved less often in patients with than without abnormal Q waves on presentation [68]. Further studies are needed to find other ECG markers that will assist in differentiation

between acutely ischemic but viable from irreversible necrotic myocardium. Regardless of the underlying mechanism, the presence of abnormal Q waves in the leads with ST elevation on the admission ECG is associated with larger final infarct size and increased in-hospital mortality [69].

Patients who have grade 3 ischemia on enrollment have larger final infarct size [26,50] but not larger initial ischemic area at risk [42,50]. In addition, patients who have grade 3 ischemia are less likely to benefit from thrombolytic therapy than patients who have grade 2 ischemia [27]. Distortion of the terminal portion of the QRS complex in leads with ST elevation is not a sign that irreversible damage had already occurred upon presentation, however, because the same ECG pattern frequently is detected in patients who have Prinzmetal's angina during ischemic episodes that are not associated with significant myocardial damage.

Some patients who have STEMI present with negative T waves (Fig. 5). Early inversion of the T waves, along with resolution of ST elevation, is a sign of reperfusion [70]; however, the significance of negative T waves in leads with ST elevation before reperfusion therapy is initiated is currently unclear. Wong and colleagues [68] reported that 90 minutes after thrombolytic therapy, TIMI flow grade 3 was seen less often in patients who presented with ST elevation and negative T waves than in those who had positive T waves. In a retrospective analysis of the HERO-1 study [49], the same authors found on multivariate analysis that the T-wave inversion grade (graded according to the depth and location of T-wave inversion) on admission in patients with first STEMI was the strongest predictor of less

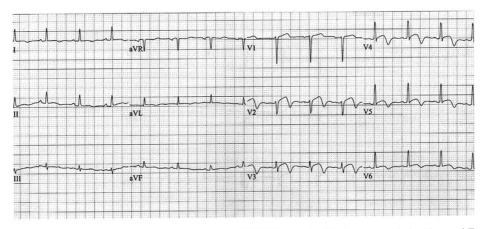

Fig. 5. Admission ECG of a patient who has anterolateral STEMI, showing ST elevation with deep inverted T waves.

myocardial salvage (r = 0.57; $P < .001$). Herz and colleagues [71] reported that among patients treated 2 to 6 hours after onset of symptoms, those who presented with inverted T waves in leads with ST elevation had higher in-hospital mortality than patients with positive T waves. In contrast, among patients treated within the first 2 hours of onset of symptoms, patients who had negative T waves had no hospital mortality (0/52 patients), as compared with a 5.0% mortality rate in patients who had positive T waves (36/726 patients; $P = .19$) [71]. Therefore, ST elevation with negative T waves, especially if it occurs in patients presenting more than 2 hours of onset of symptoms, may be used as an ECG sign of a more advanced stage of infarction or presence of irreversible damage, associated with lesser chance of achieving successful reperfusion, and subsequently leading to higher mortality.

Expected rate of progression of myocardial infarction

It currently is impossible to assess the severity of myocardial ischemia or the expected rate of progression of myocardial necrosis by direct myocardial imaging. The magnitude of ST elevation reflects mainly the severity of the subepicardial ischemia. The standard surface 12-lead ECG is less sensitive to subendocardial ischemia. Subendocardial ischemia may cause either ST depression or no change in the ST segment. ST depression, however, also may result from reciprocal changes in leads oriented away from the ischemic zone [72]. Augmentation of collateral flow ameliorates the magnitude of ST deviation during coronary balloon occlusion [73]. Moreover, ischemic preconditioning by preceding brief ischemic episodes attenuates the magnitude of ST deviation [73,74]. Data regarding the effects of myocardial preconditioning or the presence of sufficient collateral circulation on the 12-lead ECG during acute myocardial infarction are sparse, however. Collateral circulation reduces the severity of the subepicardial ischemia and hence attenuates ST elevation [38]. Indeed, Sagie and colleagues [75] showed that in patients who had acute anterior STEMI and who had good collateral circulation, only T-wave changes, without ST elevation (grade 1 ischemia) were observed. Other cardiac and noncardiac variables, such as presence of myocardial hypertrophy, the distance of the heart from the chest wall, or the width of the chest wall, may also affect the magnitude of

ST deviation. Therefore, the absolute magnitude of ST deviation can give only a rough estimation of the magnitude of myocardial protection or the severity of ischemia.

Identifying ischemia at a distance

Patients who have ST elevation in one territory often have ST depression in other territories. The additional ST deviation may represent ischemia in a myocardial region other than the area of infarction or may represent pure reciprocal changes. There is abundant literature on the significance of different types of ST depression during STEMI [72]. Most of the common patterns of remote ST depression probably represent reciprocal changes and not ischemia at a distance. In anterior STEMI, ST depression in the inferior leads is reciprocal to involvement of the basal anterolateral region, supplied by the first diagonal branch and represented by ST elevation in leads I and aVL [76,77]. In patients who have inferior STEMI, ST depression in lead aVL is a pure reciprocal change and is found in almost all patients [78], and ST depression in leads V_1 to V_3 probably does not represent ischemia at a distance but rather reciprocal changes caused by more posterior, inferoseptal, apical, or lateral left ventricular involvement [53,55,56]. In contrast, among patients who have inferior STEMI, ST depression in leads V_4 to V_6 is associated with concomitant left anterior descending (LAD) coronary artery stenosis or three-vessel disease [11,13,79]. Thus, presence of an atypical pattern of ST depression and especially ST depression in leads V_4 to V_6 in inferior STEMI may signify ischemia at a distance.

In special circumstances both types of ST depression may be present. In STEMI caused by occlusion of the first diagonal branch, in addition to ST elevation with positive T waves in leads aVL and V_2, there usually is reciprocal ST depression with negative T waves in the inferior leads (pure mirror image) and a different pattern of ST depression with tall, peaked T waves (subendocardial ischemia) in V_4 and V_5; the ST segment in lead V_3 is either isoelectric or depressed [77].

Boden and colleagues [80] reported that in patients who have non-STEMI, isolated ST-segment depression in leads V_1 to V_4 was more likely to caused by posterior wall STEMI (reciprocal changes) when it was associated with upright T waves; it was caused by anterior subendocardial ischemia when the T waves were negative., Porter and colleagues [81], however, found that the polarity of the T waves in the precordial leads with ST depression cannot be used to differentiate between the two etiologies of ST depression. In many patients who have inferior STEMI and ST depression in leads V_1 to V_3, the associated T waves in these leads are negative initially (a reciprocal image of ST elevation with positive T waves in leads facing the infarct zone), and only later do the T waves become positive and the R-wave amplitude increase (a reciprocal image of inversion of the T waves and development of Q waves in leads facing the infarction).

Identification of the exact site of the infarct-related artery

The admission ECG, by suggesting the location of the ischemic area at risk, may assist in identificating the exact site of coronary artery occlusion. Because of variability in the coronary anatomy, in some instances there may be more than one possible explanation for a specific ECG pattern. Moreover, because the size and exact location of the vascular bed supplied by the occluded artery varies considerably, occlusion in the same site of a coronary artery in different patients may result in a different size and location of the ischemic area at risk and hence different ECG changes. In addition, presence of severe preexisting narrowing in a nonculprit coronary artery may cause ischemia at a distance that may alter the classic ECG picture. Much of the work that studied the correlation between various ECG patterns and the site of the culprit lesion included only patients who had single-vessel disease and a first myocardial infarction; thus the applicability of these criteria to the general population, and especially to the patients who had prior STEMI or coronary artery bypass graft, is unclear.

Acute anterior ST-elevation myocardial infarction

Classic ECG patterns

LAD obstruction usually causes ST elevation in the precordial leads V_1 to V_4 [82]. Aldrich and colleagues [83] reported similar findings showing the frequency of ST elevation in patients who have acute STEMI caused by LAD occlusion to be, in descending order: V_2, V_3, V_4, V_5, aVL, V_1, and V_6 [83]. Uncommonly, ST elevation in leads V_1 to V_4 may be caused by proximal right coronary artery (RCA) occlusion with concomitant right

ventricular infarction [46,84,85]. In Blanke and co-workers' [82] analysis of patients who have acute STEMI caused by RCA occlusion, the frequency of ST elevation in these four precordial leads was as follows: V_1, 5%; V_2 and V_3, 15%; and V_4, 8%. These investigators found no instances of ST elevation in leads V_1 to V_4 in the patients who had acute myocardial infarction caused by LCX occlusion. Right ventricular infarction that produces ST elevation in leads V_1 to V_4 may be distinguished from anterior STEMI by observing an ST elevation in lead V_1 greater than in lead V_2, ST elevation in the right precordial leads V_3R and V_4R, ST depression in lead V_6, and ST elevation in the inferior leads II, III, and aVF [84,86]. The magnitude of ST elevation in lead V_1 correlates better with the magnitude of ST elevation in lead V_3R than with lead V_2, suggesting that ST elevation in lead V_1 reflects the right ventricle more than the left ventricle [86]. The typical ECG findings in acute anterior STEMI are presented in Box 1.

Diagnosis of anterior infarction extending to contiguous myocardial zones

Anterosuperior myocardial zone

The high anterolateral wall at the base of the left ventricle receives its coronary blood flow from the first diagonal branch of the LAD, the first obtuse marginal branch of the LCX, or, occasionally, from the ramus intermedius artery [87]. The ECG lead that most directly faces this anterosuperior myocardial zone is lead aVL [87,88]. In acute anterior STEMI, ST elevation in lead I, and particularly in lead aVL, signifies an LAD occlusion proximal to the first diagonal branch [88,89]. In contrast, ST depression in lead aVL during acute anterior STEMI signifies LAD occlusion distal to the first diagonal branch [90]. Although ST elevation in lead aVL is a very specific sign of proximal LAD occlusion, it has a relatively low sensitivity for this diagnosis. Sasaki and colleagues [91] noted that patients who have a proximal occlusion of long LAD artery that wraps around the cardiac apex have concomitant injury to the inferorapical and anterosuperior walls of the left ventricle. When this happens, no ST elevation may be seen in either anterosuperior leads (ie, I, aVL) or inferior leads (ie, II, III, aVF) because the opposing forces cancel each other. Isolated occlusion of the first diagonal branch also may result in ST elevation in lead aVL [77,88]. The ECG can be useful in distinguishing isolated diagonal branch occlusion from LAD occlusion proximal

---

Box 1. ECG findings in acute anterior STEMI

Precordial leads
- ST elevation is usually present in V_2 to V_4.
- ST elevation in V_4 to.V_6 without ST elevation in V_1 to V_3 usually is caused by LCX or distal diagonal occlusion.
- ST elevation in leads V_2 to V_6 may represent LAD occlusion proximal to the first diagonal branch.

Leads I and aVL
- ST elevation in lead I and aVL signifies

  1. Occlusion of a short LAD coronary artery before the first diagonal branch (if there is ST elevation in V_2 to V_4)
  2. Occlusion of first diagonal branch (if associated with ST elevation in V_2 and isoelectric ST or ST depression in V_3 to V_6)
  3. Occlusion of the first marginal branch of the LCX (if there is ST depression in V_2)

- ST depression in aVL signifies LAD artery occlusion distal to the first diagonal branch.

Leads II, III, and aVF
- ST depression in the inferior leads signifies

  1. Occlusion of a short LAD coronary artery before the first diagonal branch (if there is ST elevation in V_2 to V_4)
  2. Occlusion of the first diagonal branch (if associated with ST elevation in V_2 and isoelectric ST or ST depression in V_3 to V_6

- ST elevation in the inferior leads signifies occlusion of a long LAD artery (that wraps the cardiac apex) distal to the first diagonal branch.

Lead aVR
- ST elevation in aVR signifies LAD artery occlusion proximal to the first septal branch.

Right bundle-branch block (new)
- Right bundle-branch block signifies LAD artery occlusion proximal to the first septal branch.

---

to the first diagonal branch, however. Occlusion of the diagonal branch typically results in ST elevation in leads I, aVL, and V_2 with ST segments in leads V_3 and V_4 either isoelectric or depressed [77,87]. In contrast, LAD occlusion proximal to the first diagonal branch results in ST elevation extending beyond lead V_2 or V_3 and occasionally, to V_4 to V_6 [77,87]. In addition, when ST elevation in leads I and aVL are caused by occlusion of the LCX, reciprocal ST depression is usually observed in lead V_2 because the vascular bed supplied by the LCX extends more posteriorly [25].

Several ECG criteria have been reported by Engelen and colleagues [90] to indicate an LAD artery occlusion proximal to the first septal perforator branch: (1) ST elevation in lead aVR (sensitivity 43%; specificity 95%; $P = .000$); (2) right bundle branch block (sensitivity 14%; specificity 100%; $P = .004$); (3) ST depression in lead V5 (sensitivity 17%; specificity 100%; $P = .009$); and (4) ST elevation in lead V_1 greater than 2.5 mm (sensitivity 12%; specificity 100%; $P = .011$). These findings were also supported by a recent study done by Vasudevan and colleagues [92] on 50 patients who had acute anterior STEMI and underwent angiography within 3 days of the infarct. Criteria reported to indicate LAD artery occlusion distal to the first septal perforator branch include abnormal Q waves in leads V_4 to V_6 [90]. On the other hand, Birnbaum and colleagues [93] did not find an association between ST elevation in lead V_1 and LAD artery occlusion proximal to the first septal branch. Ben-Gal and colleagues [94] suggested that because the right paraseptal area is supplied by the septal branches of the LAD, alone or together with the conal branch originating from the RCA, ST elevation in lead V_1 in anterior STEMI is caused by right paraseptal ischemia in patients who have an anatomically small and nonprotective conal branch of the RCA.

Lateral and apical myocardial zones

Most patients (93%) who have an acute anterior STEMI caused by LAD occlusion have an anteroseptal pattern (ST elevation in leads V_1 to V_3) [82,83]. In contrast, isolated ST elevation in leads V_4 to V_6, without ST elevation in leads V_1 to V_3, usually is caused by an occlusion of the LCX or distal diagonal branch. Many assume that in patients who have extensive anterior myocardial infarction (ST elevation in leads V_1 to V_6), the injury extends to the distal anterolateral wall and cardiac apex caused by a long LAD artery or prominent diagonal branches, whereas patients who have an anteroseptal pattern (ST elevation confined to leads V_1 to V_3) have a short LAD or large obtuse marginal branches or ramus intermediate branch supplying these anterolateral and apical zones. A study by Shalev and colleagues [95] investigated the correlation of the ECG pattern of anteroseptal myocardial infarction with the echocardiographic and angiographic findings. They found that 48 of 52 patients (92%) who presented with ST elevation in leads V_1 to V_3 had an anteroapical infarct and a normal septal motion. The culprit narrowing was found more frequently in the mid to distal LAD (in 85% of patients). They conclude that the ECG pattern traditionally termed "anteroseptal STEMI" should be called an "anteroapical myocardial infarction"; the term "extensive anterior STEMI" should be used when associated with diffuse ST changes involving the anterior, lateral, and occasionally, inferior leads. Recently, using transthoracic echocardiography, Porter and coworkers [96] found no difference in regional wall motion abnormalities in the lateral and apical segments in patients presenting with first acute anterior STEMI, with or without ST elevation in leads V_5 and V_6.

Inferior myocardial zone

During acute anterior STEMI, injury may extend to the inferior wall, as evidenced by ST elevation in leads II, III, and aVF, if the LAD artery wraps around the cardiac apex [82,97,98]. As previously mentioned, however, anterior STEMI that is caused by a wrapping LAD occlusion proximal to

the first diagonal branch does not manifest as an anterior and inferior injury pattern because of cancellation of opposing vectors [91,98]. In theory, occlusion of an LAD artery that supplies collateral blood flow to an obstructed RCA or LCX may produce a similar anterior and inferior pattern; however, Tamura and colleagues [98] did not observe such a pattern in the 12 patients they studied with this type of ECG.

ST depression in the inferior leads II, III, and aVF during acute anterior STEMI indicates injury to the high anterolateral wall and does not signify inferior wall ischemia [99,100]. Several investigators found such reciprocal ST depression in the inferior leads to indicate LAD artery occlusion proximal to the first diagonal branch [76,90]. In patients who have a long LAD artery that wraps around the cardiac apex, however, proximal LAD artery occlusion may not produce reciprocal ST depression in the inferior leads because of extension of the infarction to the inferoapical wall [91].

Acute inferior ST-elevation myocardial infarction

Classic ECG patterns

In inferior STEMI, the leads showing the greatest magnitude of ST elevation, in descending order, are leads III, aVF, and II. Most patients who have ST elevation in these inferior leads (80%–90%) have an occlusion of the RCA; however, an occlusion of the LCX can produce a similar ECG pattern [101]. In addition to ST elevation in the inferior leads II, III, and aVF, reciprocal ST depression in lead aVL is seen in almost all patients who have acute inferior STEMI [78]. The ECG distinction between RCA- and LCX-related inferior STEMI is presented in Table 1 [101–107]. ECG confirmation of the infarct-related artery during acute inferior STEMI may be particularly valuable when coronary angiography indicates lesions in both the RCA and LCX.

Criteria in the precordial leads

Because the right ventricular branch originates from the RCA, criteria for right ventricular infarction, especially ST elevation in leads V_3R and V_4R, provide compelling evidence that the infarct-related artery in acute inferior STEMI is the proximal RCA. Kontos and colleagues [102] reported that LCX-related inferior STEMI was

Table 1
Common ECG features distinguishing the culprit artery in acute inferior wall myocardial infarction

Right Coronary Artery Occlusion			Left Circumflex Artery Occlusion		
Criterion	Sensitivity (%)	Specificity (%)	Criterion	Sensitivity (%)	Specificity (%)
ST↑ V3R, V4R	100	87	No ST↓ aVL	80	93
ST↓ V3 / ST↑ III < 0.5 = proximal RCA; 0.5–1.2 = distal RCA	91	91	ST↓ V3 / ST↑ III > 1.2	84	95
	84	93			
S:R ratio aVL > 3	76	88	S:R ratio aVL ≤ 3	88	76
ST↑; III > II	88	94			
ST↓; aVL > ST↓ I	80	94			

Abbreviation: RCA, right coronary artery.

suggested by reciprocal ST depression in leads V_1 and V_2. When Birnbaum and colleagues [13] compared patients who had inferior STEMI caused by mid or distal RCA versus LCX occlusion, however, they found no difference in the frequency of ST depression in leads V_1 to V_3. ST depression is absent in leads V_1 to V_3 only during proximal RCA occlusion, because the resultant right ventricular injury pattern cancels out such reciprocal ST depression [13]. Some investigators have reported a higher frequency of ST elevation in leads V_4 to V_6 in patients who had LCX-related acute inferior STEMI [102,103]. Hasdai and colleagues [105], however, found little difference in the frequency of ST elevation in leads V_4 to V_6 between patients who have LCX- versus RCA-related inferior STEMI. The authors state that because most cases of acute inferior STEMI are caused by RCA occlusions, the positive predictive value (PPV) of ST elevation in leads V_5 or V_6 for LCX-related infarction is only 59% [105]. Kosuge and colleagues [106] reported that the magnitude of ST depression in lead V_3 relative to the ST elevation in lead III (V_3:III ratio) was useful in distinguishing the culprit artery in inferior STEMI. They found that a V_3:III ratio of less than 0.5 indicated a proximal RCA occlusion; a V_3:III ratio of 0.5 to 1.2 indicated a distal RCA occlusion; and a V3:III ratio of more than 1.2 indicated LCX occlusion [106]. Again, these criteria are based on the fact that with RCA occlusion the vector that causes ST depression in lead V_3 is masked by the vector of right ventricular injury.

Criteria in the limb leads

ECG criteria in the limb leads also have been found to be useful in distinguishing RCA and LCX occlusion in acute inferior STEMI. For example, greater ST elevation in lead III than in lead II has been shown to indicate RCA infarction [104,108]. Additional limb lead criteria involve careful analysis of leads I and aVL. Patients who have LCX-related STEMI less frequently show reciprocal ST depression in lead aVL and more often show an isoelectric or a raised ST segment in leads I and aVL compared with patients who have RCA-related inferior infarction [102,104]. Hasdai and colleagues [105] reported that such absence of reciprocal ST depression in lead aVL indicates injury of the anterosuperior base of the heart typically caused by LCX occlusion proximal to the first obtuse marginal branch. These investigators found absence of reciprocal

ST depression in lead aVL in 86% of patients who had proximal LCX-related inferior STEMI but in none of the patients who had RCA- or distal LCX-related infarctions ($P = .0001$). An additional criterion for identifying the culprit artery in inferior STEMI is the magnitude of ST depression in lead aVL compared with lead I [104]. Greater reciprocal ST depression in lead aVL than in lead I suggests an RCA-related inferior STEMI [104]. A likely explanation for this phenomenon is that injury of the high posterolateral region caused by LCX occlusion attenuates ST depression in lead aVL more than in lead I, which has a less superior orientation. A final criterion in lead aVL to distinguish the culprit artery in inferior STEMI relates to the amplitude of the respective R and S waves in this lead [107]. In the initial stages, leads facing an infarcted wall with ST elevation tend to show QRS changes as well, including an increase in R-wave amplitude and a decrease in S-wave amplitude [109]. Therefore, in inferior STEMI, the opposite pattern (that is, decrease in R wave and increase in S wave) would be expected in lead aVL, if there is no involvement of the high posterolateral region (RCA infarction). In contrast, if there is concomitant involvement of the high posterolateral segments (as expected especially in proximal LCX infarction), these reciprocal changes in the QRS may not be apparent. Indeed, Assali and colleagues [107] found that a decrease in R-wave amplitude and an increase in S-wave amplitude with a S:R ratio greater than 3 predicted RCA occlusion, whereas a S:R ratio less than 3 predicted LCX occlusion. A summary of the criteria to distinguish the culprit artery in inferior STEMI is provided in Table 1, and an example of the criteria is shown in Fig. 6. From these criteria it is clear that the ability to differentiate RCA from LCX occlusion is greater for proximal occlusion. Because occlusion occurs more distally in the culprit artery, the distinctive characteristics are lost, and the ECG cannot be expected to distinguish between right and left posterior descending artery occlusion.

A recent study by Fiol and colleagues [110] has suggested using the following ECG criteria in a three-step algorithm to differentiate RCA from LCX occlusion as the culprit artery: (1) ST changes in lead I, (2) the ratio of ST elevation in lead III to that in lead II, and (3) the ratio of the sum ST depression in leads V_1 to V_3 divided by the sum ST elevation in leads II, III, and aVF. ST elevation in lead I has a 100% PPV for LCX occlusion, whereas ST depression of 0.5 mm

or more has a 94% PPV for RCA occlusion. A ratio of ST elevation in lead III to lead II greater than 1 has a 92% PPV for RCA occlusion, and the ratio of the sum of ST depression in leads V_1 to V_3/ST elevation in II, III, aVF of 1 or less has a 90% PPV for RCA occlusion. Application of this sensitive algorithm suggested the location of the culprit coronary artery (RCA versus LCX) in 60 of 63 patients (>95%).

Diagnosis of inferior infarction extending to contiguous myocardial zones

Right ventricular myocardial zone

Right ventricular infarction occurs almost exclusively in the setting of inferior STEMI. Although isolated right ventricular infarction has been reported, it is rare and occurs most often in patients who have right ventricular hypertrophy [111]. Several investigators have found that ST elevation in lead V_4R is diagnostic of right ventricular infarction with a sensitivity and specificity well over 90% [101,112,113]. It is important to point out that ST elevation in the right precordial leads (eg, V_4R) is most prominent in the early hours of inferior STEMI and dissipates rapidly thereafter. Hence, the window of opportunity to diagnose right ventricular infarction by ECG is limited, and right precordial leads should be recorded immediately as a patient who has ST elevation in the inferior leads presents to the emergency room. As mentioned previously, ST elevation in leads V_1 to V_3 in a patient who has inferior STEMI is a manifestation of associated right ventricular infarction caused by a proximal RCA occlusion [46,84,85]. Lopez-Sendon and colleagues [114] reported that the criterion of ST elevation in lead V_4R greater than ST elevation in any of leads V_1 to V_3 is a very specific sign of right ventricular infarction (specificity, 100%). This criterion was less sensitive (sensitivity 78.6%) than ST elevation in V_4R alone, however [114].

A recent analysis of the GUSTO-I angiographic substudy by Sadanandan and colleagues [115], in patients who had concomitant ST elevation in the anterior (V_1–V_4) and inferior (II, III, aVF) leads, revealed that the infarct-related artery was the RCA in 59% of the cases and was the LAD in 36%. More patients who had RCA occlusion had ST elevation in lead V_1 equal to or greater than the ST elevation in lead V_3 compared with those with LAD occlusion (35% versus 12%; $P = .001$). Furthermore, the progression of ST

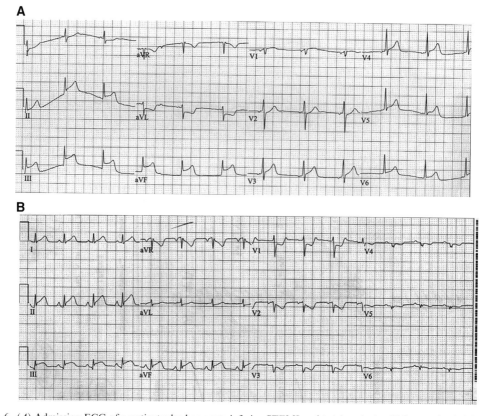

Fig. 6. (*A*) Admission ECG of a patient who has acute inferior STEMI and total occlusion if the proximal right coronary artery on immediate angiography. There is ST elevation in leads II, III, and aVF. ST elevation is greater in lead III than in lead II. There is reciprocal ST depression and deep S waves in lead aVL. The magnitude of ST depression in aVL is greater than in lead I. In addition, there is no ST depression in leads V_1 to V_3. (*B*) Admission ECG of a patient who has acute inferior STEMI caused by occlusion of the proximal LCX on immediate angiography. There is ST elevation in leads II, III, and aVF and ST depression in leads V_1 to V_3. The magnitude of ST elevation in lead III is smaller than in lead II. Of note, there is no reciprocal ST depression in lead aVL.

elevation from lead V_1 to lead V_3 was significantly greater in patients who LAD occlusion than in those who had RCA occlusion. Thus, larger ST elevation in leads II, III, and aVF and absence of progression of ST elevation from V_1 to V_3 differentiate RCA from LAD occlusion in patients who have combined anterior and inferior ST elevation. Only 35% of the patients who had RCA occlusion had ST elevation in lead V_1 equal to or greater than the ST elevation in V_3, however. Therefore, the absence of this criterion does not exclude RCA occlusion.

Lateral apical myocardial zone

In patients who have inferior STEMI, ST elevation in leads V_5 and V_6 is considered to indicate extension of the infarct to the lateral aspect of the cardiac apex; however, there is as yet no direct evidence for this extension [116]. The cause of such an extension may be occlusion of either the LCX or RCA with a posterior descending or posterolateral branch that extends to the lateral apical zone [116]. Tsuka and coworkers [58] found that ST elevation in lead V_6 during inferior STEMI was associated with a larger infarct size, a greater frequency of major cardiac arrhythmias, and a higher incidence of pericarditis during the patient's hospital course. A study by Golovchiner and colleagues [117] assessed the correlation between ST deviation in each of the six precordial leads and the presence of regional wall motion abnormalities by transthoracic echocardiography in 109 patients who had first inferior STEMI. ST elevation in lead V_5 was associated with more frequent involvement of the apical portion of the inferior wall ($P < .02$), with a specificity of 88% and a sensitivity of 33%. Global regional wall motion abnormality score was significantly worse for patients who had ST elevation than forpatients who had isoelectric ST in lead V_5 ($P = .024$). ST elevation in lead V_6 was associated with regional wall motion abnormality in the mid-posterior segment ($P < .006$), with a specificity of 91% and a sensitivity of 33%, and worse global regional wall motion abnormality score ($P = .022$).

Posterior myocardial zone

In patients who have inferior STEMI, ST depression in leads V_1 to V_3 has been shown to indicate a larger infarction with extension of the injury to the posterolateral or the inferoseptal wall [45,53–56,118–122]. Such ST depression in these anterior leads during inferior STEMI is a reciprocal change and does not indicate concomitant LAD coronary artery disease [13,79]. It may be seen in both RCA and LCX inferior infarctions [44,123]. In inferior STEMI caused by proximal RCA occlusion with concomitant right ventricular infarction, however, posterior wall injury may be masked because the two opposed electrical vectors may cancel each other (that is, ST elevation in leads V_1 to V_3 with right ventricular infarction and reciprocal ST depression in these same leads with concurrent posterior infarction) [122]. A more direct sign of posterior wall injury is ST elevation in leads V_7 to V_9 [59,124–126]. Waveform amplitudes in these posterior leads are smaller than in standard precordial leads, however. There is preliminary evidence that ST elevation of 0.5 mm should be considered a sign of injury when analyzing the posterior leads [127]. Isolated ST elevation in leads V_7 to V_9 without ST elevation in the inferior leads occurs in only 4% of patients who have acute myocardial infarction [126] and usually is caused by LCX occlusion [124]. In patients who have acute inferior STEMI, ST elevation in leads V_7 to V_9 is associated with a higher incidence of reinfarction, heart failure, and death [59].

Ischemia at a distance in acute inferior ST-elevation myocardial infarction

Most of the ST depression patterns seen during STEMI represent reciprocal changes rather than ischemia at a distance [72]. One ECG pattern, ST depression in leads V_5 and V_6 in inferior STEMI, signifies concomitant disease of the LAD with acute ischemia in a myocardial zone remote from the infarct zone [11,13,79,128]. Patients who have maximal ST depression in leads V_4 to V_6 during inferior STEMI have higher morbidity and mortality than patients without precordial ST depression or with maximal ST depression in leads V_1 to V_3 [25]. Likewise, patients who have maximal ST depression in leads V_4 to V_6 undergo multivessel revascularization (multivessel PCI or coronary artery bypass surgery) more often than do patients who do not have such an ECG pattern [128].

ST segment elevation in lead aVR has been shown to be a marker of severe diffuse coronary disease in patients who have unstable angina or non-STEMI. ST elevation in lead aVR also can be a marker of acute left main coronary (LMCA) occlusion. Yamaji and colleagues [129] studied the admission 12-lead ECG in 16 consecutive patients who had acute LMCA obstruction, 46 patients who had acute LAD obstruction, and 24 patients who had acute RCA obstruction. Lead aVR ST-segment elevation (>0.05 mV) occurred with a significantly higher incidence ($P < .01$) in the LMCA group (88%) than in the LAD (43%) or RCA (8%) groups. Lead aVR ST-segment elevation was significantly higher in the LMCA group (0.16 ± 0.13 mV) than in the LAD group (0.04 ± 0.10 mV). Lead V_1 ST-segment elevation was lower in the LMCA group (0.00 ± 0.21 mV) than in the LAD group (0.14 ± 0.11 mV). The finding of lead aVR ST-segment elevation greater than or equal to lead V_1 ST elevation distinguished the LMCA group from the LAD group with 81% sensitivity, 80% specificity, and 81% accuracy. ST segment shift in lead aVR and the inferior leads distinguished the LMCA group from the RCA group. The authors conclude that lead aVR ST-segment elevation with less ST-segment elevation in lead V_1 is an important predictor of acute LMCA obstruction [129].

Discussion

The admission ECG pattern is the most informative noninvasive tool for the diagnosis, triage, and risk stratification in patients who have STEMI. Three ECG patterns presented in this article are especially relevant: (1) right ventricular infarction accompanying acute inferior STEMI, (2) a very proximal LAD occlusion in anterior STEMI, and (3) patients at higher risk (ie, those who have grade 3 ischemia, ST depression in V_4–V_6 concomitant with inferior STEMI, and ST elevation in lead aVR).

Moreover, it is crucial to recognize cases in which opposing ECG vectors cancel each other and result in attenuation of the ischemic changes, such as occlusion of a proximal LAD that wraps the cardiac apex or a proximal dominant LCX. In terms of the first assessment, the opportunity to diagnose right ventricular infarction using the ECG is greatest in the emergency department because ST elevation in the right precordial leads resolves quickly. The admitting physician should make certain that all patients who have acute inferior STEMI have a second ECG recorded with right ventricular leads. If ST-segment elevation of 1 mm is observed in lead V_4R, the diagnosis of right ventricular infarction can be made.

Another ECG assessment of importance to the admitting physician is the identification of a very proximal LAD occlusion in acute anterior STEMI. If the occlusion site is proximal to the first diagonal branch of the LAD, a large portion of the left ventricle is at risk of irreversible damage, including the anteroseptal, anterosuperior, anterolateral, and apical regions. Such high-risk patients should be transferred urgently to a cardiac catheterization laboratory for primary PCI.

Patients who have grade 3 ischemia on the admission ECG have higher mortality [24–26,130,131] and reinfarction rates [130,132]. Retrospective analysis of the GUSTO IIB trial patients revealed that grade 3 ischemia was associated with higher mortality both in the primary PCI group and in the thrombolysis group [130]. In the grade 2 group, in-hospital mortality was similar in the thrombolysis and angioplasty subgroups (3.2% and 3.3%; $P = .941$). In patients who had grade 3 ischemia, in-hospital mortality was 6.4% and 7.3%, respectively ($P = .762$). These findings were confirmed in an analysis of the Danish multicenter randomized study on fibrinolytic therapy versus acute coronary angioplasty in acute myocardial infarction, DANAMI–2 [133]. The study showed that mortality increased significantly with symptom duration (>3 hours) in both grade 2 and grade 3 ischemia regardless of treatment strategy. For patients presenting early (<3 hours of symptom onset) who had grade 3 ischemia, however, those in the primary PCI group had a 5.5% 30-day mortality reduction (1.4% versus 6.9%) compared with the thrombolysis group.

Summary

The admission ECG in patients who have STEMI is valuable for selecting patients who are candidates for early reperfusion treatment and also for providing information regarding the location and extent of acute myocardial injury. By reflecting the pathophysiology of the myocardium during acute ischemia, the ECG conveys information not provided by coronary angiography and provides important information to guide clinical decision making.

References

[1] Keeley EC, Boura JA, Grines CL. Primary angioplasty versus intravenous thrombolytic therapy for acute myocardial infarction: a quantitative review of 23 randomised trials. Lancet 2003; 361(9351):13–20.

[2] Antman EM, Anbe DT, Armstrong PW, et al. ACC/AHA guidelines for the management of patients with ST-elevation myocardial infarction–executive summary: a report of the American College of Cardiology/American Heart Association Task Force on Practice Guidelines (Writing Committee to Revise the 1999 Guidelines for the Management of Patients With Acute Myocardial Infarction). Circulation 2004;110(5):588–636.

[3] Braunwald E, Antman EM, Beasley JW, et al. ACC/AHA guideline update for the management of patients with unstable angina and non-ST-segment elevation myocardial infarction–2002: summary article: a report of the American College of Cardiology/American Heart Association Task Force on Practice Guidelines (Committee on the Management of Patients With Unstable Angina). Circulation 2002;106(14):1893–900.

[4] Arnold AER, Simoons ML. "Expected infarct size without thrombolysis", a concept that predicts immediate and long-term benefit from thrombolysis for evolving myocardial infarction. Eur Heart J 1997;18:1736–48.

[5] Wang K, Asinger RW, Marriott HJ. ST-segment elevation in conditions other than acute myocardial infarction. N Engl J Med 2003;349(22):2128–35.

[6] Hiss RG, Lamb LE, Allen MF. Electrocardiographic findings in 67,375 asymptomatic subjects. X. Normal values. Am J Cardiol 1960;6:200–31.

[7] Surawicz B, Parikh SR. Prevalence of male and female patterns of early ventricular repolarization in the normal ECG of males and females from childhood to old age. J Am Coll Cardiol 2002;40(10): 1870–6.

[8] Dowdy L, Wagner GS, Birnbaum Y, et al. Aborted infarction: the ultimate myocardial salvage. Am Heart J 2004;147(3):390–4.

[9] Wong CK, French JK, Aylward PE, et al. Patients with prolonged ischemic chest pain and presumed-new left bundle branch block have heterogeneous outcomes depending on the presence of ST-segment changes. J Am Coll Cardiol 2005;46(1):29–38.

[10] Moshkovitz Y, Sclarovsky S, Behar S, et al. Infarct site-related mortality in patients with recurrent myocardial infarction. SPRINT Study Group. Am J Med 1993;94:388–94.

[11] Strasberg B, Pinchas A, Barbash GI, et al. Importance of reciprocal ST segment depression in leads V5 and V6 as an indicator of disease of the left anterior descending coronary artery in acute inferior wall myocardial infarction. Br Heart J 1990;63:339–41.

[12] Birnbaum Y, Sclarovsky S, Strasberg B. Critical left main stenosis [letter]. Am Heart J 1994;127:1662–3.

[13] Birnbaum Y, Wagner GS, Barbash GI, et al. Correlation of angiographic findings and right (V1 to V3) versus left (V4 to V6) precordial ST-segment depression in inferior wall acute myocardial infarction. Am J Cardiol 1999;83(2):143–8.

[14] Habib GB, Heibig J, Forman SA, et al. Influence of coronary collateral vessels on myocardial infarct size in humans. Results of phase I Thrombolysis in Myocardial Infarction (TIMI) Trial. Circulation 1991;83:739–46.

[15] Haider AW, Andreotti F, Hackett DR, et al. Early spontaneous intermittent myocardial reperfusion during acute myocardial infarction is associated with augmented thrombogenic activity and less myocardial damage. J Am Coll Cardiol 1995;26:662–7.

[16] Kloner RA, Yellon D. Does ischemic preconditioning occur in patients? J Am Coll Cardiol 1994;24(4):1133–42.

[17] Sclarovsky S, Mager A, Kusniec J, et al. Electrocardiographic classification of acute myocardial ischemia. Isr J Med Sc 1990;26:525–33.

[18] Sclarovsky S. Electrocardiography of acute myocardial ischaemic syndromes. London: Martin Dunitz Ltd.; 1999. p. 48–72.

[19] Birnbaum Y, Wagner GS. The Initial electrocardiographic pattern in acute myocardial infarction: correlation with infarct size. J Electrocardiol 1999;32(Suppl):122–8.

[20] Spekhorst H, SippensGroenewegen A, David G, et al. Body surface mapping during percutaneous transluminal coronary angioplasty. QRS changes indicating regional myocardial conduction delay. Circulation 1990;81:840–9.

[21] Wagner N, Sevilla D, Krucoff M, et al. Transient alterations of the QRS complex and ST segment during percutaneous transluminal balloon angioplasty of the left anterior descending coronary artery. Am J Cardiol 1988;62:1038–42.

[22] DeHaan R. Differentiation of the atrioventricular conducting system of the heart. Circulation 1961;24:458–70.

[23] Feldman T, Chua K, Childres R. R wave of the surface and intracoronary electrogram during acute coronary artery occlusion. Am J Cardiol 1986;58:885–90.

[24] Birnbaum Y, Sclarovsky S, Blum A, et al. Prognostic significance of the initial electrocardiographic pattern in a first acute anterior wall myocardial infarction. Chest 1993;103:1681–7.

[25] Birnbaum Y, Herz I, Sclarovsky S, et al. Prognostic significance of the admission electrocardiogram in acute myocardial infarction. J Am Coll Cardiol 1996;27:1128–32.

[26] Birnbaum Y, Kloner R, Sclarovsky S, et al. Distortion of the terminal portion of the QRS on the admission electrocardiogram in acute myocardial infarction and correlation with infarct size and long term prognosis (Thrombolysis In Myocardial Infarction 4 Trial). Am J Cardiol 1996;78:396–403.

[27] Birnbaum Y, Maynard C, Wolfe S, et al. Terminal QRS distortion on admission is better than ST-segment measurements in predicting final infarct size and assessing the potential effect of thrombolytic therapy in anterior wall acute myocardial infarction. Am J Cardiol 1999;84(5):530–4.

[28] Garcia-Rubira JC, Perez-Leal I, Garcia-Martinez JT, et al. The initial electrocardiographic pattern is a strong predictor of outcome in acute myocardial infarction. Int J Cardiol 1995;51:301–5.

[29] Rude RF, Poole KW, Muller JE, et al. Electrocardiographic and clinical criteria for recognition of acute myocardial infarction based on analysis of 3,697 patients. Am J Cardiol 1983;52:936–42.

[30] Lee TH, Rouan GW, Weisberg MC, et al. Sensitivity of routine clinical criteria for diagnosing myocardial infarction within 24 hours of hospitalization. Ann Intern Med 1987;106(2):181–6.

[31] Gibler WB, Young GP, Hedges JR, et al. Acute myocardial infarction in chest pain patients with nondiagnostic ECGs: serial CK-MB sampling in the emergency department. The Emergency Medicine Cardiac Research Group. Ann Emerg Med 1992;21(5):504–12.

[32] Hedges JR, Young GP, Henkel GF, et al. Serial ECGs are less accurate than serial CK-MB results for emergency department diagnosis of myocardial infarction. Ann Emerg Med 1992;21(12):1445–50.

[33] Menown IB, Mackenzie G, Adgey AA. Optimizing the initial 12-lead electrocardiographic diagnosis of acute myocardial infarction. Eur Heart J 2000;21(4):275–83.

[34] Birnbaum Y, Kloner RA. Clinical aspects of myocardial stunning. Coron Artery Dis 1995;6(8):606–12.

[35] Kaul S. There may be more to myocardial viability than meets the eye! Circulation 1995;92:2790–3.

[36] Aldrich H, Wagner N, Boswick J, et al. Use of initial ST-segment deviation for prediction of final electrocardiographic size of acute myocardial infarcts. Am J Cardiol 1988;61:749–53.

[37] Clemmensen P, Grande P, Aldrich H, et al. Evaluation of formulas for estimating the final size of acute myocardial infarcts from quantitative ST-

segment elevation on the initial standard 12-lead ECG. J Electrocardiol 1991;24:77–83.

[38] Christian T, Gibbons R, Clements I, et al. Estimates of myocardium at risk and collateral flow in acute myocardial infarction using electrocardiographic indexes with comparison to radionuclide and angiographic measures. J Am Coll Cardiol 1995;26: 388–93.

[39] Clements I, Kaufmann P, Bailey K, et al. Electrocardiographic prediction of myocardial area at risk. Mayo Clin Proc 1991;66:985–90.

[40] Willems JL, Willems RJ, Willems GM, et al. Significance of initial ST segment elevation and depression for the management of thrombolytic therapy in acute myocardial infarction. Circulation 1990; 82:1147–58.

[41] Vermeer F, Simoons ML, Bar FW, et al. Which patients benefit most from early thrombolytic therapy with intracoronary streptokinase? Circulation 1986;74(6):1379–89.

[42] Birnbaum Y, Criger DA, Strasberg B, et al. Prediction of the extent and severity of left ventricular dysfunction in anterior acute myocardial infarction by the admission electrocardiogram. Am Heart J 2001;141:915–24.

[43] Roberts WC, Gardin JM. Location of myocardial infarcts: a confusion of terms and definitions. Am J Cardiol 1978;42:868–72.

[44] Huey BL, Beller GA, Kaiser DL, et al. A comprehensive analysis of myocardial infarction due to left circumflex artery occlusion: comparison with infarction due to right coronary artery and left anterior descending artery occlusion. J Am Coll Cardiol 1988;12:1156–66.

[45] Sclarovsky S, Topaz O, Rechavia E, et al. Ischemic ST segment depression in leads V2–V3 as the presenting electrocardiographic feature of posterolateral wall myocardial infarction. Am Heart J 1987; 113:1085–90.

[46] Geft IL, Shah PK, Rodriguez L, et al. ST elevation in lead V1 to V5 may be caused by right coronary artery occlusion and acute right ventricular infarction. Am J Cardiol 1984;53:991–6.

[47] Juergens CP, Fernandes C, Hasche ET, et al. Electrocardiographic measurement of infarct size after thrombolytic therapy. J Am Coll Cardiol 1996;27: 617–24.

[48] Hasche ET, Fernandes C, Freedman SB, et al. Relation between ischemia time, infarct size, and left ventricular function in humans. Circulation 1995; 92:710–9.

[49] Wong CK, French JK, Andrews J, et al. Usefulness of the presenting electrocardiogram in predicting myocardial salvage with thrombolytic therapy in patients with a first acute myocardial infarction. Eur Heart J 2002;23(5):399–404.

[50] Birnbaum Y, Mahaffey KW, Criger DA, et al. Grade III ischemia on presentation with acute myocardial infarction predicts rapid progression

of necrosis and less myocardial salvage with thrombolysis. Cardiology 2002;97(3):166–74.

[51] Billgren T, Maynard C, Christian TF, et al. Grade 3 ischemia on the admission electrocardiogram predicts rapid progression of necrosis over time and less myocardial salvage by primary angioplasty. J Electrocardiol 2005;38(3):187–94.

[52] Shah PK, Pichler M, Berman DS, et al. Noninvasive identification of a high risk subset of patients with acute inferior myocardial infarction. Am J Cardiol 1980;46:915–21.

[53] Gibson RS, Crampton RS, Watson DD, et al. Precordial ST-segment depression during acute inferior myocardial infarction: clinical, scintigraphic and angiographic correlations. Circulation 1982; 66:732–41.

[54] Roubin GS, Shen WF, Nicholson M, Dunn RF, et al. Anterolateral ST segment depression in acute inferior myocardial infarction: angiographic and clinical implications. Am Heart J 1984;107:1177–82.

[55] Ruddy TD, Yasuda T, Gold HK, et al. Anterior ST segment depression in acute inferior myocardial infarction as a marker of greater inferior, apical, and posterolateral damage. Am Heart J 1986;112: 1210–6.

[56] Ong L, Valdellon B, Coromilas J, et al. Precordial S-T segment depression in inferior myocardial infarction: evaluation by quantitative thallium-201 scintigraphy and technetium-99m ventriculography. Am J Cardiol 1983;51:734–9.

[57] Birnbaum Y, Herz I, Sclarovsky S, et al. Prognostic significance of precordial ST segment depression on admission electrocardiogram in patients with inferior wall myocardial infarction. J Am Coll Cardiol 1996;28:313–8.

[58] Tsuka Y, Sugiura T, Hatada K, et al. Clinical characteristics of ST-segment elevation in lead V6 in patients with Q-wave acute inferior wall myocardial infarction. Coron Artery Dis 1999;10(7):465–9.

[59] Matetzky S, Freimark D, Chouraqui P, et al. Significance of ST segment elevations in posterior chest leads (V7 to V9) in patients with acute inferior myocardial infarction: application for thrombolytic therapy. J Am Coll Cardiol 1998;31(3):506–11.

[60] Fisch C. Electrocardiography. In: Braunwald E, editor. Heart disease. A textbook of cardiovascular medicine. 5th edition. Philadelphia: W.B. Saunders; 1997. p. 109–52.

[61] Raitt M, Maynard C, Wagner G, et al. Appearance of abnormal Q waves early in the course of acute myocardial infarction: implications for efficacy of thrombolytic therapy. J Am Coll Cardiol 1995;25: 1084–8.

[62] Goldberg S, Urban P, Greenspon A, et al. Limitation of infarct size with thrombolytic agents-electrocardiographic indexes. Circulation 1983; 68(Suppl I):I-77–82.

[63] Rechavia E, Blum A, Mager A, et al. Electrocardiographic Q-waves inconstancy during thrombolysis

in acute anterior wall myocardial infarction. Cardiology 1992;80:392–8.

[64] Bateman TM, Czer LSC, Gray RJ, et al. Transient pathologic Q waves during acute ischemic events: an electrocardiographic correlate of stunned but viable myocardium. Am Heart J 1983;106:1421–6.

[65] Gross H, Rubin IL, Laufer H, et al. Transient abnormal Q waves in the dog without myocardial infarction. Am J Cardiol 1964;14:669–74.

[66] Bar FW, Vermeer F, de Zwaan C, et al. Value of admission electrocardiogram in predicting outcome of thrombolytic therapy in acute myocardial infarction. A randomized trial conducted by The Netherlands Interuniversity Cardiology Institute. Am J Cardiol 1987;59:6–13.

[67] Timmis G. Electrocardiographic effects of reperfusion. Cardiol Clin 1987;5:427–45.

[68] Wong CK, French JK, Aylward PE, et al. Usefulness of the presenting electrocardiogram in predicting successful reperfusion with streptokinase in acute myocardial infarction. Am J Cardiol 1999; 83(2):164–8.

[69] Birnbaum Y, Chetrit A, Sclarovsky S, et al. Abnormal Q waves on the admission electrocardiogram of patients with first acute myocardial infarction: prognostic implications. Clin Cardiol 1997;20(5): 477–81.

[70] Matetzky S, Barabash GI, Shahar A, et al. Early T wave inversion after thrombolytic therapy predicts better coronary perfusion: clinical and angiographic study. J Am Coll Cardiol 1994;24(2): 378–83.

[71] Herz I, Birnbaum Y, Zlotikamien B, et al. The prognostic implications of negative T waves in the leads with ST segment elevation on admission in acute myocardial infarction. Cardiology 1999; 92(2):121–7.

[72] Becker R, Alpert J. Electrocardiographic ST segment depression in coronary heart disease. Am Heart J 1988;115:862–8.

[73] Cribier A, Korsatz L, Koning R, et al. Improved myocardial ischemic response and enhanced collateral circulation with long repetitive coronary occlusion during angioplasty: a prospective study. J Am Coll Cardiol 1992;20:578–86.

[74] Birnbaum Y, Hale SL, Kloner RA. Progressive decrease in the ST segment elevation during ischemic preconditioning: is it related to recruitment of collateral vessels? J Mol Cell Cardiol 1996;28(7): 1493–9.

[75] Sagie A, Sclarovsky S, Strasberg B, et al. Acute anterior wall myocardial infarction presenting with positive T waves and without ST segment shift. Electrocardiographic features and angiographic correlation. Chest 1989;95:1211–5.

[76] Birnbaum Y, Solodky A, Herz I, et al. Implication of inferior ST segment depression in anterior acute myocardial infarction: electrocardiographic and angiographic correlation. Am Heart J 1994;127: 1467–73.

[77] Sclarovsky S, Birnbaum Y, Solodky A, et al. Isolated mid-anterior myocardial infarction: a special electrocardiographic sub-type of acute myocardial infarction consisting of ST-elevation in non-consecutive leads and two different morphologic types of ST-depression. Int J Cardiol 1994;46:37–47.

[78] Birnbaum Y, Sclarovsky S, Mager A, et al. ST segment depression in aVL: a sensitive marker for acute inferior myocardial infarction. Eur Heart J 1993;14:4–7.

[79] Hasdai D, Birnbaum Y, Porter A, et al. Maximal precordial ST-segment depression in leads V4–V6 in patients with inferior wall acute myocardial infarction indicates coronary artery disease involving the left anterior descending coronary artery system. Int J Cardiol 1997;58:273–8.

[80] Boden WE, Kleiger RE, Gibson RS, et al. Electrocardiographic evolution of posterior acute myocardial infarction: importance of early precordial ST-segment depression. Am J Cardiol 1987;59(8): 782–7.

[81] Porter A, Vaturi M, Adler Y, et al. Are there differences among patients with inferior acute myocardial infarction with ST depression in leads V2 and V3 and positive versus negative T waves in these leads on admission? Cardiology 1998;90(4): 295–8.

[82] Blanke H, Cohen M, Schlueter GU, et al. Electrocardiographic and coronary arteriographic correlations during acute myocardial infarction. Am J Cardiol 1984;54:249–55.

[83] Aldrich HR, Hindman NB, Hinohara T, et al. Identification of the optimal electrocardiographic leads for detecting acute epicardial injury in acute myocardial infarction. Am J Cardiol 1987;59(1):20–3.

[84] Coma-Canella I, Lopez-Sendon J, Alcasena S, et al. Electrocardiographic alterations in leads V1 to V3 in the diagnosis of right and left ventricular infarction. Am Heart J 1986;112:940–6.

[85] Porter A, Herz I, Strasberg B. Isolated right ventricular infarction presenting as anterior wall myocardial infarction on electrocardiography. Clin Cardiol 1997;20:971–3.

[86] Ben-Gal T, Herz I, Solodky A, et al. Acute anterior wall myocardial infarction entailing ST-segment elevation in lead V1: electrocardiographic and angiographic correlations. Clin Cardiol 1998;21(6): 399–404.

[87] Birnbaum Y, Hasdai D, Sclarovsky S, et al. Acute myocardial infarction entailing ST segment elevation in lead aVL: electrocardiographic differentiation among occlusion of the left anterior descending, first diagonal, and first obtuse marginal coronary arteries. Am Heart J 1996;131: 38–42.

[88] Birnbaum Y, Sclarovsky S, Solodky A, et al. Prediction of the level of left anterior coronary artery obstruction during acute anterior wall myocardial infarction by the admission electrocardiogram. Am J Cardiol 1993;72:823–6.

[89] Arbane M, Goy JJ. Prediction of the site of total occlusion in the left anterior descending coronary artery using admission electrocardiogram in anterior wall acute myocardial infarction. Am J Cardiol 2000;85(4):487–91.

[90] Engelen DJ, Gorgels AP, Cheriex EC, et al. Value of the electrocardiogram in localizing the occlusion site in the left anterior descending coronary artery in acute anterior myocardial infarction. J Am Coll Cardiol 1999;34(2):389–95.

[91] Sasaki K, Yotsukura M, Sakata K, et al. Relation of ST-segment changes in inferior leads during anterior wall acute myocardial infarction to length and occlusion site of the left anterior descending coronary artery. Am J Cardiol 2001;87(12):1340–5.

[92] Vasudevan K, Manjunath CN, Srinivas KH, et al. Electrocardiographic localization of the occlusion site in left anterior descending coronary artery in acute anterior myocardial infarction. Indian Heart J 2004;56(4):315–9.

[93] Birnbaum Y, Herz I, Solodky A, et al. Can we differentiate by the admission ECG between anterior wall acute myocardial infarction due to a left anterior descending artery occlusion proximal to the origin of the first septal branch and a postseptal occlusion? American Journal of Noninvasive Cardiology 1994;8:115–9.

[94] Ben-Gal T, Sclarovsky S, Herz I, et al. Importance of the conal branch of the right coronary artery in patients with acute anterior wall myocardial infarction: electrocardiographic and angiographic correlation. J Am Coll Cardiol 1997;29(3):506–11.

[95] Shalev Y, Fogelman R, Oettinger M, et al. Does the electrocardiographic pattern of "anteroseptal" myocardial infarction correlate with the anatomic location of myocardial injury? Am J Cardiol 1995;75:763–6.

[96] Porter A, Wyshelesky A, Strasberg B, et al. Correlation between the admission electrocardiogram and regional wall motion abnormalities as detected by echocardiography in anterior acute myocardial infarction. Cardiology 2000;94(2):118–26.

[97] Sapin PM, Musselman DR, Dehmer GJ, et al. Implications of inferior ST-segment elevation accompanying anterior wall acute myocardial infarction for the angiographic morphology of the left anterior descending coronary artery morphology and site of occlusion. Am J Cardiol 1992;69(9):860–5.

[98] Tamura A, Kataoka H, Nagase K, et al. Clinical significance of inferior ST elevation during acute anterior myocardial infarction. Br Heart J 1995;74:611–4.

[99] Fletcher WO, Gibbons RJ, Clements IP. The relationship of inferior ST depression, lateral ST elevation, and left precordial ST elevation to myocardium at risk in acute anterior myocardial infarction. Am Heart J 1993;126(3 Pt 1):526–35.

[100] Haraphongse M, Tanomsup S, Jugdutt BI. Inferior ST segment depression during acute anterior myocardial infarction: clinical and angiographic correlations. J Am Coll Cardiol 1984;4(3):467–76.

[101] Braat SH, Brugada P, den Dulk K, et al. Value of lead V4R for recognition of the infarct coronary artery in acute inferior myocardial infarction. Am J Cardiol 1984;53(11):1538–41.

[102] Kontos MC, Desai PV, Jesse RL, et al. Usefulness of the admission electrocardiogram for identifying the infarct-related artery in inferior wall acute myocardial infarction. Am J Cardiol 1997;79:182–4.

[103] Bairey CN, Shah PK, Lew AS, et al. Electrocardiographic differentiation of occlusion of the left circumflex versus the right coronary artery as a cause of inferior acute myocardial infarction. Am J Cardiol 1987;60:456–9.

[104] Herz I, Assali AR, Adler Y, et al. New electrocardiographic criteria for predicting either the right or left circumflex artery as the culprit coronary artery in inferior wall acute myocardial infarction. Am J Cardiol 1997;80:1343–5.

[105] Hasdai D, Birnbaum Y, Herz I, et al. ST segment depression in lateral limb leads in inferior wall acute myocardial infarction. Implications regarding the culprit artery and the site of obstruction. Eur Heart J 1995;16(11):1549–53.

[106] Kosuge M, Kimura K, Ishikawa T, et al. New electrocardiographic criteria for predicting the site of coronary artery occlusion in inferior wall acute myocardial infarction. Am J Cardiol 1998;82(11):1318–22.

[107] Assali AR, Herz I, Vaturi M, et al. Electrocardiographic criteria for predicting the culprit artery in inferior wall acute myocardial infarction. Am J Cardiol 1999;84(1):87–9.

[108] Zimetbaum PJ, Krishnan S, Gold A, et al. Usefulness of ST-segment elevation in lead III exceeding that of lead II for identifying the location of the totally occluded coronary artery in inferior wall myocardial infarction. Am J Cardiol 1998;81(7):918–9.

[109] Birnbaum Y, Hale SL, Kloner RA. Changes in R wave amplitude: ECG differentiation between episodes of reocclusion and reperfusion associated with ST-segment elevation. J Electrocardiol 1997;30(3):211–6.

[110] Fiol M, Cygankiewicz I, Carrillo A, et al. Value of electrocardiographic algorithm based on "ups and downs" of ST in assessment of a culprit artery in evolving inferior wall acute myocardial infarction. Am J Cardiol 2004;94(6):709–14.

[111] Kopelman HA, Forman MB, Wilson BH, et al. Right ventricular myocardial infarction in patients with chronic lung disease: possible role of right

ventricular hypertrophy. J Am Coll Cardiol 1985; 5(6):1302–7.

[112] Erhardt LR, Sjogren A, Wahlberg I. Single right-sided precordial lead in the diagnosis of right ventricular involvement in inferior myocardial infarction. Am Heart J 1976;91(5):571–6.

[113] Zehender M, Kasper W, Kauder E, et al. Right ventricular infarction as an independent predictor of prognosis after acute inferior myocardial infarction. N Engl J Med 1993;328(14):981–8.

[114] Lopez-Sendon J, Coma-Canella I, Alcasena S, et al. Electrocardiographic findings in acute right ventricular infarction: sensitivity and specificity of electrocardiographic alterations in right precordial leads V4R, V3R, V1, V2, and V3. J Am Coll Cardiol 1985;6(6):1273–9.

[115] Sadanandan S, Hochman JS, Kolodziej A, et al. Clinical and angiographic characteristics of patients with combined anterior and inferior ST-segment elevation on the initial electrocardiogram during acute myocardial infarction. Am Heart J 2003;146(4):653–61.

[116] Assali AR, Sclarobsky S, Herz I, et al. Comparison of patients with inferior wall acute myocardial infarction with versus without ST-segment elevation in leads V5 and V6. Am J Cardiol 1998;81:81–3.

[117] Golovchiner G, Matz I, Iakobishvili Z, et al. Correlation between the electrocardiogram and regional wall motion abnormalities as detected by echocardiography in first inferior acute myocardial infarction. Cardiology 2002;98(1–2):81–91.

[118] Ruddy TD, Yasuda T, Gold HK, et al. Correlations of regional wall motion and myocardial perfusion in patients with and without anterior precordial ST segment depression during acute inferior myocardial infarction. American Journal of Noninvasive Cardiology 1987;1:81–7.

[119] Boden WE, Bough EW, Korr KS, et al. Inferoseptal myocardial infarction: another cause of precordial ST-segment depression in transmural inferior wall myocardial infarction? Am J Cardiol 1984; 54(10):1216–23.

[120] Haraphongse M, Jugdutt BI, Rossall RE. Significance of precordial ST-segment depression in acute transmural inferior infarction: coronary angiographic findings. Cathet Cardiovasc Diagn 1983;9(2):143–51.

[121] Hasdai D, Sclarovsky S, Solodky A, et al. Prognostic significance of maximal precordial ST-segment depression in right (V1 to V3) versus left (V4 to V6) leads in patients with inferior wall acute myocardial infarction. Am J Cardiol 1994;74:1081–4.

[122] Lew AS, Maddahi J, Shah PK, et al. Factors that determine the direction and magnitude of precordial ST-segment deviations during inferior wall acute myocardial infarction. Am J Cardiol 1985; 55(8):883–8.

[123] Salcedo JR, Baird MG, Chambers RJ, et al. Significance of reciprocal S-T segment depression in anterior precordial leads in acute inferior myocardial infarction: concomitant left anterior descending coronary artery disease? Am J Cardiol 1981; 48(6):1003–8.

[124] Agarwal JB, Khaw K, Aurignac F, et al. Importance of posterior chest leads in patients with suspected myocardial infarction, but nondiagnostic, routine 12-lead electrocardiogram. Am J Cardiol 1999;83(3):323–6.

[125] Casas RE, Marriott HJ, Glancy DL. Value of leads V7–V9 in diagnosing posterior wall acute myocardial infarction and other causes of tall R waves in V1–V2. Am J Cardiol 1997;80(4):508–9.

[126] Matetzky S, Freimark D, Feinberg MS, et al. Acute myocardial infarction with isolated ST-segment elevation in posterior chest leads V7–9: "hidden" ST-segment elevations revealing acute posterior infarction. J Am Coll Cardiol 1999; 34(3):748–53.

[127] Wung SF, Drew BJ. New electrocardiographic criteria for posterior wall acute myocardial ischemia validated by a percutaneous transluminal coronary angioplasty model of acute myocardial infarction. Am J Cardiol 2001;87 (8):970–4.

[128] Mager A, Sclarovsky S, Herz I, et al. Value of the initial electrocardiogram in patients with inferior-wall acute myocardial infarction for prediction of multivessel coronary artery disease. Coron Artery Dis 2000;11(5):415–20.

[129] Yamaji H, Iwasaki K, Kusachi S, et al. Prediction of acute left main coronary artery obstruction by 12-lead electrocardiography. ST segment elevation in lead aVR with less ST segment elevation in lead V(1). J Am Coll Cardiol 2001;38(5): 1348–54.

[130] Birnbaum Y, Goodman S, Barr A, et al. Comparison of primary coronary angioplasty versus thrombolysis in patients with ST-segment elevation acute myocardial infarction and grade II and grade III myocardial ischemia on the enrollment electrocardiogram. Am J Cardiol 2001; 88(8):842–7.

[131] Lee CW, Hong M-K, Yang H-S, et al. Determinants and prognostic implications of terminal QRS complex distortion in patients treated with primary angioplasty for acute myocardial infarction. Am J Cardiol 2001;88:210–3.

[132] Birnbaum Y, Herz I, Sclarovsky S, et al. Admission clinical and electrocardiographic characteristics predicting an increased risk for early reinfarction after thrombolytic therapy. Am Heart J 1998; 135(5 Pt 1):805–12.

[133] Sejersten M, Birnbaum Y, Ripa RS, et al. Electrocardiographic identification of patients with ST-elevation acute myocardium infarction benefiting most from primary angioplasty versus fibrinolysis: results from the DANAMI-2 Trial. Circulation 2004;110 III-409.

ELSEVIER
SAUNDERS

Cardiol Clin 24 (2006) 367–376

CARDIOLOGY
CLINICS

Electrocardiographic Markers of Reperfusion in ST-elevation Myocardial Infarction

Shaul Atar, MD, Alejandro Barbagelata, MD,
Yochai Birnbaum, MD*

Division of Cardiology, University of Texas Medical Branch, 5.106 John Sealy Annex, 301 University Boulevard, Galveston, TX 77555, USA

Reperfusion therapy with intravenous thrombolytic agents or percutaneous coronary intervention (PCI) has emerged in the past 2 decades as an effective means of reducing infarct size, preserving ventricular function and topography, reducing electrical instability, and reducing morbidity and mortality in patients who have an acute ST-elevation myocardial infarction (STEMI) [1,2]. Conversely, failure of reperfusion has been shown to portend a substantial increase in morbidity and mortality [3]. Because the outcome of patients who fail to reperfuse with reperfusion therapy may be improved with additional interventions such as rescue PCI or additional pharmacologic treatments, it becomes clinically important to recognize reperfusion or its failure at the bedside. In contrast to experimental animal models of acute myocardial infarction and reperfusion in which the coronary artery is ligated for controlled periods of time, acute myocardial infarction in humans is a dynamic process with frequent repeat episodes of coronary artery reperfusion and reocclusion, both before and after the initiation of reperfusion therapy [4–7]. Although the extent of myocardium involved can be estimated clinically by physical examination (presence of heart failure, tachycardia, hypotension, and other markers), and with various imaging techniques (echocardiography, radionuclide imaging, ventriculography), there currently is no alternative to the ECG for continuous assessment of the status of coronary and myocardial perfusion. Coronary angiography, Technetium-99m sestamibi single-photon-emission CT imaging, and contrast echocardiography can give only a snapshot of the status of coronary or myocardial perfusion.

Although urgent coronary angiography can distinguish an open from a closed culprit artery effectively, and it remains the criterion for patency, its routine continuous application for this purpose is seriously limited because of logistic reasons, cost, invasive nature with attendant risk of peri-access complications, the snapshot nature of angiographic evaluation, and the fact that epicardial vessel patency may exist despite lack of nutritive flow at the level of downstream microcirculation. For example, in numerous animal models it has been repeatedly demonstrated that immediately after opening of the occluded coronary artery there is a hyperemic phase, followed later by gradual decline of myocardial perfusion, even though the epicardial coronary artery remains open. This phenomenon of "no reflow" is currently undetected by angiograms performed immediately after recanalization of the infarct-related artery (IRA) [8,9]. Therefore several investigators have evaluated a number of noninvasive nonangiographic markers to determine the success or failure of reperfusion. Among these techniques, ECG monitoring is most suitable for routine bedside application. This article reviews the role of bedside 12-lead ECG in identifying and monitoring the perfusion state of the myocardium in STEMI.

---

* Corresponding author.
E-mail address: yobirnba@utmb.edu (Y. Birnbaum).

ECG markers of reperfusion

There are four ECG markers for prediction of the perfusion status of the ischemic myocardium: (1) ST-segment measurements, (2) T-wave configuration, (3) QRS changes, and (4) reperfusion arrhythmias.

ST resolution

Several studies showed that recanalization of the IRA results in rapid resolution ($\geq 50\%$) of ST elevation (Fig. 1) [10–14]. These results were obtained from serial ECG recordings performed on admission of the patient to the hospital and at various time intervals after initiation of therapy. Unfortunately, these studies were not unified regarding the definition of ST resolution (STR) [15] or the timing of coronary angiography and final ECG assessment [12–14,16]. Some of the studies [11,12,15,16] assessed a single ECG lead with maximal ST elevation, whereas others [10,13] have assessed the reduction in the sum of ST elevation in all 12 leads. It seems that the latter method is more useful in patients who have minimal ST elevation, whereas in cases of extensive ST elevation, assessing the reduction of ST in the single lead with maximal ST elevation is preferable [5,17].

Because reperfusion is a dynamic process, in which the IRA may recanalize and reocclude intermittently [7,18], serial ECG recording is limited in predicting the state of reperfusion. Moreover, one third of episodes of recurrent ST elevation are silent [7]. Thus, unless recorded continuously, these ECG changes may be missed completely by serial intermittent ECG recordings or misinterpreted as signs of improvement, should the re-elevation in ST be smaller than that in the initial ECG recording (Fig. 2) [5]. Moreover, because some investigators have suggested that the ECG criterion for reperfusion is 50% or greater STR compared with maximal ST elevation at any time-point (not necessarily the enrollment ECG), without continuous ECG monitoring starting immediately upon admission, interpretation of STR relative to the enrollment ECG may be misleading. A proper alternative to continuous 12-lead recording would be ECG monitoring that

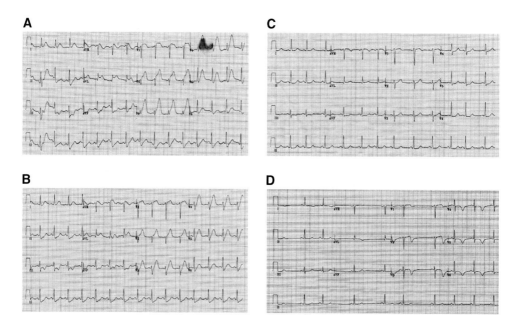

Fig. 1. (A) A 48-year-old woman with 3 hours of chest pain. The admission ECG shows ST elevation in aVL and V$_1$ to V$_3$ and reciprocal ST depression in the inferior leads. (B) After receiving aspirin and nitroglycerin, the patient developed ventricular fibrillation and was defibrillated. The ECG shows an increase in S-wave amplitude in V$_3$ to V$_6$, ST elevation resolution in V$_1$ to V$_3$, and junctional ST depression in leads V$_3$ to V$_6$ with tall, upright T waves. (C) Seventy minutes later, the patient had no chest pain. Repeat ECG shows resolution of ST elevation in leads aVL and V$_1$ to V$_3$ and less ST depression in the inferior leads. There is now mild ST depression in leads V$_4$ to V$_6$; however, T-wave amplitude in the precordial leads has decreased. (D) On the next day, after PCI, the ECG shows isoelectric ST segments with T-wave inversion in leads I, aVL, and V$_1$ to V$_6$.

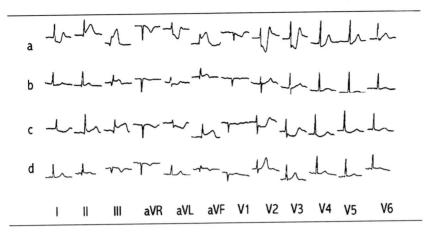

I   II   III   aVR   aVL   aVF   V1   V2   V3   V4   V5   V6

Fig. 2. Serial ECG tracings of a patient who had inferoposterior STEMI. (*a*) Before initiation of thrombolytic therapy there is ST elevation in leads II, III, and aVF and ST depression in leads I, aVL, and V_2 to V_4.(*b*) Sixty minutes after initiation of thrombolytic therapy, pain subsided, and there is 70% or greater STR in the inferior leads. (*c*) Fifteen minutes later, there is ST re-elevation relative to tracing B, but the ST elevation is less than 50% of the initial values. The patient was referred to rescue PCI. (*d*) After PCI with stent implantation in the right coronary artery, there is 70% or greater STR with inversion of the T waves in leads III and aVF. (*Adapted from* Vaturi M, Birnbaum Y. The use of the electrocardiogram to identify epicardial coronary and tissue reperfusion in acute myocardial infarction. J Thromb-Thrombolysis 2000;10:140; with permission.)

engages computer-assisted ST-segment analysis and continuous 12-lead recording (using either the single lead or the sum of ST elevation) [19]. Another technique, continuous vectorcardiographic monitoring, assesses online both the QRS complex vector and the ST elevation vector simultaneously [20,21].

Five distinct patterns of ST segment evolution were identified by using continuous ECG recording: (1) rapid STR without re-elevation, (2) rapid STR following a delayed ST re-elevation, (3) persistent ST elevation without STR, (4) rapid STR followed by rapid ST re-elevation, and (5) a delayed ST elevation peak followed by a rapid STR and recurrent ST elevation [18]. Whereas the first three patterns indicate the status of the infarct related artery, the latter two patterns are less specific regarding patency, because they suggest an unstable myocardial tissue perfusion (regardless of the IRA patency). Krucoff and colleagues [18] reported that absence of STR or presence of ST re-elevation at the time of coronary angiography predicts an occluded IRA with a sensitivity of 90% and specificity of 92%. Dellborg and colleagues [20,21] reported the role of changes in ST vectors in STEMI. The sensitivity of vector changes to predict IRA patency was 81% to 94%, and the specificity was 70% to 80%.

Additional elevation of the sum of ST of 5 mm or more during reperfusion, also termed "reperfusion syndrome," is a frequently noted phenomenon, and most studies found it to be a marker of impaired microvascular reperfusion, with lower coronary velocity reserve, reduced left ventricular function, and larger infarct size [22,23]. The significance of the reperfusion syndrome is still debatable, however, because others have reported it to be a favorable prognostic factor [24].

The Global Utilization of Streptokinase and Tissue Plasminogen Activator for Occluded Coronary Arteries (GUSTO-1) ECG ischemia-monitoring substudy [25] studied 1067 patients divided into three groups: 460 patients were monitored with vector-derived 12-lead ECG, 373 with 12-lead ECG, and 288 with a three-lead Holter system. In this study, 50% STR before either 90- or 180-minutes' angiography was considered to be a sign of reperfusion. Recurrence of ST elevation was considered to be reocclusion or reischemia. To unify the study, only a single-lead ST trend was considered. The addition of initial peak ST levels, the time to 50% STR, and various STR patterns improved the predictive accuracy of the IRA patency. This study reinforced the notion that 50% or greater STR within 90 minutes from starting thrombolysis reflected patency of the IRA. They also found that the amount of ST elevation present during recording is a major determinant of the accuracy of patency prediction.

The accuracy of prediction of IRA patency correlated with the degree of initial ST elevation. The absence of STR does not accurately predict an occluded IRA, however, because approximately 50% of patients with no (<30%) STR still have a patent IRA [26,27]. Previously, the absence of STR despite a patent IRA had been considered to be a false-negative sign of lake of reperfusion by the 12-lead ECG.

Important differences exist between anterior and inferior STEMI with regard to STR [13,14,26,28–30]. Patients who have anterior STEMI develop significantly less STR than those who have inferior infarction, despite only modest differences in epicardial blood flow, suggesting that STR is a less accurate predictor of epicardial reperfusion among patients who have anterior versus inferior STEMI [13,26,28,29]. This reduced accuracy may result from technical factors, such as the frequent (normal) presence of J-point elevation in the anterior precordial leads [31], which would serve to decrease the extent of STR that is possible. Additionally, anterior STEMI typically is associated with a larger infarct size and greater tissue injury than inferior STEMI. As a result, different threshold levels of STR may be appropriate for anterior versus inferior STEMI [26]. When sensitivity analyses are performed, 70% or greater STR seems to be the optimal threshold for patients who have inferior myocardial infarction, whereas 50% or greater STR may be optimal for anterior STEMI [26].

To detect STR, the recording must be started as early as possible (preferably before the initiation of thrombolytic therapy). Otherwise, the first episode of 50% or greater ST recovery may not be properly recorded, which may result in false assessment of the IRA patency (Fig. 2). ST monitoring then should continued, preferably for at least 3 hours, as suggested by Schroder and colleagues [32], who found that the prognostic significance of incomplete STR was better at 180 minutes after the initiation of streptokinase therapy (30-day cardiac mortality, 13.6%) than at 90 minutes (30-day cardiac mortality, 7.3%).

Use of ST resolution for evaluation of myocardial tissue reperfusion

Myocardial reperfusion is not a dichotomous phenomenon. Epicardial coronary flow is graded by the Thrombolysis in Myocardial Infarction (TIMI) flow classification. Myocardial tissue perfusion may be complete, partial, or absent, however, irrespective of the epicedial coronary TIMI flow grade [30,33]. Analysis of STR may give a better estimation of myocardial tissue perfusion over time [34,35]. Complete (≥70%) STR is associated with better outcome and preservation of left ventricular function than partial (30% to 70%) or no (<30%) STR [28,32,35,36]. Thus, whereas 50% or greater resolution of ST elevation is a reliable indicator of patency of the IRA, only complete (≥70%) STR is an indicator of restoration of myocardial tissue perfusion. The same findings apply for patients who undergo successful recanalization of the IRA by primary PCI, in whom early resolution of ST elevation predicts better outcome than incomplete or no resolution of ST elevation [35,37]. Recent studies have shown that the combination of STR with angiographic parameters, such as the myocardial blush (MB) and the corrected TIMI frame count, allow better grading of microvascular reperfusion and better prediction of cardiovascular events 30 days and 6 months after primary PCI for STEMI [38,39]. Poli and colleagues [38] combined MB and sum of STR and identified three main groups of patients: group 1 (n = 60) had both significant MB (grade 2 to 3) and STR (>50% versus baseline) and had a high rate of 7-day (65%) and 6-month (95%) left ventricular functional recovery. Group 2 (n = 21) showed MB but persistent ST elevation, and the prevalence of early left ventricular functional recovery was low (24%) but increased up to 86% in the late phase. Group 3 (n = 28) had neither significant MB nor STR and had poor early (18%) and late (32%) left ventricular functional recovery. Thus the addition of STR to angiographic parameters provides better determination of myocardial reperfusion.

T-wave configuration

Early inversion of the terminal portion of the T waves after initiation of reperfusion therapy, as shown in Figs. 1–3, is an indicator of successful reperfusion [40]. Moreover, a study by Corbalan and colleagues [41], in which inversion of T waves more than 0.5 mm below the baseline within the first 24 hours of thrombolytic therapy in all the leads with previous ST elevation was considered a marker for coronary artery reperfusion, showed that T-wave inversion was associated with the lowest in-hospital mortality rate (odds ratio, 0.25; 95% confidence interval, 0.10–0.56) [41]. When all markers of coronary artery reperfusion (resolution of chest pain, STR greater than 50%

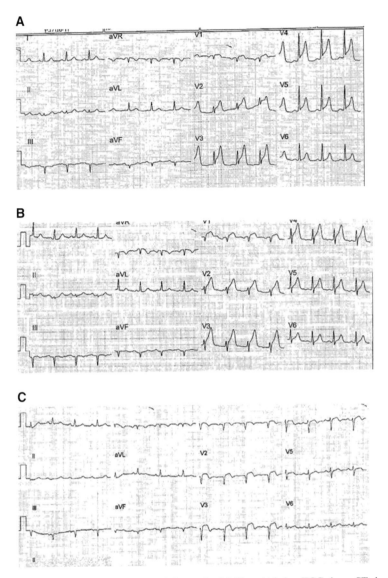

Fig. 3. A 73-year-old man presenting with 2 hours of chest pain. (*A*) The admission ECG shows ST elevation in leads V_1 to V_5. (*B*) Repeat ECG done 24 minutes later shows the same ST elevation, but now S waves appear in leads V_2 to V_6, without inversion of the T waves. Immediate angiography showed proximal left anterior descending artery stenosis, with thrombus and TIMI grade 2 flow. (*C*) An ECG done 2 hours and 50 minutes after successful PCI with stent insertion with resulting TIMI grade 3 flow, showing complete (>70%) STR, QS pattern in leads V_1 to V_3, shortening of the R wave in leads V_3 to V_6, and T-wave inversion in leads V_1 to V_4.

at 90 minutes, abrupt creatine kinase rise before 12 hours, and T-wave inversion) were included in a logistic regression model, T-wave inversion (odds ratio; 0.29; 95% confidence interval, 0.11–0.68) and abrupt creatine kinase rise (odds ratio, 0.36; 95% confidence interval, 0.16–0.77) continued to be significantly associated with better outcome, whereas STR was not [41].

Only a few studies have investigated the significance of T-wave direction in leads with ST elevation. Herz and colleagues [42] found that, before initiation of thrombolytic therapy, negative T waves in leads with ST elevation were associated with better prognosis in patients enrolled within 2 hours of symptoms onset, whereas in those enrolled 2 to 6 hours after initiation of symptoms negative T waves were associated with increased mortality. At 90 minutes after initiation of streptokinase therapy, TIMI grade 3 flow in the IRA was more commonly seen in patients who did not have T-wave inversion (50%) than in those who had T-wave inversion on the pretreatment ECG (30%; $P = .002$) [43]. Among patients treated within 3 hours of onset of symptoms, TIMI grade 3 flow was seen in 62% of those without versus 43% of those with T-wave inversion ($P = .06$). Among patients treated after 3 hours, TIMI grade 3 flow was seen in 38% of those who did not have T-wave inversion versus 23% of those who had T-wave inversion ($P = .05$) [43]. After initiation of thrombolytic therapy, early inversion of the T waves may be a sign of reperfusion [41,44]. Negative T waves on the predischarge ECG of patients who have anterior STEMI, especially if associated with complete resolution of the ST elevation, is a sign of a relatively small infarct size with preserved left ventricular ejection fraction [45]. During the following months, however, early spontaneous normalization of the T waves in the involved leads may be associated with better outcome and preservation of left ventricular function [46]. Therefore, the configuration of the T waves may carry different meanings at different stages after STEMI. Moreover, it is unclear whether partial inversion of the terminal portion of the T waves has the same significance as complete or giant T-wave inversion [47]. Furthermore, the exact underlying mechanisms and significance of various patterns of STR and T-wave inversion have not been studied. It is well known that the amplitude of the STR is influenced mostly by epicardial ischemia and is less influenced by the degree of subendocardial ischemia. Thus, STR may correlate better with amelioration of epicardial ischemia caused by restoration of flow through the IRA or by recruitment of collaterals and less with the status of the subendocardial zones. It is possible that the configuration of the T waves is related more to the subendocardial perfusion status. Because myocardial necrosis starts from the subendocardium and expands toward the epicardium, the configuration of the T waves after reperfusion therapy may correlate better with recovery of left ventricular function and prognosis [41].

QRS changes during ischemia and reperfusion

Dynamic changes in the QRS complex are detected during reperfusion therapy for STEMI,

as shown in Fig. 3. These changes have been investigated mainly by vectorcardiography [20,21,48]. It seems that the QRS vector changes are less specific than the ST-vector changes for predicting reperfusion [20]. Using standard 12-lead ECG, dynamic changes in Q-wave number, amplitude, and width, R-wave amplitude and S-wave appearance are detected. Some have reported that early pathologic Q waves develop especially after reperfusion [49,50]; however, others have found these to be associated with larger ischemic zone and ultimate necrotic area [51–53]. It has been reported that the early appearance of Q waves (within <6 hours of symptom onset) does not signify irreversible damage and does not preclude myocardial salvage by thrombolytic therapy [53]; however, Q waves on admission are associated with worse prognosis [54]. It is unclear whether dynamic changes in Q waves early after initiation of reperfusion therapy have additive prognostic significance to ST monitoring and T-wave configuration. It generally is accepted that the loss of R waves and the appearance of new Q waves in the days following STEMI represent myocardial necrosis [55]. During the first 48 hours of STEMI, however, a recovery of R wave and disappearance of new Q waves can be detected even in patients not undergoing reperfusion therapy [56]. This phenomenon usually is confined to small STEMI [57].

In an open-chest rabbit model, episodes of ST elevation caused by coronary artery occlusion were associated with an increase in R-wave amplitude, whereas ST-segment elevation during reperfusion episodes was associated with a decrease in R-wave amplitude [58]. Absence of S waves in leads V_1 to V_3 in the enrollment ECG of patients who have anterior STEMI is associated with increased mortality, larger final infarct size, higher rates of no reflow or no STR, and less benefit from thrombolytic therapy [59–61]. During thrombolytic therapy, S waves in these leads may increase or decrease in size and even disappear (see Fig. 3). It is unclear whether decrease in S-wave amplitude is a marker of more severe ischemia and whether the reappearance of an S wave is a sign of reperfusion.

Reperfusion arrhythmias

Accelerated idioventricular rhythm

Nonsustained or sustained ventricular tachycardia at rates of less than or equal to 120 beats per minute, also called accelerated idioventricular rhythm (AIVR), is a common arrhythmia in patients who have STEMI. Several studies have shown that reperfusion is accompanied by AIVR in up to 50% of patients, especially when continuous or frequent ECG monitoring is used [14,62]. Classic AIVR has been defined as a ventricular rhythm occurring at 50 to 120 beats per minute starting after a long pause resulting in a long coupling interval. This rhythm is usually regular and is terminated by the capture of ventricle by the sinus node. In a prospective study of 87 patients receiving intravenous or intracoronary thrombolysis for STEMI, Gorgels and colleagues [63] showed that classic AIVR occurred in 50% of patients with reperfusion and in only 7% of patients without reperfusion. AIVR is a specific but relatively insensitive indicator of reperfusion occurring in only in 50% of reperfused patients.

Cardioinhibitory (Bezold-Jarisch) reflex

Several investigators have shown that sudden appearance of sinus bradycardia accompanied by hypotension can signal reperfusion of the artery supplying inferior wall of the myocardium, (ie, in most instances, the right coronary artery). This phenomenon is believed to be a type of Bezold-Jarisch reflex provoked by stimulation of cardiac baroreceptors with increased vagal input and withdrawal of sympathetic tone [64]. This phenomenon is observed in 23% to 65% of cases of right coronary artery reperfusion, thus providing corroborative evidence of reperfusion [14,65].

Signal-averaged electrocardiography for detection of late potentials

Signal-averaged electrocardiography (SAECG) has been used to detect late potentials as markers of increased vulnerability for inducible and spontaneous ventricular arrhythmias following acute STEMI. Several studies have demonstrated that in patients who have acute STEMI a patent IRA is associated with a reduced frequency of positive late potentials compared with patients who have persistent occlusion [66,67]. Tranchesi and colleagues [68] have examined the significance of late potentials in SAECG as a marker of reperfusion. In 54 patients who had acute STEMI and an angiographically documented occlusion, a baseline SAECG was recorded before initiation of thrombolysis. Coronary angiogram and SAECG were recorded again 90 minutes after thrombolytic infusion. In 50% of the patients who had successful reperfusion the late potentials disappeared after reperfusion (from 16/35 to 8/35; *P* = .03),

whereas in patients who had a closed artery there was no change in the prevalence of positive late potentials (8/19 before to 7/19 after attempted but failed thrombolysis). These preliminary findings, although interesting, demonstrate the limited accuracy of late potentials and their changes following thrombolytic therapy for the bedside diagnosis of reperfusion.

Summary

At present, bedside recognition of reperfusion in patients presenting with acute STEMI can be accomplished best by assessment of several objective and subjective signs of termination of ischemia (ie, resolution of chest pain or rapid STR). A study by Oude Ophuis and colleagues [69] of 230 patients who had STEMI suggested that the combination of ECG and clinical markers may better predict the patency of the IRA and the status of myocardial reperfusion. They found that a sudden decrease in chest pain was the most common sign of reperfusion (36%), followed by STR of 50% or more (30%), and the development of a terminal negative T wave (20%) in the lead with the highest ST elevation. STR of 50% or more and the appearance of AIVR had the highest positive predictive value for reperfusion. For TIMI grade 3 flow, the positive predictive value of STR was 66% and for AIVR it was 59%. The presence of three or more noninvasive markers of reperfusion predicted TIMI grade 3 flow accurately in 80% of cases.

Because ST segments may fluctuate dramatically before and during thrombolytic therapy, an accurate determination of progressive decrease (by ≥ 50%) relative to the highest ST elevation requires frequent (every 5–15 minutes) or continuous monitoring of ST (in either a selected lead or all 12 leads). Although other bedside signs such as AIVR and Bezold-Jarisch reflex also indicate reperfusion, their limited sensitivity restricts their usefulness. Biochemical markers related to accelerated washout associated with reperfusion, although promising, are still limited in their usefulness because the results are difficult to obtain in a timely fashion. Acute coronary angiography, although useful, is not practical, and it may turn out not to be the reference standard for reperfusion. Because the goal of reperfusion is to achieve termination of ongoing ischemia, noninvasive markers of ischemia termination may be a better standard than the anatomic evidence obtained by coronary angiography. The favorable prognostic impact of early STR in reperfusion trials supports the clinical relevance and importance of signs of ischemia termination.

It is necessary, however, to improve the understanding of the pathophysiologic mechanisms leading to the ECG changes during reperfusion, namely the significance of STR, T-wave configuration, and early and terminal QRS complex changes. Better understanding of the pathophysiology may help in the design of studies to examine specific interventions (ie, intravenous glycoprotein IIb/IIIa inhibitors, clopidogrel, nitrates, adenosine, and other drugs) that may be beneficial in patients who have not reached complete ECG signs of reperfusion (STR with complete T-wave inversion).

References

[1] Gruppo Italiano per lo Studio della Sopravvivenza nell'Infarto Miocardico. GISSI-2. A factorial randomised trial of alteplase versus streptokinase and heparin versus no heparin among 12,490 patients with acute myocardial infarction. Lancet 1990; 336(8707):65–71.

[2] Third International Study of Infarct Survival Collaborative Group. ISIS-3. A randomised comparison of streptokinase vs tissue plasminogen activator vs anistreplase and of aspirin plus heparin vs aspirin alone among 41,299 cases of suspected acute myocardial infarction. Lancet 1992;339(8796):753–70.

[3] The GUSTO Angiographic Investigators. The effects of tissue plasminogen activator, streptokinase, or both on coronary-artery patency, ventricular function, and survival after acute myocardial infarction. N Engl J Med 1993;329(22):1615–22.

[4] Haider AW, Andreotti F, Hackett DR, et al. Early spontaneous intermittent myocardial reperfusion during acute myocardial infarction is associated with augmented thrombogenic activity and less myocardial damage. J Am Coll Cardiol 1995;26(3):662–7.

[5] Klootwijk P, Cobbaert C, Fioretti P, et al. Noninvasive assessment of reperfusion and reocclusion after thrombolysis in acute myocardial infarction. Am J Cardiol 1993;72(19):75G–84G.

[6] Krucoff MW, Croll MA, Pope JE, et al. Continuous 12-lead ST-segment recovery analysis in the TAMI 7 study. Performance of a noninvasive method for real-time detection of failed myocardial reperfusion. Circulation 1993;88(2):437–46.

[7] Kwon K, Freedman SB, Wilcox I, et al. The unstable ST segment early after thrombolysis for acute infarction and its usefulness as a marker of recurrent coronary occlusion. Am J Cardiol 1991;67(2):109–15.

[8] Kloner RA, Ganote CE, Jennings RB. The "no-reflow" phenomenon after temporary coronary occlusion in the dog. J Clin Invest 1974;54(6):1496–508.

[9] Reffelmann T, Kloner RA. The "no-reflow" phenomenon: basic science and clinical correlates. Heart 2002;87(2):162–8.

[10] Clemmensen P, Ohman EM, Sevilla DC, et al. Changes in standard electrocardiographic ST-segment elevation predictive of successful reperfusion in acute myocardial infarction. Am J Cardiol 1990;66(20):1407–11.

[11] Hogg KJ, Hornung RS, Howie CA, et al. Electrocardiographic prediction of coronary artery patency after thrombolytic treatment in acute myocardial infarction: use of the ST segment as a non-invasive marker. Br Heart J 1988;60(4):275–80.

[12] Saran RK, Been M, Furniss SS, et al. Reduction in ST segment elevation after thrombolysis predicts either coronary reperfusion or preservation of left ventricular function. Br Heart J 1990;64(2):113–7.

[13] Barbash GI, Roth A, Hod H, et al. Rapid resolution of ST elevation and prediction of clinical outcome in patients undergoing thrombolysis with alteplase (recombinant tissue-type plasminogen activator): results of the Israeli Study of Early Intervention in Myocardial Infarction. Br Heart J 1990;64(4): 241–7.

[14] Shah PK, Cercek B, Lew AS, et al. Angiographic validation of bedside markers of reperfusion. J Am Coll Cardiol 1993;21(1):55–61.

[15] Kircher BJ, Topol EJ, O'Neill WW, et al. Prediction of infarct coronary artery recanalization after intravenous thrombolytic therapy. Am J Cardiol 1987; 59(6):513–5.

[16] Richardson SG, Morton P, Murtagh JG, et al. Relation of coronary arterial patency and left ventricular function to electrocardiographic changes after streptokinase treatment during acute myocardial infarction. Am J Cardiol 1988;61(13):961–5.

[17] Syed MA, Borzak S, Asfour A, et al. Single lead ST-segment recovery: a simple, reliable measure of successful fibrinolysis after acute myocardial infarction. Am Heart J 2004;147(2):275–80.

[18] Krucoff MW, Croll MA, Pope JE, et al. Continuously updated 12-lead ST-segment recovery analysis for myocardial infarct artery patency assessment and its correlation with multiple simultaneous early angiographic observations. Am J Cardiol 1993; 71(2):145–51.

[19] Krucoff MW, Wagner NB, Pope JE, et al. The portable programmable microprocessor-driven real-time 12-lead electrocardiographic monitor: a preliminary report of a new device for the noninvasive detection of successful reperfusion or silent coronary reocclusion. Am J Cardiol 1990;65(3):143–8.

[20] Dellborg M, Topol EJ, Swedberg K. Dynamic QRS complex and ST segment vectorcardiographic monitoring can identify vessel patency in patients with acute myocardial infarction treated with reperfusion therapy. Am Heart J 1991;122(4 Pt 1):943–8.

[21] Dellborg M, Steg PG, Simoons M, et al. Vectorcardiographic monitoring to assess early vessel patency

after reperfusion therapy for acute myocardial infarction. Eur Heart J 1995;16(1):21–9.

[22] Feldman LJ, Himbert D, Juliard JM, et al. Reperfusion syndrome: relationship of coronary blood flow reserve to left ventricular function and infarct size. J Am Coll Cardiol 2000;35(5):1162–9.

[23] Yokoshiki H, Kohya T, Tateda K, et al. Abrupt augmentation of ST segment elevation associated with successful reperfusion: a sign of diminished myocardial salvage. Am Heart J 1995;130(4):698–704.

[24] Shechter M, Rabinowitz B, Beker B, et al. Additional ST segment elevation during the first hour of thrombolytic therapy: an electrocardiographic sign predicting a favorable clinical outcome. J Am Coll Cardiol 1992;20(7):1460–4.

[25] Klootwijk P, Langer A, Meij S, et al. Non-invasive prediction of reperfusion and coronary artery patency by continuous ST segment monitoring in the GUSTO-I trial. Eur Heart J 1996;17(5):689–98.

[26] de Lemos JA, Antman EM, Giugliano RP, et al. ST-segment resolution and infarct-related artery patency and flow after thrombolytic therapy. Thrombolysis in Myocardial Infarction (TIMI) 14 investigators. Am J Cardiol 2000;85(3):299–304.

[27] Zeymer U, Schroder R, Tebbe U, et al. Non-invasive detection of early infarct vessel patency by resolution of ST-segment elevation in patients with thrombolysis for acute myocardial infarction; results of the angiographic substudy of the Hirudin for Improvement of Thrombolysis (HIT)-4 trial. Eur Heart J 2001;22(9):769–75.

[28] Schroder R, Dissmann R, Bruggemann T, et al. Extent of early ST segment elevation resolution: a simple but strong predictor of outcome in patients with acute myocardial infarction. J Am Coll Cardiol 1994;24(2):384–91.

[29] Schroder R, Wegscheider K, Schroder K, et al. Extent of early ST segment elevation resolution: a strong predictor of outcome in patients with acute myocardial infarction and a sensitive measure to compare thrombolytic regimens. A substudy of the International Joint Efficacy Comparison of Thrombolytics (INJECT) trial. J Am Coll Cardiol 1995; 26(7):1657–64.

[30] Matetzky S, Freimark D, Chouraqui P, et al. The distinction between coronary and myocardial reperfusion after thrombolytic therapy by clinical markers of reperfusion. J Am Coll Cardiol 1998; 32(5):1326–30.

[31] Willems JL, Willems RJ, Willems GM, et al. Significance of initial ST segment elevation and depression for the management of thrombolytic therapy in acute myocardial infarction. European Cooperative Study Group for Recombinant Tissue-Type Plasminogen Activator. Circulation 1990;82(4):1147–58.

[32] Schroder R, Zeymer U, Wegscheider K, et al. Comparison of the predictive value of ST segment elevation resolution at 90 and 180 min after start of streptokinase in acute myocardial infarction. A substudy of

the hirudin for improvement of thrombolysis (HIT)-4 study. Eur Heart J 1999;20(21):1563–71.

[33] van 't Hof AW, Liem A, Suryapranata H, et al. Angiographic assessment of myocardial reperfusion in patients treated with primary angioplasty for acute myocardial infarction: myocardial blush grade. Zwolle Myocardial Infarction Study Group. Circulation 1998;97(23):2302–6.

[34] Santoro GM, Valenti R, Buonamici P, et al. Relation between ST-segment changes and myocardial perfusion evaluated by myocardial contrast echocardiography in patients with acute myocardial infarction treated with direct angioplasty. Am J Cardiol 1998;82(8):932–7.

[35] van 't Hof AW, Liem A, de Boer MJ, et al. Clinical value of 12-lead electrocardiogram after successful reperfusion therapy for acute myocardial infarction. Zwolle Myocardial Infarction Study Group. Lancet 1997;350(9078):615–9.

[36] de Lemos JA, Braunwald E. ST segment resolution as a tool for assessing the efficacy of reperfusion therapy. J Am Coll Cardiol 2001;38(5):1283–94.

[37] Matetzky S, Novikov M, Gruberg L, et al. The significance of persistent ST elevation versus early resolution of ST segment elevation after primary PTCA. J Am Coll Cardiol 1999;34(7):1932–8.

[38] Poli A, Fetiveau R, Vandoni P, et al. Integrated analysis of myocardial blush and ST-segment elevation recovery after successful primary angioplasty: real-time grading of microvascular reperfusion and prediction of early and late recovery of left ventricular function. Circulation 2002;106(3):313–8.

[39] Haager PK, Christott P, Heussen N, et al. Prediction of clinical outcome after mechanical revascularization in acute myocardial infarction by markers of myocardial reperfusion. J Am Coll Cardiol 2003; 41(4):532–8.

[40] Doevendans PA, Gorgels AP, van der Zee R, et al. Electrocardiographic diagnosis of reperfusion during thrombolytic therapy in acute myocardial infarction. Am J Cardiol 1995;75(17):1206–10.

[41] Corbalan R, Prieto JC, Chavez E, et al. Bedside markers of coronary artery patency and short-term prognosis of patients with acute myocardial infarction and thrombolysis. Am Heart J 1999;138(3 Pt 1): 533–9.

[42] Herz I, Birnbaum Y, Zlotikamien B, et al. The prognostic implications of negative T waves in the leads with ST segment elevation on admission in acute myocardial infarction. Cardiology 1999;92(2):121–7.

[43] Wong CK, French JK, Aylward PE, et al. Usefulness of the presenting electrocardiogram in predicting successful reperfusion with streptokinase in acute myocardial infarction. Am J Cardiol 1999; 83(2):164–8.

[44] Matetzky S, Barabash GI, Shahar A, et al. Early T wave inversion after thrombolytic therapy predicts better coronary perfusion: clinical and angiographic study. J Am Coll Cardiol 1994;24(2):378–83.

[45] Adler Y, Zafrir N, Ben-Gal T, et al. Relation between evolutionary ST segment and T-wave direction and electrocardiographic prediction of myocardial infarct size and left ventricular function among patients with anterior wall Q-wave acute myocardial infarction who received reperfusion therapy. Am J Cardiol 2000;85(8):927–33.

[46] Tamura A, Nagase K, Mikuriya Y, et al. Significance of spontaneous normalization of negative T waves in infarct-related leads during healing of anterior wall acute myocardial infarction. Am J Cardiol 1999;84(11):1341–4.

[47] Agetsuma H, Hirai M, Hirayama H, et al. Transient giant negative T wave in acute anterior myocardial infarction predicts R wave recovery and preservation of left ventricular function. Heart 1996;75(3):229–34.

[48] Dellborg M, Riha M, Swedberg K. Dynamic QRS-complex and ST-segment monitoring in acute myocardial infarction during recombinant tissue-type plasminogen activator therapy. The TEAHAT Study Group. Am J Cardiol 1991;67(5):343–9.

[49] Goldberg S, Urban P, Greenspon A, et al. Limitation of infarct size with thrombolytic agents–electrocardiographic indexes. Circulation 1983;68(2 Pt 2): I77–82.

[50] Rechavia E, Blum A, Mager A, et al. Electrocardiographic Q-waves inconstancy during thrombolysis in acute anterior wall myocardial infarction. Cardiology 1992;80(5–6):392–8.

[51] Raitt MH, Maynard C, Wagner GS, et al. Relation between symptom duration before thrombolytic therapy and final myocardial infarct size. Circulation 1996;93(1):48–53.

[52] Raitt MH, Maynard C, Wagner GS, et al. Appearance of abnormal Q waves early in the course of acute myocardial infarction: implications for efficacy of thrombolytic therapy. J Am Coll Cardiol 1995;25(5):1084–8.

[53] Bar FW, Vermeer F, de Zwaan C, et al. Value of admission electrocardiogram in predicting outcome of thrombolytic therapy in acute myocardial infarction. A randomized trial conducted by The Netherlands Interuniversity Cardiology Institute. Am J Cardiol 1987;59(1):6–13.

[54] Birnbaum Y, Chetrit A, Sclarovsky S, et al. Abnormal Q waves on the admission electrocardiogram of patients with first acute myocardial infarction: prognostic implications. Clin Cardiol 1997;20(5): 477–81.

[55] Selwyn AP, Ogunro E, Shillingford JP. Loss of electrically active myocardium during anterior infarction in man. Br Heart J 1977;39(11):1186–91.

[56] von Essen R, Merx W, Doerr R, et al. QRS mapping in the evaluation of acute anterior myocardial infarction. Circulation 1980;62(2):266–76.

[57] Kalbfleisch JM, Shadaksharappa KS, Conrad LL, et al. Disappearance of the Q-deflection following myocardial infarction. Am Heart J 1968;76(2):193–8.

[58] Birnbaum Y, Hale SL, Kloner RA. Changes in R wave amplitude: ECG differentiation between episodes of reocclusion and reperfusion associated with ST-segment elevation. J Electrocardiol 1997; 30(3):211–6.

[59] Birnbaum Y, Maynard C, Wolfe S, et al. Terminal QRS distortion on admission is better than ST-segment measurements in predicting final infarct size and assessing the potential effect of thrombolytic therapy in anterior wall acute myocardial infarction. Am J Cardiol 1999;84(5):530–4.

[60] Birnbaum Y, Herz I, Sclarovsky S, et al. Prognostic significance of the admission electrocardiogram in acute myocardial infarction. J Am Coll Cardiol 1996;27(5):1128–32.

[61] Birnbaum Y, Kloner RA, Sclarovsky S, et al. Distortion of the terminal portion of the QRS on the admission electrocardiogram in acute myocardial infarction and correlation with infarct size and long-term prognosis (Thrombolysis in Myocardial Infarction 4 trial). Am J Cardiol 1996;78(4): 396–403.

[62] Cercek B, Lew AS, Laramee P, et al. Time course and characteristics of ventricular arrhythmias after reperfusion in acute myocardial infarction. Am J Cardiol 1987;60(4):214–8.

[63] Gorgels AP, Vos MA, Letsch IS, et al. Usefulness of the accelerated idioventricular rhythm as a marker for myocardial necrosis and reperfusion during thrombolytic therapy in acute myocardial infarction. Am J Cardiol 1988;61(4):231–5.

[64] Wei JY, Markis JE, Malagold M, et al. Cardiovascular reflexes stimulated by reperfusion of ischemic myocardium in acute myocardial infarction. Circulation 1983;67(4):796–801.

[65] Esente P, Giambartolomei A, Gensini GG, et al. Coronary reperfusion and Bezold-Jarisch reflex (bradycardia and hypotension). Am J Cardiol 1983; 52(3):221–4.

[66] Vatterott PJ, Hammill SC, Bailey KR, et al. Late potentials on signal-averaged electrocardiograms and patency of the infarct-related artery in survivors of acute myocardial infarction. J Am Coll Cardiol 1991;17(2):330–7.

[67] Hong M, Peter T, Peters W, et al. Relation between acute ventricular arrhythmias, ventricular late potentials and mortality in acute myocardial infarction. Am J Cardiol 1991;68(15):1403–9.

[68] Tranchesi B Jr, Verstraete M, Van de Werf F, et al. Usefulness of high-frequency analysis of signal-averaged surface electrocardiograms in acute myocardial infarction before and after coronary thrombolysis for assessing coronary reperfusion. Am J Cardiol 1990;66(17):1196–8.

[69] Ophuis AJ, Bar FW, Vermeer F, et al. Angiographic assessment of prospectively determined non-invasive reperfusion indices in acute myocardial infarction. Heart 2000;84(2):164–70.

ELSEVIER
SAUNDERS

CARDIOLOGY
CLINICS

Cardiol Clin 24 (2006) 377–385

Electrocardiographic Diagnosis of Myocardial Infarction during Left Bundle Branch Block

S. Serge Barold, MD*, Bengt Herweg, MD

*Division of Cardiology, University of South Florida College of Medicine and Tampa General Hospital,
Tampa, FL 33606, USA*

The diagnosis of myocardial infarction (MI) in the presence of left bundle branch block (LBBB) has long been considered problematic or even almost impossible. Many proposed ECG markers in the old literature have now been discarded. However, the advent of reperfusion therapy has generated greater interest in the ECG diagnosis of acute MI (based on ST-segment abnormalities) [1–4], although criteria for old MI (based on QRS changes) have not been reevaluated for almost 20 years [5,6]. Furthermore, analysis of the some of the published data is compounded by the considerable interobserver variability in the interpretation of ECGs [6–8].

Acute myocardial infarction

ST-segment deviation is the only useful electrocardiographic sign for the diagnosis of acute MI in the presence of LBBB. In uncomplicated LBBB, ECG leads with a predominantly negative QRS complex show ST-segment elevation with positive T waves, a pattern similar to the current of injury observed during acute myocardial ischemia or MI. Studies of patients with LBBB during either acute MI [9–11], or occlusion of a coronary artery by an angioplasty balloon [12,13] have shown that further ST-segment elevation occurs in these leads. Electrocardiographic signs involving the QRS complex are not diagnostically useful in the acute setting.

Sgarbossa and colleagues [1] studied 131 patients (enrolled in the GUSTO-1 trial) with acute

MI (documented by serum enzyme changes) and LBBB on their baseline ECG. The following definition of LBBB was used: a QRS duration of at least 0.125 seconds in the presence of sinus or supraventricular rhythm, a QS or rS complex in lead V_1, and an R-wave peak time of at least 0.06 seconds in lead I, V_5, or V_6 associated with the absence of a Q or q wave in the same leads. Patients with ECGs showing intermittent LBBB were excluded from the study. The control group consisted of 131 patients randomly selected from the Duke Databank for Cardiovascular Disease, who had complete LBBB and stable, angiographically documented coronary artery disease. These patients did not have acute chest pain at the time of the recorded ECGs.

The maximal sensitivity with the target specificity (>90%) was achieved in the following situations: (1) at least one lead exhibiting ST-segment elevation ≥1 mm concordant with (in the same direction as) a predominantly positive QRS complex. (2) Discordant ST-segment elevation 5 mm with (in the opposite direction from) a predominantly negative QRS complex. (3) ST-segment depression ≥1 mm in V_1, V_2, or V_3 (Figs. 1 and 2). Electrocardiographic criteria with statistical significance for the diagnosis of acute MI and their sensitivities, specificities, and likelihood ratios from the study of Sgarbossa and colleagues are listed in Table 1. The likelihood ratios indicate to what extent a particular criterion will increase or decrease the probability of infarction. The ECG criterion with the highest likelihood ratio was ST-segment elevation of at least 1 mm in leads with a QRS complex in the same direction. Similarly, the absence of this criterion was associated with the lowest likelihood ratio.

---

* Corresponding author.
E-mail address: ssbarold@aol.com (S.S. Barold).

cardiology.theclinics.com

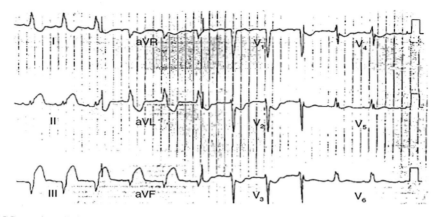

Fig. 1. ECG meeting all three independent criteria of Sgarbossa and colleagues for the diagnosis of acute MI with LBBB. The ECG shows at least 1-mm concordant ST-elevation in lead II, at least 1-mm ST depression in leads V_2 and V_3, as well as discordant ST-elevation of at least 5 mm in leads III and aVF (*Reproduced from* Sgarbossa EB, Pinski SL, Barbagelata A, et al, for the GUSTO-1 investigators. Electrocardiographic diagnosis of evolving acute myocardial infarction in the presence of left bundle branch block. N Engl J Med 1996;334:481–7; © 1996 Massachusetts Medical Society. Used with permission.)

With regard to the weakest criterion (ST-segment elevation ≥5 mm discordant with the QRS), Madias [14,15] warned that this sign may occur in clinically stable patients with LBBB without an acute MI (6%) in the presence of unusually large QRS complexes in V_1 to V_3 in which leads the ST-segment elevations are also large. Such patients frequently have severe left ventricular hypertrophy or markedly dilated hearts.

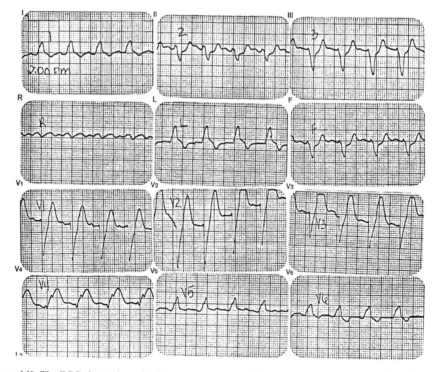

Fig. 2. Acute MI. The ECG shows sinus rhythm, and complete LBBB, and an acute anterolateral MI. There is concordant ST-elevation obvious in lead aVL, and less prominent in lead I. The right precordial leads (V_1–V_4) show marked discordant ST-elevation.

Table 1
Results of the univariate analysis of the electrocardiographic criteria in the study of Sgarbossa and colleagues [1]

Criterion	Sensitivity percent (95% CI)	Specificity percent (95% CI)	Positive likelihood ratio (95% CI)	Negative likelihood ratio (95% CI)
ST-segment elevation ≥1 mm and concordant with the QRS complex	73 (64–80)	92 (86–96)	9.54 (3.1–17.3)	0.3 (0.22–0.39)
ST-segment depression ≥1 mm in lead V_1, V_2, or V_3	25 (18–34)	96 (91–99)	6.58 (2.6–16.1)	0.78 (0.7–0.87)
ST-segment elevation ≥5 mm and discordant with QRS complex	31 (23–39)	92 (85–96)	3.63 (2.0–6.8)	0.75 (0.67–0.86)
Positive T wave in lead V_5 or V_6	26 (19–34)	92 (86–96)	3.42 (0.18–6.5)	0.8 (0.72–0.9)
Left-axis deviation	72 (63–79)	48 (39–57)	1.38 (1.13–9.8)	0.59 (0.25–1.39)

Abbreviation: CI, confidence interval.

Positive likelihood (LR) ratio: the percentage of acute myocardial infarction (MI) patients positive by a stated ECG sign for diagnosis divided by the percentage of patients without MI but showing a similar positive ECG sign. LR>1 indicates an increased probability that the target disorder is present, and an LR<1 indicates a decreased probability that the target disorder is present. A likelihood ratio of 9 means that the criterion in question is nine times as likely to occur in acute MI as it is in a patient without an MI.

$$LR+ = \frac{\text{probability of an individual } with \text{ acute MI having a positive sign}}{\text{probability of an individual } without \text{ acute MI having a positive sign}}$$

$$LR- = \frac{\text{probability of an individual } with \text{ acute MI having a negative sign}}{\text{probability of an individual } without \text{ acute MI having a negative sign}}$$

Reproduced from Sgarbossa EB, Pinski SL, Barbagelata A, et al, for the GUSTO-1 investigators. Electrocardiographic diagnosis of evolving acute myocardial infarction in the presence of left bundle branch block. N Engl J Med 1996;334:481–7. © 1996 Massachusetts Medical Society. Used with permission.

Scoring system

Sgarbossa and colleagues [1] developed an algorithm where an ECG is considered positive for MI if its score is at least three points on the basis of three criteria: ST-segment elevation of at least 1 mm in the lead with concordant QRS complex–a score of five points; ST-segment depression of at least 1 mm in leads V_1, V_2, or V_3—a score of three points; and ST-segment elevation of at least 5 mm in the lead with discordant QRS complex—a score of two points (Table 2). The scoring system represents the fact that ST-segment elevation of at least 1 mm that is concordant with the QRS complex or ST-segment depression of at least 1 mm in lead V_1, V_2, or V_3 is a specific marker of infarction, even when no other ECG change is observed. On the other hand, the sole presence of ST-segment elevation of at least 5 mm that is discordant with the QRS complex (with a score of 2)

indicates a moderate-to-high probability of MI, and further procedures should be undertaken to confirm the diagnosis. Sgarbossa and colleagues [1] indicated that their algorithm based on ST-segment changes (index score of at least 3) had a sensitivity of 78% and a specificity of 90% for the diagnosis of MI in patients with LBBB.

Hirulog and Early Reperfusion or Occlusion Trial (HERO-2)

The recently reported Hirulog and Early Reperfusion or Occlusion Trial (HERO-2) study [4] involved 300 patients presenting with >30 min of ischemic chest discomfort and presumed new-onset LBBB according to the criteria of Sgarbossa and colleagues [1]. Enzymatically confirmed acute MI occurred in 80.7% of the LBBB patients. Ninety-two patients exhibited positive ST-segment

Table 2

Odds ratios and scores for independent electrocardiographic criteria from Sgarbossa and colleagues [1]

Criterion	Odds ratio (95% CI)	Score
ST-segment elevation ≥ 1 mm and concordant with QRS complex	25.2 (11.6–54.7)	5
ST-segment depression ≥ 1 mm in lead V_1, V_2, or V_3	6.0 (1.9–19.3)	3
ST-segment elevation ≥ 5 mm and discordant with QRS complex	4.3 (1.8–10.6)	2

The odds ratio is a way of comparing whether the probability of a certain event is the same for two groups. An odds ratio of 1 implies that the event is equally likely in both groups. An odds ratio >1 implies that the event is more likely in the first group. An odds ratio <1 implies that the event is less likely in the first group. The table shows the ratio of the odds of having the ECG sign in the acute myocardial infarction group relative to the odds of having the sign in the control group. (*Reproduced from* Sgarbossa EB, Pinski SL, Barbagelata A, et al, for the GUSTO-1 investigators. Electro+cardiographic diagnosis of evolving acute myocardial infarction in the presence of left bundle branch block. N Engl J med 1996;334:481–7.)

abnormalities for the diagnosis of acute MI according to the criteria of Sgarbossa and colleagues [1]. The study confirmed the findings of Sgarbossa and colleagues [1] in terms of the following results (Table 3): (1) concordant ST-segment elevation ≥ 1 mm: high specificity (98.3%) but low sensitivity (33.5%). (2) ST-segment depression measuring ≥ 1 mm in any of the V_1 to V_3 leads had similarly high specificity, but only 14.1% sensitivity. Lowering the cutoff for ST-segment changes to ≥ 0.5 mm for each of the criteria in 1 and 2 did not improve sensitivity. When both criteria were combined (ie, concordant ST-segment elevation *or* lead V_1 to V_3 ST-segment depression), the specificity for detection of enzymatically confirmed acute MI was 96.6%, and the sensitivity was 37.2%. (3) Discordant ST-segment elevation measuring ≥ 5 mm was neither sensitive (29.3%) nor specific (58.6%).

Clinical implications of the Sgarbossa criteria

The clinical utility of the criteria and scoring system of Sgarbossa and colleagues [1] have been validated by other studies, all of which have also demonstrated a high specificity, but some have shown an even lower sensitivity than the original data of Sgarbossa and colleagues [1] in terms of the three individual ST-segment criteria and the scoring algorithm [8,16–21]. As such, although the criteria and the algorithm cannot be used to rule out MI, it can help to rule it in. Patients with an acute MI and LBBB have a high mortality rate, but this is significantly related to age and co-morbidities [22–24]. Thus, these markers should be used together with the clinical findings because the ECG markers alone miss acute MI in many patients who would benefit from aggressive

Table 3

Application of ST-segment criteria for the diagnosis of AMI in the 300 patients with LBBB at randomization from Wong and colleagues [4]

	n	Sensitivity (%)	Specificity (%)	Positive predictive value (%)	Negative predictive value (%)
Concordant ST-segment elevation ≥ 1 mm	82	33.5 (27.6–39.8)	98.3 (89.5–99.9)	98.8 (92.5–99.9)	26.1 (20.6–32.6)
Lead V_1 to V_3 ST-segment depression ≥ 1 mm	35	14.1 (10.1–19.2)	98.4 (89.5–99.9)	97.1 (83.4–99.9)	21.5 (16.8–27.0)
Concordant ST-segment elevation ≥ 1 mm or lead V_1 to V_3 ST-segment depression ≥ 1 mm	92	37.2 (31.1–43.6)	96.6 (87.0–99.4)	97.8 (91.6–99.6)	26.9 (21.1–33.6)

Abbreviations: AMI, acute myocardial infarction; LBBB, left bundle branch block. (*Reproduced from* Wong CK, French JK, Aylward PE, et al, and the HERO-2 Trial Investigators. Patients with prolonged ischemic chest pain and presumed-new left bundle branch block have heterogeneous outcomes depending on the presence of ST-segment changes. J Am Coll cardiol 2005;46:29–38; with permission from American College of Cardiology Foundation.)

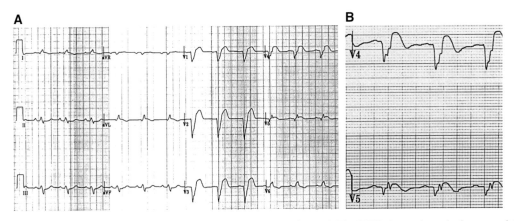

Fig. 3. Anterior MI of undetermined age with double Cabrera's sign. (*A*) The ECG shows sinus rhythm, complete LBBB, and qR complexes in leads I, aVL, and V$_4$. Note the double Cabrera's sign in lead V$_4$. The presence of sinus rhythm with a normal PR interval rules out a retrograde P wave as the cause of one of the notches on the ascending limb of the S wave. (*B*) Magnified ECG of leads V$_4$ and V$_5$.

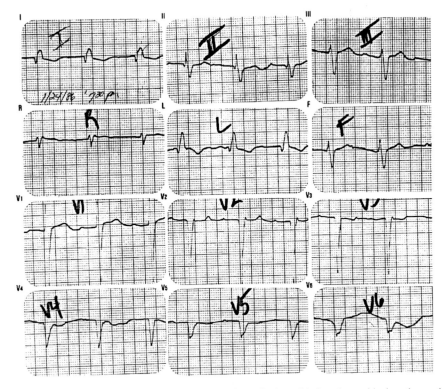

Fig. 4. Anterior MI of undetermined age. The ECG shows sinus rhythm with first-degree block and complete LBBB. Note the rather tall first deflection in lead V$_1$, which is an R wave. This finding in complete LBBB is very typical of anteroseptal MI of undetermined age. Poor R-wave progression V$_1$ toV$_6$ is also consistent with anterior MI.

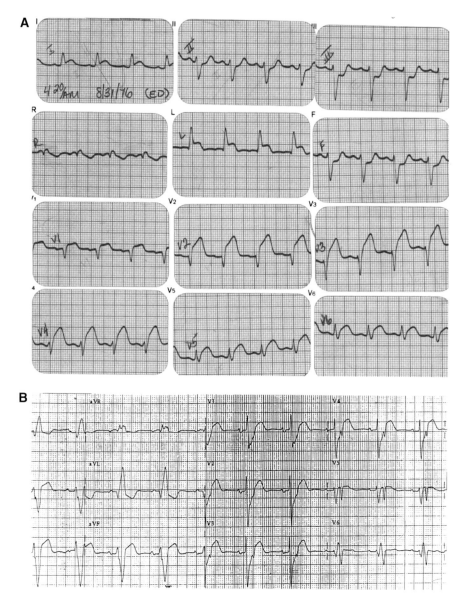

Fig. 5. ECG pattern of MI after development of complete LBBB. (*A*) ECG showing sinus rhythm and an extensive acute anterior MI. (*B*) ECG 1 month later showing sinus rhythm, new complete LBBB, and many of the signs of anterior MI: tall initial positive deflection (R wave) in lead V_1, Cabrera's sign in leads V_2– V_4, q wave in leads 1 and aVL, and poor r-wave progression in leads V_4–V_6.

treatment. The published studies showing poor sensitivity of the ECG markers support the recommendations of the American College of Cardiology and the American Heart Association that all patients with LBBB irrespective of ECG features and symptoms of acute MI should receive reperfusion therapy (angioplasty may be preferable to fibrinolytic therapy if there are no contraindications) [25,26].

Old (remote) myocardial infarction

In uncomplicated LBBB, septal activation occurs from right to left because the left septal mass cannot be activated via the left bundle. Consequently, LBBB does not generate a q wave in the lateral leads (I and V_6). Lead V_1 may show an initial r wave because of the anterior component of right-to-left septal activation but

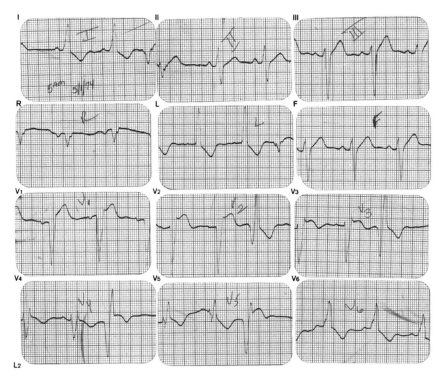

Fig. 6. Possible anterior MI unmasked by ventricular extrasystole during complete LBBB. Leads V_2–V_5 show ventricular extrasystoles with a qR or Qr comlexes consistent with anterior MI.

leads V_1 to V_3 may also show QS complexes. After crossing the ventricular septum, the activation reaches the left ventricle, which is depolarized via ordinary myocardium, QS complexes may be seen in leads III and aVF. Secondary ST segment, and T-wave abnormalities are oriented in the opposite direction compared with the QRS complex. The ECG manifestations of the old MI may remain concealed, probably more commonly than those of acute MI with LBBB [2].

During LBBB, an *extensive* anteroseptal MI will alter the initial QRS vector, with forces pointing to the right because of unopposed activation of the right ventricle. This causes (initial) q waves in leads I, aVL, V_5, and V_6, producing an Qr or qR pattern.

A number of old studies reported that the presence of a Q wave in lead 1 was a highly specific and relatively sensitive sign for the diagnosis of anterior infarction in the presence of complete LBBB [27,28]. Cabrera and Friedland [29] described the diagnostic value of late notching of the S wave in leads V_3 to V_5 (Fig. 3) in anterior infarction in terms of very high sensitivity and specificity.

With regard to the QRS complex in the diagnosis of MI in LBBB, Wackers [6] also found that an abnormal Q wave in leads I, aVL, or V_6 (duration not stated) may be of diagnostic value in anteroseptal MI with a sensitivity of 53% and specificity of 91% (Figs. 4 and 5). A highly specific criterion (100%) was the combination of an abnormal Q wave in V_6 and an increased sharp R wave in V_1. This combination occurred only in patients with an anteroseptal MI, but the sensitivity was low (20%). Cabrera's sign (defined as notching of 0.05 sec in duration in the ascending limb of the S wave in leads V_3 or V_4) was also useful with a specificity of 47% for anteroseptal MI and a specificity of 87% (see Fig. 3). Wackers [6] also found that a number of other previously proposed QRS signs were disappointing for the diagnosis of MI. Wackers [6] also found that so-called primary T-wave changes (T wave in the same direction as the QRS complex) carry no important diagnostic value.

The most recent study involving the QRS complex was published in 1989 by Hands and colleagues [5]. They confirmed that Q waves (≥ 30 msec) in two or more lateral leads (I, aVL, V_5, and

V_6) and R-wave regression from V_1 to V_4 each had a poor sensitivity (21%) but high specificity (100%) for the diagnosis of anterior infarction (see Figs. 3–5). A Q wave of any size in the lateral leads yielded a sensitivity of 29% and specificity of 91%. Pathologic studies have confirmed the presence of septal infarction in patients with LBBB and Q waves in the lateral leads (I, aVL, V_5, and V_6). Late notching of the upstroke of the S wave (Cabrera's sign) in at least two leads V_3 to V_5 provided a sensitivity of 29% and specificity of 91% (see Figs. 3 and 5). Other previously proposed signs of MI involving the QRS complex in LBBB were found to have poor sensitivity, specificity, and predictive value. The significance of a tall R wave in lead V_1 during LBBB as a sign of anterior MI was not studied in the report of Hands and colleagues (see Figs. 4 and 5) [5]. This may be a rare but very specific sign of MI corresponding to a q wave possibly in leads V_7 or V_8.

Ventricular extrasystoles

Ventricular extrasystoles may unmask the pattern of an underlying MI in patients with LBBB, but this sign is not absolutely specific [30]. Such ventricular extrasystoles must satisfy two conditions. (1) The configuration must be either qR or qRs but not QS, because a QS complex can be generated by an extrasystole originating in an area underlying the recording electrode. (2) The qR or qRs complex must be registered in a lead that would ordinarily be expected to reflect left ventricular epicardial potentials in the precordial leads (Fig. 6). According to Coumel [31], who analyzed the significance of QR complexes during ventricular tachycardia in patients with coronary artery disease, the QR, qR, or qRs patterns reflect an MI, although its exact site cannot be determined. Josephson and Miller [32] disagree with Coumel [31] because they observed qR patterns in ventricular tachycardia with a LBBB pattern in patients with cardiomyopathy. They emphasized that a QR complex could originate from a fixed scar (infarct) or a conduction disturbance secondary to fibrosis regardless of etiology.

References

[1] Sgarbossa EB, Pinski SL, Barbagelata A, et al, for the GUSTO-1 investigators. Electrocardiographic diagnosis of evolving acute myocardial infarction in the presence of left bundle branch block. New Engl J Med 1996;334:481–7.

[2] Sgarbossa EB. Recent advances in the electrocardiographic diagnosis of myocardial infarction: left bundle branch block and pacing. Pacing Clin Electrophysiol 1996;19:1370–9.

[3] Sgarbossa EB. Value of the ECG in suspected acute myocardial infarction with left bundle branch block. J Electrocardiol 2000;33(Suppl):87–92.

[4] Wong CK, French JK, Aylward PE, et al, and HERO-2 Trial Investigators. Patients with prolonged ischemic chest pain and presumed-new left bundle branch block have heterogeneous outcomes depending on the presence of ST-segmentchanges. J Am Coll Cardiol 2005;46:29–38.

[5] Hands ME, Cook EF, Stone PH, et al, and the MILIS Study Group. Electrocardiographic diagnosis of myocardial infarction in the presence of complete left bundle branch block. Am Heart J 1988; 116:23–32.

[6] Wackers FJ. The diagnosis of myocardial infarction in the presence of left bundle branch block. Cardiol Clin 1987;5:393–401.

[7] Wellens HJ. Acute myocardial infarction and left bundle-branch block—can we lift the veil? N Engl J Med 1996;334:528–9.

[8] Gula LJ, Dick A, Massel D. Diagnosing acute myocardial infarction in the setting of left bundle branch block: prevalence and observer variability from a large community setting. Coronary Artery Dis 2003;14:387–93.

[9] Kennamer R, Prinzmetal M. Myocardial infarction complicated by left bundle branch block. Am Heart J 1956;51:78–90.

[10] Wackers FJ. Complete left bundle branch block: is the diagnosis of myocardial infarction possible? Int J Cardiol 1983;2:521–9.

[11] Sclarovsky S, Sagie A, Strasberg B, et al. Ischemic blocks during early phase of anterior myocardial infarction: correlation with ST-segment shift. Clin Cardiol 1988;11:757–62.

[12] Cannon A, Freedman SB, Bailey BP, et al. ST-segment changes during transmural myocardial ischemia in chronic left bundle branch block. Am J Cardiol 1989;64:1216–7.

[13] Stark KS, Krucoff MW, Schryver B, et al. Quantification of ST-segment changes during coronary angioplasty in patients with left bundle branch block. Am J Cardiol 1991;67:1219–22.

[14] Madias JE, Sinha A, Ashtiani R, et al. A critique of the new ST-segment criteria for the diagnosis of acute myocardial infarction in patients with left bundle-branch block. Clin Cardiol 2001;24: 652–5.

[15] Madias JE, Sinha A, Agarwal H, et al. ST-segment elevation in leads V1–V3 in patients with LBBB. J Electrocardiol 2001;34:87–8.

[16] Li SF, Walden PL, Maccrilla O, et al. Electrocardiographic diagnosis of myocardial infarction in patients with left bundle branch block. Ann Emerg Med 2000;36:561–5.

[17] Sokolove PE, Sgarbossa EB, Amsterdam EA, et al. Interobserver variability in the electrocardiographic diagnosis of acute myocardial infarction in patients with left bundle branch block. Ann Emerg Med 2000;36:566–71.

[18] Gunnarsson G, Eriksson P, Dellborg M. ECG criteria in diagnosis of acute myocardial infarction in the presence of left bundle branch block. Int J Cardiol 2001;78:167–74.

[19] Kontos MC, McQueen RH, Jesse RL, et al. Can myocardial infarction be rapidly identified in Emergency Department patients who have left bundle branch block? Ann Emerg Med 2001;37:431–8.

[20] Shlipak MG, Lyons WL, Go AS, et al. Should the electrocardiogram be used to guide therapy for patients with left bundle-branch block and suspected myocardial infarction? JAMA 1999;281:714–9.

[21] Edhouse JA, Sakr M, Angus J, et al. Suspected myocardial infarction and left bundle branch block: electrocardiographic indicators of acute ischaemia. J Accid Emerg Med 1999;16:331–5.

[22] Stenestrand U, Tabrizi F, Lindback J, et al. Comorbidity and myocardial dysfunction are the main explanations for the higher 1-year mortality in acute myocardial infarction with left bundle-branch block. Circulation 2004;110(14):1896–902.

[23] Haywood LJ. Left bundle branch block in acute myocardial infarction: benign or malignant? J Am Coll Cardiol 2005;46:39–41.

[24] Moreno R, Garcia E, Lopez de Sa E, et al. Implications of left bundle branch block in acute myocardial infarction treated with primary angioplasty. Am J Cardiol 2002;90:401–3.

[25] Fibrinolytic Therapy Trialists' (FTT) Collaborative Group. Indications for fibrinolytic therapy in suspected myocardial infarction: collaborative overview of early mortality and major morbidity results from all randomised trials of more than 1000 patients. Lancet 1994;343:311–22.

[26] Antman EM, Anbe DT, Armstrong PW, et al. ACC/AHA guidelines for the management of patients with ST-elevation myocardial infarction; a report of the American College of Cardiology/American Heart Association Task Force on Practice Guidelines (Committee to Revise the 1999 Guidelines for the Management of patients with acute myocardial infarction). J Am Coll Cardiol 2004;44(3):E1–211.

[27] Besoaín-Santander M, Gómez-Ebensperguer G. Electrocardiographic diagnosis of myocardial infarction in cases of complete left bundle branch block. Am Heart J 1960;60:886–97.

[28] Doucet P, Walsh TJ, Massie E. A vectorcardiographic and electrocardiographic study of left bundle branch block with myocardial infarction. Am J Cardiol 1966;17:171–9.

[29] Cabrera E, Friedland C. La onda de activación ventricular en el bloqueo de rama izquierda con infarto: un nuevo signo electrocardiográfico. Arch Inst Cardiol Mex 1953;23:441–60.

[30] Dressler W. A case of myocardial infarction masked by bundle branch block but revealed by occasional premature ventricular beats. Am J Med Sci 1943; 206:361.

[31] Coumel P. Diagnostic significance of the QRS wave form in patients with ventricular tachycardia. Cardiol Clin 1987;5:527–40.

[32] Josephson ME, Miller JM. Endocardial and epicardial recordings. Correlation of twelve-lead electrocardiograms at the site of origin of ventricular tachycardia. Ann N Y Acad Sci 1990;601:128–47.

Electrocardiographic Diagnosis of Myocardial Infarction and Ischemia during Cardiac Pacing

S. Serge Barold, MD*, Bengt Herweg, MD, Anne B. Curtis, MD

*Division of Cardiology, University of South Florida College of Medicine
and Tampa General Hospital, Tampa, FL, USA*

The ECG diagnosis of myocardial infarction (MI) and ischemia in pacemaker patients can be challenging. Many of the criteria are insensitive, but the diagnosis can be made in a limited number of cases because of the high specificity of some of the criteria.

Old myocardial infarction

Box 1 outlines the difficulties in the diagnosis of MI, and Box 2 lists a number of signs of no value in the diagnosis of MI. Generally, when using the QRS complex, the sensitivity is low (25%) and the specificity is close to 100%. One cannot determine the age of the MI from the QRS complex.

Anterior myocardial infarction

St-qR pattern

Because the QRS complex during right ventricular (RV) pacing resembles (except for the initial forces) that of spontaneous left bundle branch block (LBBB), many of the criteria for the diagnosis of MI in LBBB also apply to MI during RV pacing [1–4]. RV pacing almost invariably masks a relatively small anteroseptal MI.

During RV pacing, as in LBBB, an extensive anteroseptal MI close to the stimulating electrode will alter the initial QRS vector, with forces pointing to the right because of unopposed activation of the RV. This causes (initial) q waves in leads I, aVL, V_5, and V_6, producing an St-qR pattern (Fig. 1). The abnormal q wave is usually 0.03 seconds or more, but a narrower one is also diagnostic.

Occasionally the St-qR complex is best seen in leads V_2 to V_4, and it may even be restricted to these leads. Finding the (initial) q wave may sometimes require placing the leads one intercostal space higher or perhaps lower. Ventricular fusion may cause pseudoinfarction patterns (Fig. 2).

The sensitivity of the St-qR pattern varies from 10% to 50% according to the way data are analyzed [5,6]. Patients who require temporary pacing in acute MI represent a preselected group with a large MI, so that the overall sensitivity is substantially lower than 50% in the patient population with implanted pacemakers. The specificity is virtually 100%.

Late notching of the ascending S wave (Cabrera's sign)

As in LBBB, during RV pacing an extensive anterior MI may produce notching of the ascending limb of the S wave in the precordial leads usually V_3 and V_4—Cabrera's sign ≥ 0.03 seconds and present in two leads (Fig. 3) [1]. The sign may occur together with the St-qR pattern in anterior MI (see Fig. 1). The sensitivity varies from 25% to 50% according to the size of the MI, but the specificity is close to 100% if notching is properly defined [1,5]. Interestingly, workers [7] that placed little diagnostic value on q waves, found a 57% sensitivity for Cabrera's sign (0.04-second notching) in the diagnosis of extensive anterior MI. Box 3 outlines the causes of "false" Cabrera's signs and the highly specific variants of Cabrera's sign (Fig. 4).

Inferior myocardial infarction

The paced QRS complex is often unrevealing. During RV pacing in inferior MI diagnostic Qr,

---

* Corresponding author.
  E-mail address: ssbarold@aol.com (S.S. Barold).

Box 1. Difficulties in the diagnosis
of MI during ventricular pacing

1. Large unipolar stimuli may obscure
   initial forces, cause a pseudo Q
   wave and false ST segment current
   of injury.
2. QS complexes are of no diagnostic
   value. Only qR or Qr complexes may
   be diagnostically valuable.
3. Fusion beats may cause
   a pseudoinfarction pattern (qR/Qr
   complex or notching of the upstroke
   of the S wave).
4. Cabrera's sign can be easily
   overdiagnosed.
5. Retrograde P waves in the terminal
   part of the QRS complex may mimic
   Cabrera's sign.
6. Acute MI and ischemia may be
   difficult to differentiate.
7. Differentiation of acute MI
   and old or indeterminate age MI
   may not be possible on the basis
   of abnormalities of the
   ST segment.
8. Signs in the QRS complex are not
   useful for the diagnosis of acute MI.
9. ST segment changes usually but not
   always indicate an acute process.
10. Recording QRS signs of MI may
    require different sites of the left V
    leads such as a different intercostals
    space.
11. Biventricular pacing can mask an
    MI pattern in the QRS complex
    evident during RV pacing.
12. qR or Qr complexes are common
    during biventricular pacing and do
    not represent an MI.
13. Cardiac memory. Repolarization
    ST-T wave abnormalities (mostly T
    wave inversion) in the spontaneous
    rhythm may be secondary to RV
    pacing per se and not related to
    ischemia or non–Q wave MI.
14. QRS abnormalities have low
    sensitivity (but high specificity).
15. Beware that not all the diagnostic
    criteria of MI in left bundle branch
    block are applicable during RV
    pacing.

Box 2. QRS criteria of no value
in diagnosis of MI

- QS complexes V_1 to V_6
- RS or terminal S wave in V_5 and V_6
- QS complexes in the inferior leads
- Slight notching of R waves
- Slight upward slurring of the
  ascending limb of the S wave

QR, or qR complexes provide a sensitivity of 15% and specificity of 100% (Fig. 5) [1,5]. The St-qR pattern must not be confused with an overshoot of the QRS complex due to overshoot of massive ST elevation creating a diminutive terminal r wave or ventricular fusion (see Fig. 5). Cabrera's sign in *both* leads III and aVF is very specific, but even less sensitive than its counterpart in anterior MI (S.S. Barold, unpublished observations).

Myocardial infarction at other sites

A posterior MI should shift the QRS forces anteriorly and produce a dominant R wave in the right V leads, but the diagnosis cannot be made during RV pacing because of the many causes of a dominant R wave in V_1. An RV MI could conceivably be reflected in V_3R with prominent ST elevation. Klein and colleagues [8] suggested that the diagnosis of RV infarction could be made when there is prominent ST elevation in lead V_4R in the first 24 hours, but such a change should be interpreted cautiously unless it is associated with obvious abnormalities suggestive of an acute inferior MI.

Conflicting views on the diagnosis of myocardial infarction of uncertain age

Kochiadakis and colleagues [9] studied ECG patterns of ventricular pacing in 45 patients with old MI and 26 controls (without angiographic evidence of coronary artery disease) during temporary RV apical at the time of routine cardiac catheterization (Fig. 6). In 15 of the 26 controls, a Q wave was observed in leads I, aVL, or V_6. However, it was not specified whether the Q waves were part of a qR (Qr) or a QS complex (their Fig. 1E shows a QS complex). This differentiation is important because a QS complex carries no diagnostic value during RV pacing in any of the

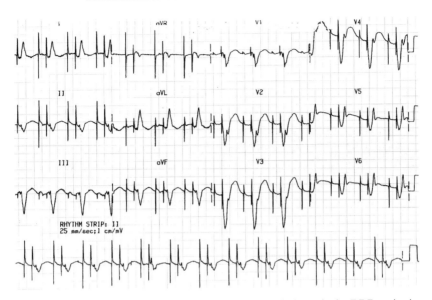

Fig. 1. Twelve-lead ECG showing old anteroseptal myocardial infarction during unipolar DDD pacing in a patient with complete AV block. The ventricular stimulus does not obscure or contribute to the qR pattern in leads I, aVL, and V_6. Leads V_2 to V_4 show Cabrera's sign and a variant in lead V_5. The lack of an underlying rhythm because of complete AV block excluded the presence of ventricular fusion.

standard 12 leads (QS complexes can be normal in leads I, II, III, aVF, V_5, and V_6). A well-positioned lead at the RV apex rarely generates a qR complex in lead I, and in our experience never produces a qR complex in V_5 and V_6 in the absence of an MI. It is also possible that in the study of Kochiadakis and colleagues [9], the pacing catheter in some of the controls might

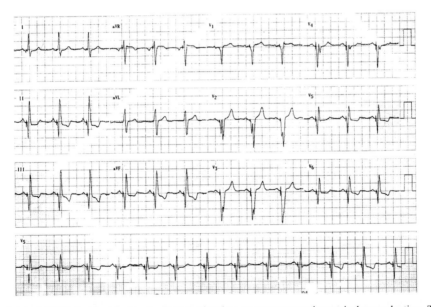

Fig. 2. Twelve-lead ECG showing ventricular fusion related to spontaneous atrioventricular conduction. The pattern simulates myocardial infarction during DDD pacing (atrial sensing-ventricular pacing) in a patient with sick sinus syndrome, relatively normal AV conduction, and no evidence of coronary artery disease. The spontaneous ECG showed a normal QRS pattern. Note the QR complexes in leads II, III, aVF, V_5, and V_6.

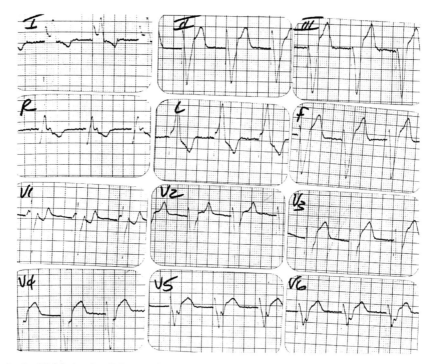

Fig. 3. Twelve-lead ECG showing Cabrera's sign during VVI pacing in a patient with an old extensive anterior myocardial infarction. Note the typical notching of the S wave in leads V_4 to V_6. There is no qR pattern.

Box 3. Cabrera's sign

Specific Cabrera variants
- Small, narrow r wave deforming the terminal QRS.
- Series of tiny notches giving a serrated appearance along the ascending S wave.
- Similar series of late notches on QRS during epicardial pacing.

Notches are probably due to a gross derangement of intraventricular conduction.

False Cabrera's signs
- Slight notching of the ascending S wave in V leads is normal during RV apical pacing. It is usually confined to 1 lead, shows a sharp upward direction on the S wave and usually <0.03 seconds; no shelflike or downward notch typical of true Cabrera's sign.
- Ventricular fusion beats.
- Early retrograde P waves deforming the late part of the QRS complex.

have been slightly displaced away from RV apex and produced qR ventricular complexes in leads I and aVL (but not V_6) with preservation of superior axis deviation in the frontal plane. On this basis, we cannot accept the authors' claim of the poor diagnostic accuracy and specificity of Q waves in the diagnosis of MI.

Furthermore, Kochiadakis and colleagues [9] published an ECG example of Cabrera's sign (their Fig. 1A), but the tracing showed unimpressive slight slurring (with a rapid upward deflection—dv/dt or slope) of the ascending limb of the S wave (see Fig. 6). In our experience, this pattern is commonly seen during uncomplicated RV apical pacing. A true Cabrera's sign is more prominent, with a markedly different dv/dt beyond the notch, making the sign unmistakable as seen in Figs. 1 and 3. We believe that the ECG in their Fig. 1B [4] showing Chapman's sign (notching with minimal slurring of the upstroke of the R wave) is also consistent with uncomplicated RV apical pacing (see Fig. 6).

Another group [7] has claimed that Q waves (qR or Qr complexes were not specified) in leads I, aVL, or V_6 are not diagnostically useful, but their conclusions are also questionable because of problematic methodology: (1) the number

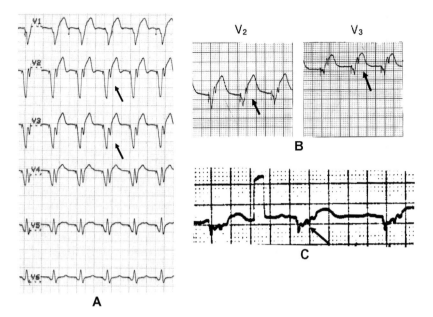

Fig. 4. Cabrera Variants. (*A, B*) There are small and narrow terminal R waves in leads V_2 and V_3, respectively, during ventricular pacing. (*C*) Series of tiny notches representing gross derangement of intraventricular conduction during ventricular pacing in a patient with an extensive anterior myocardial infarction. (*From* Barold SS, Falkoff MD, Ong LS, et al. Normal and abnormal patterns of ventricular depolarization during cardiac pacing. In: Barold SS, editor. Modern cardiac pacing. Mt Kisco [NY]: Futura; 1985; with permission.)

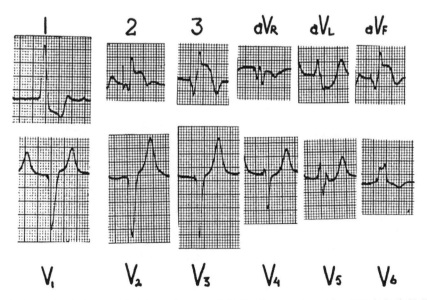

Fig. 5. Ventricular pacing during acute inferior wall myocardial infarction showing a qR pattern in leads II, III, and aVF associated with ST segment elevation. The R wave in the inferior leads is substantial and, therefore, not due to an overshoot of the QRS complex by marked ST-segment elevation. (*Reproduced from* Barold SS, Ong LS, Banner RL. Diagnosis of inferior wall myocardial infarction during right ventricular right apical pacing. Chest 1976;69:232–5; with permission.)

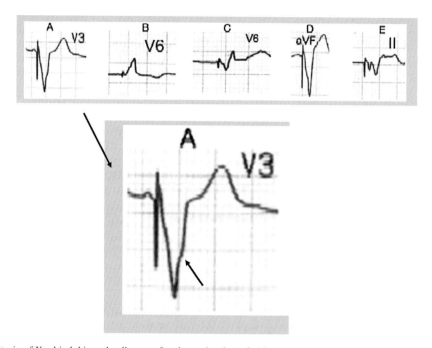

Fig. 6. Criteria of Kochiadakis and colleagues for the evaluation of old myocardial infarction during ventricular pacing [9]. (*A*) Notching 0.04 seconds in duration on the ascending limb of the S wave of leads V_3, V_4, or V_5 (Cabrera's sign). (*A* is shown at the bottom in a magnified form). (*B*) Notching of the upstroke of the R wave in leads I, aVL, or V_6 (Chapman's sign). (*C*) Q waves >0.03 seconds in duration in leads I, aVL, or V_6. (*D*) Notching of the first 0.04 seconds of the QRS complex in leads II, III, and aVF. (*E*) Q wave >0.03 seconds in duration in leads II, III, and aVF. (*From* Kochiadakis GE, Kaleboubas MD, Igoumenidis NE, et al. Electrocardiographic diagnosis of acute myocardial infarction in the presence of ventricular paced rhythm. PACE 2001;24:1289–90; with permission.)

of "abnormal" patients with Q waves only in the two frontal plane leads and not in V_6 was not specified. (2) The protocol called for a LBBB pattern with left axis deviation (more negative than −30 degrees). Normal subjects might have been included in the "abnormal" group because a pacing lead somewhat away from the RV apex can cause left-axis deviation with q waves in I and aVL in the absence of MI.

Based on the above arguments, we believe that the findings of Kachiadakis and colleagues [4] and Kindwall and colleagues [5] are questionable and probably not valid.

Acute myocardial infarction

Leads V_1 to V_3 sometimes show marked ST elevation during ventricular pacing in the absence of myocardial ischemia or infarction [10]. The diagnosis of myocardial ischemia or infarction should therefore be based on the new development of ST elevation. Sgarbossa and colleagues

[11,12] recently reported the value of ST segment abnormalities in the diagnosis of acute MI during ventricular pacing and their high specificity. ST elevation ≥5 mm in predominantly negative QRS complexes is the best marker, with a sensitivity of 53% and specificity of 88%, and was the only criterion of statistical significance in their study (Figs. 7 and 8). Other less important ST changes with high specificity include ST depression = or > 1 mm in V_1, V_2, and V_3 (sensitivity 29%, specificity 82%), and ST elevation ≥1 mm in leads with a concordant QRS polarity. ST depression concordant with the QRS complex may occur in leads V_3 to V_6 during uncomplicated RV pacing [11,12]. Patients who present with discordant ST elevation ≥5 mm have more severe coronary artery disease than other MI patients without such ST elevation [13,14]. Patients with an acute MI, the primary ST changes may persist as the MI becomes old. So-called primary T-wave abnormalities (concordant) are not diagnostically useful during RV pacing if they are not accompanied by primary ST abnormalities (Fig. 9) [11].

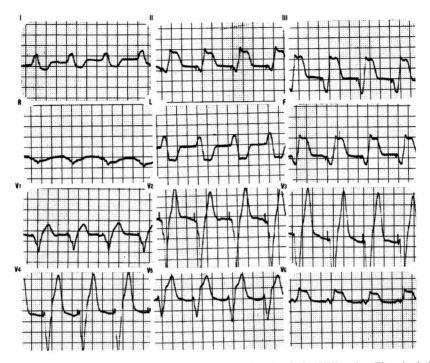

Fig. 7. Twelve-lead ECG showing acute inferolateral myocardial infarction during VVI pacing. There is obvious discordant ST-elevation in leads II, III, aVF, and V$_6$ that meets the criterion of Sgarbossa and colleagues [11] for the diagnosis of acute infarction. (*From* Barold SS, Falkoff MD, Ong LS, et al. Normal and abnormal patterns of ventricular depolarization during cardiac pacing. In: Barold SS, editor. Modern cardiac pacing. Mt Kisco [NY]: Futura; 1985; with permission.)

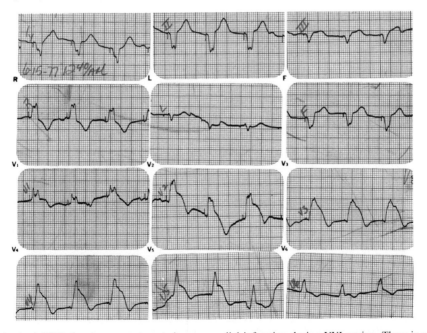

Fig. 8. Twelve-lead ECG showing an acute anterior myocardial infarction during VVI pacing. There is marked ST-elevation in leads V$_1$ to V$_5$ that meets the criterion of Sgarbossa and colleagues [11] for the diagnosis of acute infarction. The ST-elevation drags the QRS complex upwards. Note the right superior frontal plane axis occasionally seen with right ventricular apical pacing.

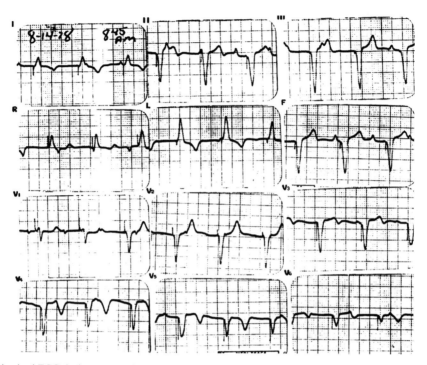

Fig. 9. Twelve-lead ECG during uncomplicated right ventricular apical pacing showing concordant T-wave inversion in leads V_4 to V_6. So-called primary T-wave abnormalities are of no diagnostic value without accompanying ST changes.

Cardiac ischemia

Discordant ST elevation

Marked discordant ST elevation (>5 mm) during ventricular pacing, a recently described sign (with good specificity and moderate sensitivity) for the diagnosis of myocardial infarction [9], could also be used for the diagnosis of severe reversible transmural myocardial ischemia as recently reported in a case of anterior ischemia (Fig. 10) [15]. Two similar cases of ischemia with discordant ST elevation during ventricular pacing have been published [16,17]. Both affected the *inferior* wall. A report in the French literature [17] involved a temporary pacing lead in the RV in a patient who demonstrated transient but massive ST elevation of unspecified duration in the inferior leads during Prinzmetal's angina, possibly superimposed on an inferior infarction of undetermined age. During these ischemic episodes, the ECG documented reversible second-degree type I (Wenckebach) atrioventricular block and reversible type I second-degree exit block from the pacemaker stimulus to the myocardium. The latter probably occurred because the tip of the lead was in direct contact with

the area of severe transmural ischemia. The other case is less impressive because the patient had a unipolar VVI system (unclear degree of overshoot into the ST segment) and exhibited during chest pain of uncertain duration only about 5 mm of additional discordant ST elevation in a Holter recording with an unspecified lead [16]. Transient massive ST elevation (>10 mm) in paced beats and spontaneous beats in lead III was precipitated during an ergonovine-induced spasm of a dominant right coronary artery in the presence of otherwise normal coronary arteries angiographically [16]. In this patient, the associated ST elevation in spontaneously conducted beats diminished the diagnostic value of the changes during pacing.

Discordant ST abnormalities

ST depression in leads V_1 and V_2 is rarely normal, and should be considered abnormal and indicative of anterior or inferior MI or ischemia.

Exercise-induced ST changes

Exercise-induced ST abnormalities are in all likelihood nondiagnostic, as in complete LBBB.

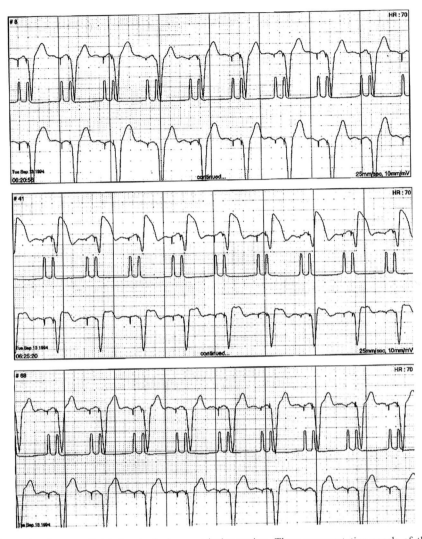

Fig. 10. Diagnosis of myocardial ischemia during ventricular pacing. Three representative panels of three-channel Holter recordings of lead V_1 on top and V_5 at the bottom, together with a special pacemaker channel in the middle displaying the pacemaker stimuli.The top control panel was recorded before chest pain. The second panel shows marked ST-elevation (>5 mm) in V1 and to a lesser degree in V_5. The bottom panel was recorded about 3.5 minutes after the middle panel.The ST-elevation has partially resolved. (*From* Barold SS. Diagnosis of myocardial ischemia during ventricular pacing. Pacing Clin Electrophysiol 2000;23:1060–1; with permission.)

The two cases reported by Diaz and colleagues [18] are questionable on the basis of the criteria of Sgarbossa and colleagues [11,12].

Cardiac memory

Abnormal depolarization causes altered repolarization. Cardiac memory refers to T-wave abnormalities that manifest on resumption of a normal ventricular activation pattern after a period of abnormal ventricular activation, such as ventricular pacing, transient LBBB, ventricular arrhythmias, or Wolf-Parkinson-White syndrome [19–22]. Pacing-induced T-wave inversion is usually localized to precordial and inferior leads. The direction of the T wave of the memory effect in sinus rhythm is typically in the same direction as the QRS complex. In other words, the T wave tracks the QRS vector of the abnormal impulse. Thus, inhibition of a pacemaker may

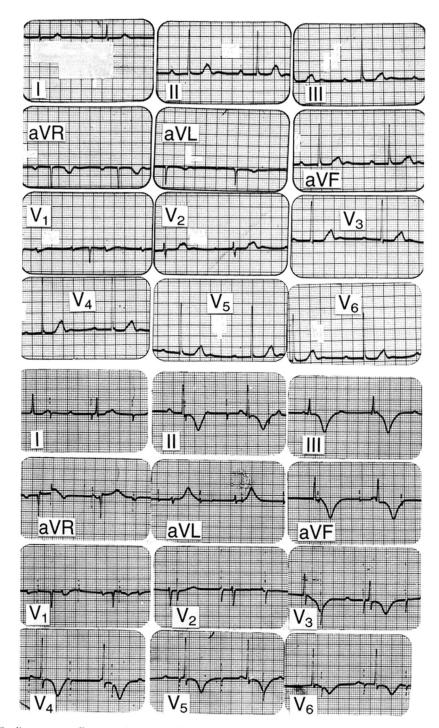

Fig. 11. Cardiac memory effect secondary to ventricular pacing recorded in the ECG of a patient with complete heart block from a lesion in the His bundle (confirmed by His bundle recordings). (Top) The tracing is normal except for the rhythm. (Bottom) Chest wall stimulation was performed to inhibit a VVI pacemaker implanted several months previously. There was no clinical evidence of heart disease apart from AV block. Note the striking T-wave inversions in leads II, III, aVF, and V_3 to V_6. (*From* Barold SS, Falkoff MD, Ong LS, et al. Electrocardiographic diagnosis of myocardial infarction during ventricular pacing. Cardiol Clin 1987;5:403–17; with permission.)

allow the emergence of the spontaneous rhythm with a diagnostic Q wave, but pacing per se may produce prominent repolarization abnormalities that do not represent ischemia, a non-ST elevation, or non-Q wave MI (Fig. 11) [19–22]. It may occur even after 1 minute of RV pacing in humans, with T-wave abnormalities visible after 20 minutes [23]. The marked repolarization abnormalities reach a steady state in a week with RV endocardial pacing at physiologic rates. The repolarization abnormalities related to cardiac memory persist when normal depolarization is restored, and they resolve completely in a month. The changes and their duration are proportional to the amount of delivered ventricular pacing [24]. Cardiac memory is associated with complex biochemical abnormalities. Angiotensin inhibitors and AT-1 receptor blockers attenuate the effects of short-term memory. Calcium blockers reduce the impact of short-term

and long term-memory [25]. Long-term cardiac memory involves de novo protein synthesis [26].

Differentiation of cardiac memory from ischemia

Shvilkin and colleagues [27] recently reported that cardiac memory induced by RV pacing results in a distinctive T-vector pattern that allows discrimination from ischemic precordial T-wave inversions regardless of the coronary artery involved. T-wave axis, polarity, and amplitude on a 12-lead ECG during sinus rhythm were compared between cardiac memory and ischemic patients (Fig. 12). The cardiac memory group included 13 patients who were paced in the DDD mode with a short entricular delay for 1 week after elective pacemaker implantation. The ischemic group consisted of 47 patients with precordial T-wave inversion identified among 228 consecutive patients undergoing percutaneous

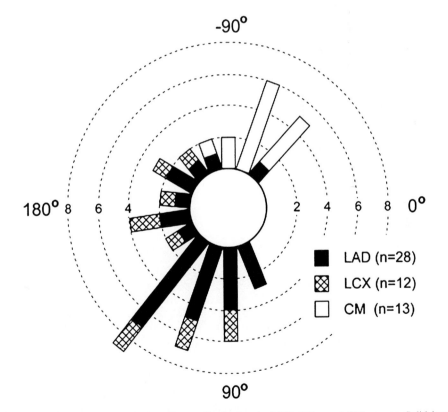

Fig. 12. Circular histogram of frontal plane T-axes distribution in LAD, LCx, and CM groups. Solid bars indicate LAD; hatched bars, LCx; open bars, CM. Difference in T-vector axis between CM and LAD/LCx is statistically significant (*P* < 0.01). (*From* Shvilkin A, Ho KK, Rosen MR, et al. T-vector direction differentiates postpacing from ischemic T-wave inversion in precordial leads. Circulation 2005;111:969–74; with permission.)

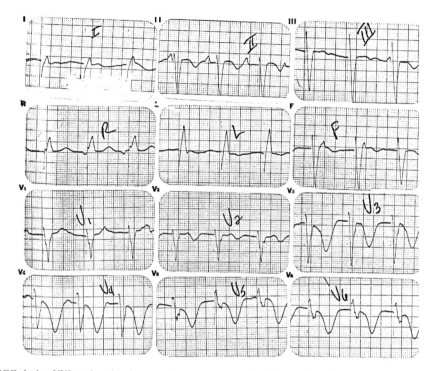

Fig. 13. ECG during VVI pacing showing very deep and symmetrical T-wave inversion in leads V_3 to V_6 in a patient who presented with chest pain. These impressive abnormalities suggest ischemia or infarction and urgent coronary angiography should be considered with a view to performing angioplasty.

coronary intervention for an acute coronary syndrome. The combination of (1) positive T wave in aVL, (2) positive or isoelectric T wave in lead I, and (3) maximal precordial T wave inversion >T-wave inversion in lead III was 92% sensitive and 100% specific for cardiac memory, discriminating it from ischemic precordial T-wave inversion regardless of the coronary artery involved.

Summary

Electrocardiographic criteria involving the paced QRS complex are less sensitive but more specific than primary ST abnormalities for MI diagnosis during ventricular pacing. Although one cannot determine with certainty the age of an MI (hours, days, or even years), from a single ECG, the presence of primary ST-segment abnormalities strongly suggests the diagnosis of acute MI or severe ischemia and need for possible emergency revascularization. Patients with a history of chest pain and a nondiagnostic paced ECG should also be considered for emergency cardiac catheterization with a view to performing

revascularization. A patient with the ECG shown in Fig. 13 should certainly be a candidate for this strategy.

References

[1] Barold SS, Falkoff MD, Ong LS, et al. Electrocardiographic diagnosis of myocardial infarction during ventricular pacing. Cardiol Clin 1987;5:403–17.

[2] Hands ME, Cook EF, Stone PH, et al. Electrocardiographic diagnosis of myocardial infarction in the presence of complete left bundle branch block. Am Heart J 1988;116:23–31.

[3] Castellanos A Jr, Zoble R, Procacci PM, et al. St-qR pattern. New sign of diagnosis of anterior myocardial infarction during right ventricular pacing. Br Heart J 1973;35:1161–5.

[4] Brandt RR, Hammil SC, Higano ST. Electrocardiographic diagnosis of acute myocardial infarction during ventricular pacing. Circulation 1998;97:2274–5.

[5] Kafka W. ECG and VCG diagnosis of infarction in pacemaker dependent patients [abstract]. Pacing Clin Electrophysiol 1985;8:A-16.

[6] Kaul U, Anand IS, Bidwai PS, et al. Diagnosis of myocardial infarction in patients during right ventricular pacing. Indian J Chest Dis Allied Sci 1981;23:68–72.

[7] Kindwall KE, Brown JP, Josephson ME. Predictive accuracy of criteria for chronic myocardial infarction in pacing-induced left bundle branch block. Am J Cardiol 1985;57:1255–60.

[8] Klein HO, Becker B, DiSegni E, et al. The pacing electrogram. How important is the QRS complex configuration? Clin Prog Electrophysiol 1986;4: 112–36.

[9] Kochiadakis GE, Kaleboubas MD, Igoumenidis NE, et al. Electrocardiographic appearance of old myocardial infarction in paced patients. Pacing Clin Electrophysiol 2002;25:1061–5.

[10] Madias JE. The nonspecificity of ST-segment elevation > or = 5.0 mm in V1–V3 in the diagnosis of acute myocardial infarction in the presence of ventricular paced rhythm. J Electrocardiol 2004;37: 135–9.

[11] Sgarbossa EB, Pinski SL, Gates KB, et al, for the Gusto-1 Investigators. Early electrocardiographic diagnosis of acute myocardial infarction in the presence of a ventricular paced rhythm. Am J Cardiol 1996;77:423–4.

[12] Sgarbossa EB. Recent advances in the electrocardiographic diagnosis of myocardial infarction: left bundle branch block and pacing. Pacing Clin Electrophysiol 1996;19:1370–9.

[13] Caldera AE, Bryce M, Kotler M, et al. Angiographic significance of a discordant ST-segment elevation of ≥5 millimeters in patients with ventricular-paced rhythm and acute myocardial infarction. Am J Cardiol 2002;90:1240–3.

[14] Kochiadakis GE, Kaleboubas MD, Igoumenidis NE, et al. Electrocardiographic diagnosis of acute myocardial infarction in the presence of ventricular paced rhythm. Pacing Clin Electrophysiol 2001;24: 1289–90.

[15] Barold SS. Diagnosis of myocardial ischemia during ventricular pacing. Pacing Clin Electrophysiol 2000; 23:1060–1.

[16] Manyari DE, Klein GJ, Kostuk WJ. Electrocardiographic recognition of variant angina during permanent pacing. Pacing Clin Electrophysiol 1983;6:99–103.

[17] Mery D, Dagran O, Bailly E, et al. First and second degree blocks (Wenckebach type) during right ventricular stimulation in the course of Prinzmetal's angina. Arch Mal Coeur Vaiss 1979;72: 385–90.

[18] Diaz CF, Ganim MS, Ellestad MH. Electrocardiographic evidence of ischemia during ventricular paced rhythms. Clin Cardiol 1996;19:520–2.

[19] Chaterjee K, Harris A, Davies G, et al. Electrocardiographic changes subsequent to artificial ventricular depolarization. Br Heart J 1969;31:770–9.

[20] Goldberger JJ, Kadish AH. Cardiac memory. Pacing Clin Electrophysiol 1999;22:1672–9.

[21] Rosen MR. What is cardiac memory? J Cardiovasc Electrophysiol 2000;11:1289–93.

[22] Patberg KW, Shvilkin A, Plotnikov A, et al. Cardiac memory. Mechanisms, and clinical application. Heart Rhythm 2005;2:1376–82.

[23] Goyal R, Syed ZA, Mukhopadhyay PS, et al. Changes in cardiac repolarization following short periods of ventricular pacing. J Cardiovasc Electrophysiol 1998;9:269–80.

[24] Wecke L, Gadler F, Linde C, et al. Temporal characteristics of cardiac memory in humans: vectorcardiographic quantification in a model of cardiac pacing. Heart Rhythm 2005;2:28–34.

[25] Plotnikov AN, Yu H, Geller JC, et al. Role of L-type calcium channels in pacing-induced short-term and long-term cardiac memory in canine heart. Circulation 2003;107:2844–9.

[26] Patberg KW, Obreztchikova MN, Giardina SF, et al. The cAMP response element binding protein modulates expression of the transient outward current: implications for cardiac memory. Cardiovasc Res 2005;68:259–67.

[27] Shvilkin A, Ho KK, Rosen MR, et al. T-vector direction differentiates postpacing from ischemic T-wave inversion in precordial leads. Circulation 2005;111:969–74.

ELSEVIER
SAUNDERS

Cardiol Clin 24 (2006) 401–411

CARDIOLOGY
CLINICS

Is Electrocardiography Still Useful in the Diagnosis of Cardiac Chamber Hypertrophy and Dilatation?

Peter W. Macfarlane, DSc, FESC, FRCP[a,b]

[a]Division of Cardiovascular and Medical Sciences, University of Glasgow, Glasgow G12 8QQ, Scotland, UK
[b]Royal Infirmary, 10 Alexandra Parade, Glasgow G31 2ER, Scotland, UK

With the ubiquitous availability of the echocardiograph, it is nowadays the case that a hospital physician will seek to obtain an echocardiogram for detailed information on ventricular function when appropriate and in so doing obtain information on the presence or absence of cardiac chamber hypertrophy or enlargement. In addition, family practitioners are more easily able to refer patients to a local hospital or cardiology practice for an echocardiogram, although steps are having to be taken, at least in the United Kingdom, to minimize unnecessary referrals, particularly in patients who have suspected heart failure, by first assessing the ECG and measuring B-type natriuretic peptide (BNP). In other health care systems, it is possible that patients may be referred directly to a cardiologist for echocardiographic investigation as required.

Notwithstanding, an ECG is always part of a cardiologic work-up, and the question posed is whether there is still value in reviewing the ECG for evidence of changes related to chamber enlargement when an echocardiogram can be obtained if required.

Atrial enlargement

The P wave of the ECG is one of the smallest components of the ECG waveform. For this reason, accurate measurement is difficult, and many criteria for P-wave abnormality are nonspecific as a result. It is generally accepted that right atrial depolarization contributes to the initial part of the P wave, whereas left atrial depolarization is responsible for the terminal P-wave appearances. Thus, if there is any form of right atrial abnormality, the P- wave duration should not be increased, and the initial component of the P wave may be increased in amplitude. On the other hand, if there is a left atrial abnormality, the duration of the P wave may be lengthened, and in some leads there will be a more obvious division of the P wave into two components. Fig. 1 shows in schematic form how these different changes may appear in lead II and lead V1 of the 12-lead ECG.

There is some dispute over the terminology to be used in cases of atrial abnormality. Left atrial enlargement is said to arise from atrial dilatation or pressure overload [1] or indeed from abnormal intra-atrial conduction [2]. Thus, a term such as "left atrial abnormality" can be used to cover different forms of atrial pathology.

Waggoner and colleagues [3] reviewed ECG criteria for left atrial enlargement and compared findings against two-dimensional echocardiograph measures. They found that of 39 patients who had false-positive ECG diagnoses of left atrial abnormality according to echocardiograph criteria, only 2 (5%) were free of organic heart disease. Thus, their conclusion was that the ECG detected left atrial abnormality rather than left atrial enlargement. Waggoner and colleagues [3] had used criteria such as P duration in lead II of 120 milliseconds or longer, (negative P duration in V1)/(PR segment duration) of 1.0 or longer, and the P terminal force in V1 greater than 3 mVms. The second of these criteria is a form of modified Macruz index, defined as P duration/PR segment (ie, end P to QRS onset) [4]. P terminal force in V1 is defined as the duration

E-mail address: peter.w.macfarlane@clinmed.gla.ac.uk

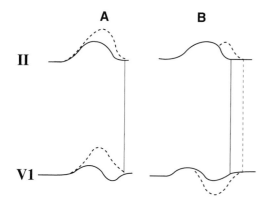

Fig. 1. Atrial abnormalities. (*A*) If there is right atrial enlargement, then the initial component of the P wave is enlarged. (*B*) If there is left atrial enlargement, there may be P-wave widening with an M-shaped P wave in lead II and an increased P terminal force in V1.

of the negative (terminal) component of the P wave times the amplitude of this component referred to baseline.

P mitrale is defined as an M-shaped P wave in lead II with an increased P duration (Fig. 1). The name suggests that this abnormality is found in mitral valve disease, which is sometimes the case, but this type of P wave also can be found in patients who have constrictive pericarditis or when there is an intra-atrial conduction defect.

In a study of 53 patients who had uncomplicated essential hypertension [5], ECG criteria of left atrial abnormality such as P duration greater than 0.12 milliseconds, P amplitude greater than 0.25 mV in lead II, Macruz index greater than 1.6 in lead II, and P terminal force in V1 of −4 mVms or less were assessed. (P terminal force more negative than −4 mVms where the P terminal amplitude is expressed as a negative value.) Echocardiograph measurements of left atrial dimensions were obtained together with Doppler estimates of left ventricular (LV) filling. The Macruz index had a sensitivity of 58.5% in detecting left atrial abnormality and was the best of the ECG measures. The authors concluded that ECG signs of left atrial abnormality were related more to an increased atrial workload, possibly secondary to impaired ventricular filling, than to left atrial enlargement [5].

Right atrial abnormality

Right atrial abnormality is not commonly reported on an ECG. It can manifest as a tall P wave in V1 with the P amplitude being greater

than an age-dependent value around 0.2 mV. It may be found in patients who have congenital heart disease, pulmonary hypertension, or obstructive airways disease.

Classically, a patient who has chronic obstructive airways disease may have so-called "P pulmonale" characterized by a tall, peaked P wave of at least 0.25-mV amplitude in lead II. There have been few studies in patients who have this abnormality, and most ECG criteria for right atrial abnormality are nonspecific and somewhat insensitive [6–8].

On occasions peaked P waves may be found in inferior leads in the absence of any demonstrable right atrial enlargement or dilatation, and in this case the term "pseudo P pulmonale" is used. It has been suggested that if left-sided heart disease is present, such an ECG finding might reflect an increase in left atrial dimensions [9].

Kaplan and colleagues [10] evaluated ECG criteria for right atrial enlargement against two-dimensional echocardiograms in 100 patients who had right atrial enlargement according to echocardiography and in 25 control patients. The most powerful predictors of right atrial enlargement were QRS axis greater than 90°, P amplitude in V2 greater than 0.15 mV, and R/S greater than 1 in V1 in the absence of complete right bundle-branch block (RBBB). The combined sensitivity of these criteria was 49% with 100% specificity. On the other hand, classic criteria for P pulmonale were only 6% sensitive.

Bi-atrial enlargement

Occasionally an ECG may show P-wave abnormalities suggestive of both right and left atrial enlargement, and in this case the term "bi-atrial enlargement" may be used. Thus, criteria for bi-atrial enlargement are essentially a combination of those for right and left atrial enlargement.

Use of the signal-averaged ECG

In the last decade, there has been interest in using the signal-averaged ECG to measure P-wave duration and in using this parameter as an indicator of atrial enlargement and even as a prognostic index for the development of atrial fibrillation. Dixen and colleagues [11] showed that the signal-averaged P-wave duration was significantly correlated with the left atrial diameter in 74 patients in whom a signal-averaged ECG and echocardiogram had been recorded. The left atrial volume, the right atrial volume, and in particular the total atrial volume were more strongly correlated to the signal-averaged P-wave duration, however.

On the other hand, Merckx and colleagues [12] looked at correlations between the P-wave duration on the signal-averaged ECG and estimates of atrial activation time derived from Doppler tissue imaging. They showed that there was a significant correlation between the signal-averaged ECG P-wave duration and atrial activation times determined from the Doppler method, which was much quicker to use than a signal-averaged ECG when an echocardiogram was being recorded in any event. Approximately 1 additional minute was required. The conclusion was that this echocardiographic estimate of atrial activation time could be useful in detecting those patients prone to develop atrial fibrillation.

In an interesting study using fractal measures, Peters [13] showed that course F waves in patients who had atrial fibrillation seemed to be more related to a larger left atrial size (≥ 4.6 cm) than were smaller fibrillatory waves.

Atrial abnormalities—conclusion

There are few areas where the ECG holds any advantage over an echocardiogram in elucidating atrial enlargement. Widened P waves as found in intra-atrial conduction defects may, however, be the only way of determining that there is some form of atrial abnormality. Furthermore, the signal-averaged ECG may be of some prognostic value in predicting those patients at increased risk of developing atrial fibrillation when an echocardiogram is not available.

Left ventricular enlargement

No ECG criteria have ever successfully separated the different forms of LV abnormality (ie, LV hypertrophy [LVH] caused by an increase in muscle thickness or LV dilatation with increased LV cavity volume). Huwez and colleagues [14] introduced a new classification of LV geometry using M mode ECG. This classification was based on the use of an indexed LV mass greater than 131 g/m^2 in men and 108 g/m^2 in women together with a knowledge of indexed LV volume, which was regarded as abnormal if it exceeded 90 mL/m^2. This classification led to four groupings based on normal or abnormal indexed LV mass and normal or abnormal indexed LV volume. Table 1 shows the classifications. Extensive investigation of ECG

Table 1
Classification of left ventricular enlargement

Left Ventricular Volume[a]	Left Ventricular Mass[b]	
	Normal	Abnormal
Normal	Normal	Concentric left ventricular hypertrophy
Abnormal	Isolated left ventricular volume overload	Eccentric left ventricular hypertrophy

[a] Abnormal left ventricular volume is defined as volume greater than 90 mL/m^2.

[b] Abnormal left ventricular mass is defined as mass greater than 131 g/m^2 in men and mass greater than 108 g/m^2 in women where indexing is with respect to body surface area.

From Huwez FU, Pringle SD, Macfarlane PW. A new classification of left ventricular geometry in patients with cardiac disease based on M-mode echocardiography. Am J Cardiol 1992;70:687.

appearances in a group of 202 cardiac patients failed to elicit any ECG criteria that could separate the different types of LV geometry, however [15].

Echocardiography itself is not without its difficulties in estimating LV mass. On the other hand, Rautaharju and colleagues [16] introduced several equations for the calculation of LV mass from the ECG. One set of equations for white men and women is as follows:

$$\text{LV mass (men)} = 0.026 \times \text{CV} + 1.25 \times \text{W} + 34.4$$

$$\text{LV mass (women)} = 0.020 \times \text{CV} + 1.12 \times \text{W} + 36.2$$

where LV mass equals LV mass in grams, CV equals Cornell voltage (RaVL + SV$_3$) in microvolts [17], and W equals weight in kilograms. By using these equations, Padmanabhan and colleagues [18] have shown that there are significant heritable effects for ECG measures used in LV mass estimation.

Influence of constitutional variables on ECG criteria for left ventricular hypertrophy

Age and sex

It has been known for many years that normal ECG voltages vary both with age and sex (eg, see

[19]). Voltages are highest in adolescence, particularly in males, and decrease with increasing age, with a leveling beyond approximately 50 years of age. A similar trend can be seen for women, although this is less marked. Significant differences in upper limits of normal QRS voltages exist between men and women of similar age, as can be seen in Fig. 2. These differences mean that any criteria for ECG LVH and ECG right ventricular hypertrophy (RVH) should be age and sex dependent and explains why some ECG criteria for ventricular hypertrophy that are not age and sex adjusted perform in a suboptimal way.

QRS duration is approximately 7 milliseconds longer in women than in men, but criteria that use QRS widening as an index of LVH generally fail to acknowledge this simple observation [19]. A fuller discussion of normal limits of ECG measures can be found elsewhere [19].

Other factors

Other factors that may affect voltage include race. Blacks tend to have higher precordial voltages than whites [20], and in turn it has been shown that Chinese individuals have lower voltages than whites [21–23] and hence also lower

voltages than blacks. Furthermore, increasing body mass index is inversely linked with precordial voltage, resulting in lower sensitivity and higher specificity of precordial voltage criteria for LVH in overweight individuals [24].

Selected criteria for left ventricular hypertrophy

Sokolow and Lyon index

Perhaps the best known of all ECG criteria for LVH is that of Sokolow and Lyon introduced in 1949 [25]. These authors actually listed four criteria, but the most commonly used amplitude criterion is SV1 plus maximum (RV5, RV6) of 3.5 mV or greater. It will be seen that this simple criterion is neither age nor sex dependent and probably has remained in use because the majority of patients in whom LVH is likely to be found are over 50 years of age. It therefore is a very nonspecific criterion in younger individuals, particularly men. More recently, Alfakih and colleagues [26] suggested new thresholds of 3.8 mV for men and 3.4 mV for women for reporting LVH, giving a combined sensitivity of 20.3% at 95% specificity. In the same study, the Cornell product (as discussed later) was 24.5% sensitive at the same specificity of 95%. The author and colleagues' data [27] suggest that in persons older than 50 years the upper limit of normal should be 4.6 mV for men and 3.6 mV for women. Clearly, application of such thresholds would reduce sensitivity even further. Interestingly, the same data indicate that SV1 plus RV5 always has a higher mean value in men and women than SV1 plus RV6 (ie, for all age ranges and both sexes). This could explain why the Sokolow and Lyon criterion is often reduced to SV1 + RV5 ≥ 3.5 mV.

Cornell index

Two sets of criteria for LVH were published by the group at Cornell University [17,28]. The second of these, published in 1987, provided a simpler set of criteria, as follows:

RaVL + SV3 > 2.8 mV in men

RaVL + SV3 > 2.0 mV in women

The Cornell group then introduced a voltage times duration product known as the Cornell product. In this case, the Cornell voltage was multiplied by the overall QRS duration, and this product showed improved accuracy in reporting LVH [29,30]. Of particular importance is the fact

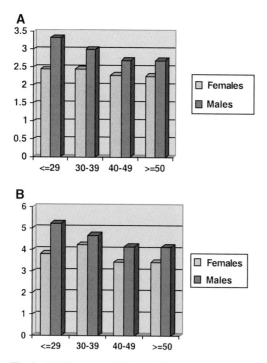

Fig. 2. (*A*) The mean of SV1 + RV5 in 725 male and 585 female adult healthy volunteers. (*B*) The upper normal limits in the same data set.

that these ECG criteria can follow changes in echocardiographic LV mass [31] and accurately assess prognosis [32]. The opportunity to use this more readily available index to track LV mass may reduce the need for repeat echocardiograms. Note that in the Losartan Intervention for Endpoint (LIFE) reduction in hypertension study, the actual criteria used were adjusted on the basis of recruitment experience to use a differential of 600 μV (rather than 800 μV, as given previously) between men and women; that is, in women 600 μV was added to RaVL plus SV3 before deriving the Cornell product. The threshold for abnormality was set at 244 mVms [32].

Secondary ST-T changes and left ventricular hypertrophy

Although it is possible to diagnose LVH on the basis of QRS changes only, as is evident from the foregoing criteria, one particularly important aspect of the ECG in assessing LVH is the presence of so-called "secondary ST-T wave changes," which have a classic morphology as shown in Fig. 3. Patients who have such abnormalities caused by LVH have been shown to have a lengthened time interval from minimum cavity dimension to mitral valve opening and a reduced rate of early diastolic wall thinning and dimension increase [33]. The importance of these ECG changes is that they are well known to affect prognosis adversely [34–36]. In fact, these changes can add significantly to the Cornell product as well as to the Sokolow and Lyon voltage for the prediction of cardiovascular mortality and

myocardial infarction in hypertensive patients [36]. Furthermore, ST depression itself in V5 and V6 has been shown to be a strong independent predictor of LVH and increased LV mass [37]. In short, the presence of secondary ST-T changes on the ECG is an independent predictor of a poorer prognosis than might exist in the absence of such a finding and shows that the ECG can provide information that is complementary to the echocardiogram.

In many hypertensive patients who have secondary ST-T changes, coronary artery disease is present. Pringle and colleagues [38] in a study involving 23 such patients, 20 of whom had concentric LVH, found that 8 (40%) had significant coronary artery disease at cardiac catheterization. This finding suggests that secondary ST-T changes in ECGs from hypertensive patients need to be interpreted as caused by hypertrophy with or without myocardial ischemia.

Composite criteria for left ventricular hypertrophy

Romhilt Estes criteria

The fact that ST-T changes are additive to voltage criteria was recognized many years ago by Romhilt and Estes [39] who introduced a point scoring system for the ECG diagnosis of LVH. Their criteria, although difficult to apply manually, can be used by computer programs, which can also adapt voltage criteria for age and sex. Table 2 shows in summary form the main criteria used in this point score system. The Romhilt Estes criteria also make use of the frontal plane QRS axis, QRS duration, and intrinsicoid deflection

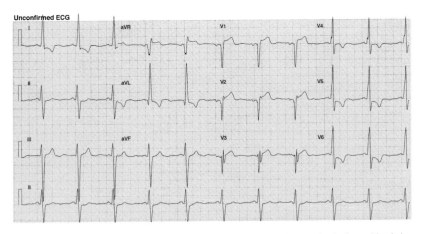

Fig. 3. An ECG showing the typical features of LVH with secondary ST-T changes in the lateral leads in an 87-year-old woman. Note the broad, deep, inverted terminal portion of the P wave in V1, left axis deviation, the very high Cornell voltage, and the typical secondary ST-T changes, particularly in I and aVL. The QS in V2 may be caused by the LVH.

Table 2
Romhilt-Estes point score system for ECG diagnosis of
left ventricular hypertrophy*

Criteria	Points
Any limb-lead R or S $\geq$ 2.0 mV	3
or SV_1 or SV_2 $\geq$ 3.0 mV	
or RV_5 or RV_6 $\geq$ 3.0 mV	
ST-T is typical of LVH[a]	
no digitalis	3
with digitalis	1
Left atrial involvement	3
P terminal force V1 > 4 mVms	
LAD $\geq$ 30°	2
QRS duration $\geq$ 90 ms	1
Intrinsicoid deflection V_5 or V_6 $\geq$ 50 ms	1

* Five points indicates definite left ventricular hypertrophy; 4 points indicates probable left ventricular
hypertrophy.
[a] ST-T configuration as in leads I, aVL of Fig. 3.

in V5 or V6 measured as the time from QRS onset
to the peak of the R wave.

Voltage- and interval-based criteria

More recently Salles and colleagues [40]
showed that a combination of QT-interval prolongation and Cornell product resulted in increased
detection of LVH in patients who had resistant
hypertension. A prolonged QTc interval greater
than 440 milliseconds or prolonged QT dispersion
greater than 60 milliseconds together with a Cornell product greater than 240 mVms was associated with a 5.3- to 9.3-fold higher chance of
having LVH compared with individuals who did
not have increased QTc or Cornell product.

*Effect of echocardiographic criteria for increased
left ventricular mass on ECG criteria*

Selection of echocardiographic criteria for increased LV mass used as the reference standard
can undoubtedly influence the sensitivity of ECG
criteria for LVH. Cuspidi and colleagues [41]
showed in 100 untreated hypertensive patients
that the sensitivity of ECG criteria ranged from
9% to 25% depending on whether the LV mass
index was 126 g/m^2 in men and 105 g/m^2 in
women or 125 g/m^2 in both men and women.
ECG LVH was based on either the Sokolow and
Lyon or the Cornell index being present. The first
criterion for increased echocardiographic LV
mass was indexed by height alone, whereas the
second was indexed by body surface area. Surprisingly, the higher sensitivity was obtained in a criterion that was not sex dependent.

*Bundle-branch block and left ventricular
hypertrophy*

An accurate diagnosis of LVH or LV mass in
patients who have left bundle-branch block
(LBBB) is essentially impossible. On the other
hand, in a large series of over 1400 hearts examined
at post mortem, Havelda and colleagues [42] noted
that 93% of 70 hearts with ECG LBBB had LVH.
Thus, the presence of LBBB itself in many ways is
indicative of the presence of LVH with high specificity. In the presence RBBB, some ECG criteria
for LVH can still be applied, notably those involving left atrial abnormality [43,44].

Regression

Regression of LVH in patients receiving antihypertensive therapy has been detected by assessing the Cornell product after 1 year of treatment.
Those patients in whom the Cornell product
reduced in value had a higher probability of
regression of echocardiographic LVH independent of changes in the systolic and diastolic blood
pressure [31]. Thus, the ECG can indeed also be
used to monitor LVH underlining the value of
a baseline ECG in patients with newly diagnosed
hypertension.

Prognosis of ECG left ventricular hypertrophy

More recent data on the prognostic value of
the ECG have come from the LIFE study [36] in
which the presence of secondary ST-T changes
was associated with a 1.5-fold increase in risk of
myocardial infarction or cardiovascular death
over a 5-year follow-up period. Conversely, Levy
and colleagues [45] found that a reduction in Cornell voltage was linked with a lower risk of cardiovascular disease.

In the Heart Outcomes Prevention Evaluation
Study [46], the combined endpoint of either regression of ECG LVH or prevention of progression by Sokolow Lyon voltage criteria following
ramipril-based therapy was associated with a reduced risk of myocardial infarction, stroke, congestive heart failure, and death.

In a study of 19,434 veterans, composite
criteria were shown to be better predictors of
cardiovascular mortality than voltage-only criteria [47]. In particular, a Romhilt Estes score of 5
or greater had a hazard ratio of 3.7 (95% confidence interval, 3.0–4.4) after adjustment for age,
body mass index, and heart rate. This hazard ra-
tion compares with hazard ratios of 3.1 and 2.7
for Cornell voltage and product respectively.

ECG in heart failure

Heart failure is regarded as unlikely to be present in the absence of dyspnea and an abnormal ECG or chest radiograph [48]. The ECG has a high sensitivity (94%) when used in the diagnosis of heart failure but a low specificity (61%); it has, however, an excellent negative predictive value (98%) [49]. On the other hand, when a measurement of plasma BNP or NTproBNP is available, a simple classification of the ECG into normal and abnormal was found to be of little value [50]. Future studies may clarify the role of the ECG in avoiding unnecessary referrals for echocardiography.

Left ventricular hypertrophy—conclusion

Although clearly the echocardiogram gives information on LV volume, wall thickness, and LV function in particular, there is still much of value that can be gained from the ECG in the evaluation of LVH. The simplicity of the approach to recording the ECG, particularly in clinical trials where patients can be followed for several years, leads to the use of ECG abnormalities as markers of risk. Indeed, in the Framingham study, increased QRS voltage together with ST-T abnormalities conferred a risk similar to that of a previous myocardial infarction [51]. In many situations where a simple approach to treatment is required, such as in essential hypertension, a baseline ECG is of value in monitoring the patient's condition at least on an annual basis. Such an investigation can be undertaken in the community, thereby avoiding an unnecessary visit to hospital for an echocardiogram recording.

Right ventricular hypertrophy

The ECG is notoriously inadequate in detecting right ventricular enlargement or hypertrophy. In an early study of Flowers and Horan [52], it was shown that criteria using V1 were very specific in detecting RVH, at 90%, but were insensitive (2%–18%).

The vectorcardiogram is rarely used these days, but Chou and Helm [53] described three types of RVH patterns. Essentially these patterns broadly translate to the 12-lead ECG as follows:

Type A: Tall R in V1, prominent S in V6 (counterclockwise inscription of the transverse QRS loop)

Type B: R/S greater than 1 in V1 with R greater than 0.5 mV (clockwise inscription of the transverse plane QRS loop)

Type C: Prominent S in V5 and V6 with R/S less than 1 in V5 (clockwise inscription of the transverse plane QRS loop)

The first of these criteria essentially relates to severe RVH, as in pulmonary stenosis. The second may be associated with rheumatic heart disease. On the other hand, type C is more linked with chronic obstructive pulmonary disease and sometimes mitral stenosis.

Secondary ST-T changes and right ventricular hypertrophy

In a fashion similar to LVH, secondary ST-T changes caused by right ventricular enlargement may be encountered. A similar pattern of ST depression with asymmetric T wave inversion is typical in V1 and V2 (Fig. 4). This pattern is encountered most frequently in patients who have congenital heart disease.

Other factors

An increased R/S ratio in V1 can sometimes be caused by posterior myocardial infarction. In such a case, the R-wave duration in V1 generally exceeds 40 milliseconds, and the T wave is upright. In the presence of inferoposterior myocardial infarction or even lateral myocardial infarction, an increased R/S in V1 should not be misinterpreted as being caused by RVH.

Right bundle-branch block and right ventricular hypertrophy

The presence of RBBB in general terms makes it difficult to report RVH. The combination of known RVH with RBBB is most often seen in congenital heart disease, but a tall R in V1 and V2 in patients who have RBBB is indeed nonspecific for RVH.

Right ventricular hypertrophy—conclusion

The ECG criteria for RVH are so poor that an echocardiogram normally will be more valuable than an ECG in patients who have congenital heart disease or pulmonary disease. In pulmonary embolism, however, the right ventricular volume may increase, leading to ECG changes, such as T-wave inversion in V1 to V3, which are more readily followed on the ECG.

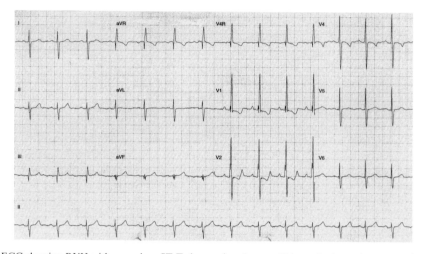

Fig. 4. An ECG showing RVH with secondary ST-T changes in a 3-year-old boy who has pulmonary valvular stenosis. Note that V4R is used to the exclusion of V3. The upright P waves in V1 and V2 have an abnormally high amplitude for age, as do the R waves in V1 and V2. T-wave inversion may be normal in V4R–V4 in infants and children, but the ST depression and overall ST-T configuration in this illustration is that of a secondary ST-T change.

Biventricular hypertrophy

In general terms, criteria for biventricular hypertrophy essentially are a combination of the individual criteria for LVH or RVH. There have been a number of studies linking ECGs with anatomic biventricular hypertrophy as determined at post mortem. The best of these showed a sensitivity of 20%, although the specificity was high at 94% [6].

Athlete's heart

With the increased advocacy of participation in sport, there has been an increase in the number of deaths associated with a variety of athletic activities. In one recent half-marathon in the northeast of England (The Great North East Run, September, 2005), four men died as a result of participating. It would seem to be prohibitive to consider undertaking an echocardiogram in all asymptomatic younger individuals with a view to detecting cardiomyopathy unless they are likely to be serious athletes. Data from Italy indicate one sudden death per year in 100,000 individuals aged 12 to 35 years in the general population, with an increase to 2.3 sudden deaths per 100,000 in those who participated in sporting activities [54]. Under these circumstances, an ECG or an echocardiogram is not likely to be cost effective in terms of the yield of abnormalities detected. The matter of screening young athletes is topical and controversial [55]. Some athletes may have

arrhythmogenic right ventricular dysplasia. This condition may rarely manifest as an epsilon wave on the ECG; additional criteria relating to differences in the sum of QRS durations in V1 + V2 + V3 versus V4 + V5 + V6 have been suggested as being of value [56]. An MRI is more informative in skilled hands, however. On the other hand, when individuals are known to have heart disease, guidelines for advising patients wishing to take part in competitive sport have recently been issued [57,58].

Summary

The echocardiogram undoubtedly is part of the cardiologist's armamentarium in the diagnosis and elucidation of cardiac abnormalities. The numbers of echocardiograms recorded annually are almost certainly increasing in every hospital and private practice, but the ECG still continues to be the most frequently recorded noninvasive test in medicine. Except in extreme cases, the ECG can almost always be recorded, whereas it is generally accepted that the echocardiogram may be unsatisfactory in an admittedly diminishingly small percentage of individuals referred. For many patients, particularly those who have newly diagnosed hypertension, a 12-lead ECG recording may be the only test that is required as a baseline measure. For those who have possible heart failure, an ECG and BNP measurement may be sufficient to obviate the need for an echocardiogram. On the other hand, there is no point in denying that an echocardiogram is recorded as part of the routine investigation of many patients, including those who have had a recent myocardial infarction, which may of course in the first place have been diagnosed by an ECG! Thus the two techniques will continue to live side-by-side for the foreseeable future.

Acknowledgments

The author wishes to thank Dr. David P Macfarlane, of Glasgow Royal Infirmary, and Dr. Peter Okin, of Cornell University, New York, who provided many relevant references of interest.

References

[1] Josephson ME, Kastor JA, Morganroth J. Electrocardiographic left atrial enlargement. Electrophysiologic, echocardiographic and hemodynamic correlates. Am J Cardiol 1977;39:967–71.

[2] Chandraratna PAN, Langevin E. On the significance of an abnormal P-terminal force in lead VI. Am Heart J 1978;95:267–8.

[3] Waggoner AD, Adyanthaya AV, Quinones MA, et al. Left atrial enlargement. Echocardiographic assessment of electrocardiographic criteria. Circulation 1976;54:553–7.

[4] Macruz R, Perloff JK, Case RH. A method for the electrocardiographic recognition of atrial enlargement. Circulation 1958;17:882–9.

[5] Genovesi-Ebert A, Marabotti C, Palombo C, et al. Electrocardiographic signs of atrial overload in hypertensive patients: indexes of abnormality of atrial morphology or function. Am Heart J 1991;121:1113–8.

[6] Murphy ML, Thenabadu PN, de Soyza N, et al. Reevaluation of electrocardiographic criteria for left, right and combined cardiac ventricular hypertrophy. Am J Cardiol 1984;53:1140–7.

[7] Cacho A, Prakash R, Sarma R, et al. Usefulness of two-dimensional echocardiography in diagnosing right ventricular hypertrophy. Chest 1983;84:1547.

[8] Kushner FG, Lam W, Morganroth J. Apex sector echocardiography in evaluation of the right atrium in patients with mitral stenosis and atrial septal defect. Am J Cardiol 1978;42:7337.

[9] Chou T-C, Helm RA. The pseudo P pulmonale. Circulation 1965;32:96–105.

[10] Kaplan JD, Evans GT Jr, Foster E, et al. Evaluation of electrocardiographic criteria for right atrial enlargement by quantitative two-dimensional echocardiography. J Am Coll Cardiol 1994;23:747–52.

[11] Dixen U, Joens C, Rasmussen BV, et al. Signal-averaged P wave duration and the dimensions of the atria. Ann Noninvasive Electrocardiol 2004;9:309–15.

[12] Merckx KL, De Vos CB, Palmans A, et al. Atrial activation time determined by transthoracic Doppler tissue imaging can be used as an estimate of the total duration of atrial electrical activation. The Journal of the American Society of Echocardiography 2005;18:940–4.

[13] Peters RM. The fractal dimension of atrial fibrillation: a new method to predict left atrial dimension from the surface electrocardiogram. Cardiology 1999;92:17–20.

[14] Huwez FU, Pringle SD, Macfarlane PW. A new classification of left ventricular geometry in patients with cardiac disease based on M-mode echocardiography. Am J Cardiol 1992;70:681–8.

[15] Huwez FU. Electrocardiography of the left ventricle in coronary artery disease and hypertrophy [Ph D thesis]. Glasgow (Scotland): University of Glasgow; 1990.

[16] Rautaharju PM, Parks LP, Gottdiener JS, et al. Race- and sex-specific ECG models for left ventricular mass in older populations. Factors influencing overestimation of left ventricular hypertrophy prevalence by ECG criteria in African-Americans. J Electrocardiol 2000;33:205–18.

[17] Casale PN, Devereux RB, Alonso DR, et al. Improved sex specific criteria of left ventricular hypertrophy for clinical and computer interpretation of electrocardiograms: validation with autopsy findings. Circulation 1987;75:565–72.

[18] Padmanabhan S, Connell JMC, Dominiczak AF, et al. Heritability and genetic determinants of electrocardiographic measures of left ventricular mass—a two generation family study. J Hypertens 2004;22:S180–1.

[19] Macfarlane PW, Lawrie TDV. The normal electrocardiogram and vectorcardiogram. In: Macfarlane PW, Lawrie TDV, editors. Comprehensive electrocardiology. Oxford (UK): Pergamon Press; 1989. p. 407–57.

[20] Rautaharju PM, Zhou SH, Calhoun HP. Ethnic differences in ECG amplitudes North American white, black and Hispanic men and women. J Electrocardiol 2004;27(Suppl):20–31.

[21] Chen CY, Chiang B, Macfarlane PW. Normal limits of the electrocardiogram in a Chinese population. J Electrocardiol 1989;22:1–15.

[22] Yang T-F, Macfarlane PW. Comparison of the derived vectorcardiogram in apparently healthy whites and Chinese. Chest 1994;106:1014–20.

[23] Wu J, Kors JA, Rijnbeek PR, et al. Normal limits of the electrocardiogram in Chinese subjects. Int J Cardiol 2003;87:37–51.

[24] Okin PM, Roman MJ, Devereux RB, et al. Electrocardiographic identification of left ventricular hypertrophy: test performance in relation to definition of hypertrophy and presence of obesity. J Am Coll Cardiol 1996;27:124–31.

[25] Sokolow M, Lyon T. The ventricular complex in left ventricular hypertrophy as obtained by unipolar precordial and limb leads. Am Heart J 1949;37:161–86.

[26] Alfakih K, Walters K, Jones T, et al. New gender-specific partition values for ECG criteria of left

ventricular hypertrophy. Recalibration against cardiac MRI. Hypertension 2004;44:175–9.

[27] Macfarlane PW, Lawrie TDV, editors. Comprehensive electrocardiology, vol. 3. Oxford (UK): Pergamon Press; 1989.

[28] Casale PN, Devereux RB, Kligfield P, et al. Electrocardiographic detection of left ventricular hypertrophy: development and prospective validation of improved criteria. J Am Coll Cardiol 1985;6:572–80.

[29] Molloy TJ, Okin PM, Devereux RB, et al. Electrocardiographic detection of left ventricular hypertrophy by the simple QRS voltage-duration product. J Am Coll Cardiol 1992;20:1180–6.

[30] Okin PM, Roman MJ, Devereux RB, et al. Electrocardiographic identification of increased left ventricular mass by simple voltage-duration products. J Am Coll Cardiol 1995;25:417–23.

[31] Okin PM, Devereux RB, Liu JE, et al. Regression of electrocardiographic left ventricular hypertrophy predicts regression of echocardiographic left ventricular mass: The LIFE Study. J Human Hypertens 2004;18:403–9.

[32] Okin PM, Devereux RB, Jern S, et al. Regression of electrocardiographic left ventricular hypertrophy during antihypertensive treatment and prediction of major cardiovascular events: The LIFE Study. JAMA 2004;292:2343–9.

[33] Moore RB, Shapiro LM, Gibson DG. Relation between electrocardiographic repolarisation changes and mechanical events in left ventricular hypertrophy. Br Heart J 1984;52:516–23.

[34] Verdecchia P, Schillaci G, Borgioni C, et al. Prognostic value of a new electrocardiographic method for diagnosis of left ventricular hypertrophy in essential hypertension. J Am Coll Cardiol 1998;31:383–90.

[35] Kannel WB, Gordon T, Offut D. Left ventricular hypertrophy by electrocardiogram: prevalence, incidence, and mortality in the Framingham Study. Ann Intern Med 1969;71:89–105.

[36] Okin PM, Devereux RB, Nieminen MS, et al. Electrocardiographic strain pattern and prediction of cardiovascular morbidity and mortality in hypertensive patients. Hypertension 2004;44:48–54.

[37] Okin PM, Devereux RB, Fabsitz RR, et al. Quantitative assessment of electrocardiographic strain predicts increased left ventricular mass: The Strong Heart Study. J Am Coll Cardiol 2002;40:1395–400.

[38] Pringle SD, Macfarlane PW, McKillop JH, et al. Pathophysiologic assessment of left ventricular hypertrophy and strain in asymptomatic patients with essential hypertension. J Am Coll Cardiol 1989;13:1377–81.

[39] Romhilt DW, Estes EH Jr. A point-score system for the ECG diagnosis of left ventricular hypertrophy. Am Heart J 1968;75:752–8.

[40] Salles G, Leocadio S, Bloch K, et al. Combined QT interval and voltage criteria improve left ventricular

hypertrophy detection in resistant hypertension. Hypertension 2005;46:1207–12.

[41] Cuspidi C, Macca G, Sampieri L, et al. Influence of different echocardiographic criteria for detection of left ventricular hypertrophy on cardiovascular risk stratification in recently diagnosed essential hypertensives. J Hum Hypertens 2001;15:619–25.

[42] Havelda CJ, Sohi GS, Flowers NC, et al. The pathologic correlates of the electrocardiogram: complete left bundle branch block. Circulation 1982;65:445–51.

[43] Murphy ML, Thenabadu PN, de Soyza N, et al. Left atrial abnormality as an electrocardiographic criterion for the diagnosis of left ventricular hypertrophy in the presence of right bundle branch block. Am J Cardiol 1983;52:381–3.

[44] Vandenberg B, Sagar K, Romhilt D. Electrocardiographic criteria for the diagnosis of left ventricular hypertrophy in the presence of complete right bundle branch block. J Am Coll Cardiol 1985;5:511.

[45] Levy D, Salomon M, D'Agostino RB, et al. Prognostic significance of baseline electrocardiographic features and their serial changes in subjects with left ventricular hypertrophy. Circulation 1994;90:1786–93.

[46] Matthew J, Sleight P, Lonn E, et al. Reduction of cardiovascular risk by regression of electrocardiographic markers of left ventricular hypertrophy by the angiotensin-converting enzyme inhibitor ramipril. Circulation 2001;104:1615–21.

[47] Hsieh BP, Pham MX, Froelicher VF. Prognostic value of electrocardiographic criteria for left ventricular hypertrophy. Am Heart J 2005;150:161–7.

[48] Struthers AD. The diagnosis of heart failure. Heart 2000;84:334–8.

[49] Zaphiriou A, Robb S, Murray-Thomas T, et al. The diagnostic accuracy of plasma BNP and NTproBNP in patients referred from primary care with suspected heart failure: results of the UK natriuretic peptide study. Eur J Heart Fail 2005;7:537–41.

[50] Kannel WB, Abbott RD. Comparison of ECG-LVH and unrecognised myocardial infarction as predictors of overt cardiovascular events: The Framingham study [abstract]. Circulation 1984;70(Suppl. II):434.

[51] Dosh SA. Diagnosis of heart failure in adults. Am Fam Physician 2004;70:2145–52.

[52] Flowers NC, Horan LG. Subtle signs of right ventricular enlargement and their relative importance. In: Schlant RC, Hurst JW, editors. Advances in electrocardiography. New York: Grune and Stratton; 1972. p. 297–308.

[53] Chou T-C, Helm R. Clinical vectorcardiography. New York: Grune and Stratton; 1967.

[54] Corrado D, Basso C, Rizzoli G, et al. Does sport activity enhance the risk of sudden death in adolescents and young adults? J Am Coll Cardiol 2003;42:1959–63.

[55] Fuller C. Physical examinations for young athletes [letter]. Cleve Clin J Med 2005;72:176.

[56] A multidisciplinary study of right ventricular dysplasia. Available at: www.arvd.org. Accessed June 9, 2006.

[57] Maron BJ, Zipes DP. 36th Bethesda Conference: Introduction Eligibility recommendations for competitive athletes with cardiovascular abnormalities. J Am Coll Cardiol 2005;45:1318–21.

[58] European Society of Cardiology consensus document. Recommendations for competitive sports participation in athletes with cardiovascular disease. Eur Heart J 2005;26:1422–45.

**ELSEVIER
SAUNDERS**

Cardiol Clin 24 (2006) 413–426

**CARDIOLOGY
CLINICS**

Electrocardiography of the Failing Heart

Vinzenz Hombach, MD

*Department of Internal Medicine II, University Hospital of Ulm,
Robet-Koch Strasse 8, Ulm D-89081, Germany*

Structural heart disease, electrical instability, and increased sympathetic activity can generate a number of specific and nonspecific ECG changes and arrhythmias in patients with congestive heart failure (CHF). This review describes direct alterations of the P–QRS–T complex and ECG-derived parameters in CHF, together with the significance of cardiac arrhythmias, markers of atrial and ventricular electrical instability, and the parameters of sympathetic nervous system activity.

General ECG alterations in the failing heart

Patients with CHF may display specific ECG alterations such as Q-waves after myocardial infarction (MI) or persistent ST-segment elevation in MI-related leads consistent with a left ventricular (LV) aneurysm. ST-segment alterations may also occur in chronic recurrent ischemia. ECG patterns of significant LV hypertrophy (LVH) may indicate chronic decompensation from aortic valvular disease, arterial hypertension, or hypertrophic cardiomyopathy. LVH also carries prognostic significance as documented in the Heart Outcomes Prevention Evaluation Study of 9541 patients. Electrocardiographic LVH was present in 793 (8.3%), and of these, 19.0% sustained a major cardiovascular event (MI, stroke, or cardiovascular death); 15.6% died, and 6.1% developed CHF after a follow-up of 4.5 years, compared with 15.6%, 10.8%, and 2.9%, respectively, in those without ECG evidence of LVH ($P = 0.0023$, $P < 0.0001$, and $P < 0.0001$). In multivariate analysis, ECG-LVH was an independent predictor of cardiovascular and all-cause

mortality and CHF [1]. Left bundle branch block (LBBB) in CHF patients almost always reflects diffuse myocardial damage as a result of ischemic or nonischemic dilated cardiomyopathy. Incomplete or complete right bundle branch block with right axis deviation and P-wave-alteration strongly suggests cor pulmonale. Finally, nonspecific ECG changes may be induced by digitalis or antiarrhythmic drugs.

The conventional ECG may be used as a first-line diagnostic tool for CHF, as shown in the Epidemiologia da Insufficiencia Cardiaca study [2]. In this investigation, 6300 subjects in a general population were screened for CHF by symptoms or signs, chest X-ray, ECG, and echocardiography. The diagnosis was confirmed in 551 cases. Patients with right atrial enlargement, atrial flutter or fibrillation, first degree and second degree Mobitz type II atrio-ventricular (AV)-block, LBBB, interstitial lung edema, and bilateral pleural effusion were more likely to be diagnosed with CHF. An abnormal ECG had an estimated sensitivity of 81% and a negative predictive value of 75%, and for an abnormal chest X-ray the numbers were 57% and 83%, respectively [2].

Atrial depolarization and repolarization in the conventional and signal-averaged ECG

P-wave-duration (PWD) in the conventional or signal-averaged ECG and P-wave-dispersion (Pd) on the standard ECG are considered noninvasive markers of intra-atrial conduction disturbances that predispose to atrial fibrillation (AF). Sanders and colleagues [3] using electroanatomic mapping, compared electrophysiologic markers such as right and left atrial refractory periods, conduction times, corrected sinus node recovery time, PWD, and conduction of the crista terminalis in 21

E-mail address: vinzenz.hombach@uniklinik-ulm.de

patients with symptomatic CHF and 21 age-matched controls. CHF patients demonstrated an increase in atrial effective refractory period, no change in the heterogeneity of refractoriness, an increase of atrial conduction time along the low right atrium and coronary sinus, prolongation of the PWD, and corrected sinus node recovery times as well as a greater number and duration of double potentials along the crista terminalis. CHF patients also demonstrated an increased propensity to AF with single extrastimuli and induced AF was more often sustained. Thus, simple PWD measurement of >20 milliseconds in the conventional ECG may be a helpful parameter for the increased susceptibility of AF in CHF patients.

PWD may be related to the clinical status of CHF patients. Song and colleagues [4] measured minimum and maximum PWD and Pd in 21 patients with decompensated CHF before and after 40 ± 23 hours of diuresis with the removal of 3 ± 1 L of fluid. There was a significant correlation between average PWD and the amount of removed fluid ($r = -0.59$, $P = 0.015$) and the average and maximum PWD decreased significantly with diuresis ($P = 0.001$ and 0.022, respectively). Diuresis may, therefore, attenuate the electrophysiologic atrial changes caused by fluid overload. Beta-blockade may also influence maximum PWD and Pd according to Camsari [5] in a study of 41 New York Heart Association (NYHA) class III and IV patients. At the 6-month follow-up, maximum PWD and Pd decreased significantly with the administration of metoprolol, a finding that may correlate with the effect of beta-blockade in reducing the incidence of AF in CHF.

In the study of Faggiano and colleagues [6] an increased PWD within the signal-averaged ECG (SAECG) correlated with an increased pulmonary capillary wedge (PCW) pressure), and an acute reduction of PCW pressure-reduced PWD. However, the left atrial end-systolic dimension did not vary significantly with the PCW pressure. In the recent study of Yamada and colleagues [7] involving 75 patients without a history of paroxysmal AF and a LV ejection fraction (LVEF) <40%, an abnormal P-SAECG was found in 29 of 75 patients. After a follow-up of 21 ± 9 months, attacks of paroxysmal AF occurred more frequently in patients with (32%) than in those without an abnormal P-SAECG (2%, $P = 0.0002$). Plasma Atrial Natriuretic Peptide (ANP)-levels were significantly higher in patients with than in those without paroxysmal AF

attacks. Multivariate analysis identified an abnormal P-SAECG (hazard ratio 19.1, $P = 0.0069$) and elevated ANP levels of 60 pg/mL (hazard ratio 8.6, $P = 0.018$) as important predictors of paroxysmal AF. Yamada and colleagues [7] concluded that an abnormal P-SAECG and elevated ANP levels might be predictors of paroxysmal AF in patients with chronic CHF. In a recent study, Dixen and colleagues [8] evaluated the prognostic role of prolonged signal-averaged PWD, raised levels of natriuretic peptide in 43 consecutive patients with stable CHF. Over a 438-day median follow-up, time to death, hospitalization for CHF exacerbation, and ECG-documented AF were investigated. Seventeen patients met these endpoints. Proportional hazard regression showed that only prolonged signal averaged PWD ≥ 49 milliseconds was associated with a increased risk of meeting an early endpoint (hazard ratio 3.94 with 95% confidence interval [CI], 1.50–10.42, $P = 0.006$). These workers concluded that in patients starting with stable CHF, a prolonged single averaged P-wave duration predicts early death, development of AF, or hospitalization for decompensated CHF.

Interventricular septal activation—absence of septal Q waves

It has been argued that the absence of septal Q waves may be a marker of LV disease. In a recent study on 110 elderly patients >65 years, Shamim and colleagues [9] analyzed standard 12-lead ECGs for the presence or absence of Q waves in leads I, aVL, V5, and V6, and patient survival from hospital and outpatient records for a mean follow-up of 4 years. Septal Q waves were absent in 71 and present in 39 patients. The overall mortality rate was 47% (43 patients), and the incidence of death was 49% (36 patients) in the group with no septal Q waves and 18% (7 patients) in those with Q waves. On univariate analysis (Cox proportional hazard method) the absence of septal Q waves was found to be a strong marker of a poor prognosis in chronic CHF (hazard ratio [HR] 1.40, 95% CI, 1.10–1.67, $P = 0.003$). Kaplan-Meier curves in the two groups showed a significant difference in survival independenly of age, NYHA functional class, peak VO_2, and QRS duration. Septal Q waves reflect early septal activation (20 milliseconds) from left to right across the mid-portion of the interventricular septum. Such normal septal Q waves are often absent in LBBB and after left coronary artery occlusion. Thus, absent septal Q waves are considered an indicator of structural heart disease and myocardial fibrosis, and may therefore serve as an independent predictor of poor prognosis in elderly CHF patients [9].

QRS duration

Measurement of QRS duration may be diagnostically useful in systolic LV dysfunction, as indicated by Krüger and colleagues [10] in a cohort of 128 consecutive patients with suspected cardiac disease. Sixty-six patients had LV systolic dysfunction judged by LVEF <50% determined echocardiographically. The QRS duration was longer in the group with LV dysfunction compared with the 62 patients without LV systolic dysfunction, and Brain Natriuretic Peptide (BNP) (normal value <75 pg/mL) was higher in the group with LV systolic dysfunction compared with the control group. A QRS duration of >0.1, >0.11, or >0.12 was highly specific (63%, 90%, and 98%) but less sensitive (84%, 81%, and 75%) for predicting LV systolic dysfunction. A QRS cutoff value of 106 milliseconds was moderately sensitive (65%) but very specific (87%) for predicting LV systolic dysfunction, whereas a BNP cutoff value >84 pg/mL was highly sensitive (89%) but only modestly specific (58%). The positive likelihood ratio for LV systolic dysfunction of an abnormal BNP (2.0) and QRS prolongation >100 milliseconds (2.3) was improved by the combination of both criteria to 5.1. In multivariate analysis, BNP and QRS duration were independent predictors of LV systolic dysfunction.

QRS duration also plays a significant role in the prognostic assessment of CHF. In a group of 165 patients with implantable cardioverter-defibrillators (ICD) with CHF NYHA functional Class III the prognostic significance of a QRS duration of ≥150 milliseconds (n = 26, group 1) was compared with a QRS duration ≤150 milliseconds (n = 139, group 2). At the 12-month follow-up the mortality in group 1 was significantly higher (31.3%) compared with 9.5% in group 2, and after 24 months the mortality rate was 46.6% in group 1 compared with 10.2% in group 2 ($P = 0.04$). A QRS duration of ≥150 milliseconds in ICD recipients with CHF appears to provide a simple noninvasive prognostic index [11].

Iuliano and colleagues [12] undertook a retrospective analysis of 669 CHF patients according to QRS duration <120 milliseconds or ≥120

milliseconds. They found that a prolonged QRS was associated with a significant increase in mortality (49.3% versus 34.0%, $P = 0.01$) and sudden death (24.8% versus 17.4%, $P = 0.004$). LBBB was associated with a worse survival ($P = 0.006$) but not sudden death. In patients with LVEF <30%, QRS prolongation was associated with a significant increase in mortality (51.6% versus 41.1%, $P = 0.01$) and sudden death (28.8% versus 21.1%, $P = 0.02$). In patients with an LVEF of 30% to 40% QRS prolongation was associated with a significant increase in mortality (42.7% versus 23.3%, $P = 0.036$), but not in sudden death. After adjustment for baseline variables independent predictors of mortality included prolongation of QRS (risk ratio 1.46, $P = 0.028$) and depressed LVEF (risk ratio 0.965, $P = 0.001$). The results indicated that QRS prolongation of ≥120 milliseconds was an independent predictor of increased total mortality and sudden death in CHF patients. Morgera and colleagues [13] reported similar observations in a study of 78 consecutive patients with idiopathic dilated cardiomyopathy who were investigated with signal averaged ECG, 24- to 48-hour ECG monitoring and electrophysiologic study. During a follow-up of 85 months, nine patients died: six of cardiac death, two of CHF. The independent predictors for death and cardiac transplantation included an his-ventricular (HV) interval >55 milliseconds and a combination of frequent and repetitive ventricular ectopic beats and poor LV function. The association of a prolonged HV interval with a wide (>110 milliseconds) QRS complex yielded a strong index of future arrhythmic events (ratio 4, 53, 95% CI, 1.75–13.4, $P = 0.05$). These results were confirmed by Shenkman and colleagues [14], who selected a subgroup of 3471 CHF patients with full echocardiographic and ECG data. The QRS duration was ≥120 milliseconds in 20.8% of the subjects. There was a linear relationship between increased QRS duration and decreased LVEF ($P < 0.01$). A prolonged QRS duration of 120 to 149 milliseconds was associated with an increased mortality at 60 months ($P = 0.001$), when adjusted for age, sex, and race ($P = 0.001$), and LV systolic dysfunction. A graded increase in mortality was correlated with ascending degrees of QRS prolongation. The study confirmed that 20% of a general CHF population can be expected to have a prolonged QRS duration within the first year of diagnosis reflecting a worse prognosis, and pointing to possible candidates for biventricular pacing.

In elderly patients the prognostic significance of a prolonged QRS complex was also shown by Shamim and colleagues [15] in 112 patients (mean age of 73.3 ± 4.4 years). During a follow-up of 12 ± 5 months, 45 patients died, and QRS duration ($P = 0.001$) and heart rate ($P = 0.03$) at baseline were found by Cox proportional hazard analysis to predict adverse outcomes. Kaplan-Meier survival analysis revealed that patients with <5% change of QRS duration had fewer complications than patients with a 5% to 20% change and a >20% change was associated with the worst prognosis. Thus, a single measurement of prolonged QRS duration or more importantly an increase in QRS duration over time predicts adverse outcomes in elderly patients [15].

Can simple ECG parameters select patients who might benefit from ICD therapy? Bloomfield and colleagues [16] selected patients for Multicenter Automatic Defibrillator Implantation Trial-II (MADIT-II) criteria using QRS duration >120 milliseconds. Of the 177 MADIT-II- like patients, 32% had a QRS duration >120 milliseconds, and 68% had an abnormal (positive or indeterminate) microvolt T-wave alternans test. Twenty patients died during an average follow-up of 20 ± 6 months, Patients with an abnormal T-wave alternans test were compared with those with a normal test and patients with QRS duration >120 milliseconds were compared with those that had a QRS ≤ 120 milliseconds. The odds ratios for 2-year mortality were 4.8 ($P = 0.020$) and 1.5 ($P = 0.367$), respectively. The actual mortality rate was substantially lower in patients with a normal microvolt T-wave alternans test than in patients with a narrow QRS. The results suggested that in MADIT-II-like patients, a microvolt T-wave alternans test is better than QRS duration at identifying a high-risk group and at identifying a low-risk group unlikely to benefit from ICD therapy.

Left bundle branch block and right axis deviation

The presence of LBBB combined with right axis deviation (RAD) in the frontal plane is extremely rare, and occurs in less than 1% of patients with LBBB. According to a study of 53 patients, (3 new patients, and 50 reviewed from the literature), Nicolic and colleagues [17] concluded that LBBB and RAD is an insensitive but very specific marker of diffuse myocardial disease. In their survey, 18 patients had cardiomyopathy (15 with primary cardiomyopathy and another 3 had alcoholic heart disease, acromegaly, and Duchenne muscular dystrophy, respectively). Twelve patients had arterial hypertension, 10 had miscellaneous disorders (congenital or valvular disease, cardiac surgery, myocarditis, or traumatic systemic AV fistula), 9 "aortomyocardiosclerosis," and 3 had presumptive coronary artery disease. In 13 cases, the RAD was observed to develop de novo or was intermittent. No clear-cut explanation for the change of axis was proposed in terms of clinical events or heart rate. Childers and colleagues [18] independently reported another cohort of 36 patients with LBBB and RAD from a database of 636,000 ECGs. The majority of patients had dilated cardiomyopathy, and in 30 of 36 RAD was episodic. The combination of LBBB and RAD in four cases was manifested as a rare form of QRS aberration with atrial premature impulses. The combination of LBBB and RAD is interesting but rare. It primarily reflects widespread conduction system involvement in diffuse myocardial disease, particularly (dilated) biventricular cardiomyopathy.

Left bundle branch block and cardiac resynchronization

The LV normally contracts rapidly and synchronously with little variation in the onset of electrical and mechanical activation throughout the wall. LBBB causes asynchronous (and delayed) electrical and mechanical LV activation. This produces an inefficient dyssynchronous pattern of LV activation with segments contracting at different times with resultant aggravation of the baseline LV systolic dysfunction [19–22]. Endocardial catheter mapping studies have unequivocally demonstrated that RV pacing mimics the endocardial activation patterns of LBBB [23]. Chronic LBBB produces structural changes, resulting in chronic systolic and diastolic LV dysfunction that contribute to reduced LV pumping function on a long-term basis. The changes include paradoxical septal wall motion, delayed LV lateral wall contraction, a shorter diastolic filling time (and/or overlapping systole/diastole), development or aggravation of functional mitral regurgitation, reduced LV pressure, increased left atrial diameters, and distorted LV geometry.

LV conduction delay in the form of classic LBBB or nonspecific intraventricular conduction delay occurs in about 20% to 30% of patients with CHF. Biventricular pacing works by reducing the degree of electromechanical asynchrony.

The improved sequence of electrical activation (a process known as resynchronization) translates into beneficial acute and long-term hemodynamic effects by virtue of producing a more coordinated and efficient LV contraction and reduction of functional mitral regurgitation. The clinical value of long-term resynchronization with biventricular stimulation has now been established in CHF patients with LV dyssynchrony with a better response in idiopathic cardiomyopathy than ischemic disease [24–30]. Growing experience with cardiac resynchronization therapy has highlighted the limitations of a wide QRS complex as a surrogate for mechanical LV dyssynchrony. About 30% to 40% of patients with a wide QRS complex (predominantly reflecting left-sided conduction delay) fail to exhibit mechanical LV dyssynchrony [31]. For this reason, echocardiographic assessment with quantification of LV dyssynchrony is emerging as a better predictor of cardiac resynchronization outcome than the widened QRS complex [32].

ST-segment and T-wave alterations in acute coronary syndromes

ST-segment and T-wave alterations are important regarding myocardial salvage, development of CHF, and prognosis following an ST-elevation MI (STEMI). In a study of 432 patients with a first MI [33] the detection of ST-segment depression in two or more lateral (I, aVL, V5, V6) leads revealed higher rates of death (14.3% versus 3.6%, $P < 0.01$), more severe CHF (14.3% versus 4.1%, $P < 0.01$) and angina with ECG changes (20.0% versus 11.6%, $P = 0.04$) than ST-segment depression in the other ECG leads. Similar findings were reported by Mager and colleagues [34] in 238 consecutive patients with acute inferior MI where patients with ST-segment depression in the left precordial leads tended to be older and had a higher incidence of hypertension, previous MI (45.8 versus 20.1%, $P = 0.01$) and CHF (21.7 versus 3.7%, $P = 0.00008$). Therefore, left precordial or left lateral ST-segment depression in acute MI heralds a poor outcome with higher rates of cardiac death and CHF. In a more extended study, Barrabes and colleagues [35] analyzed the initial ECG in 775 consecutive patients with a first MI without ST-segment elevation in leads other than aVR or V1 (non-STEMI). The rates of in-hospital death in patients without (n = 525) and with 0.05 to 0.1 mV (n = 116) or ≥0.1 mV (n = 134) of ST-segment elevation in a lead VR were 1.3%, 8.6%,

and 19.4%, respectively ($P < 0.001$). After adjustment for baseline clinical predictors and for ST-segment depression on admission, the odds ratios for death in the last two groups (those with ST-segment elevation) were 4.2 (95% CI, 1.5–12.2) and 6.6 (95% CI, 2.5–17.6), respectively. The rates of recurrent ischemic events and CHF during hospital stay also increased in a stepwise fashion among the groups according to the degree of ST-segment abnormality. The results indicated that ST-segment elevation in lead aVR provides important short-term prognostic information in patients with a first non-STEMI.

The ST-segment resolution pattern can also be used to predict CHF, as was reported in 258 patients from the TIMI-7 (Thrombolysis In Myocardial Infarction) and GUSTO-I (Global Utilization of Strategies To Open Occluded Coronary Arteries) Trials: by logistic regression analysis, ST-segment resolution patterns were an independent predictor of the combined outcome of mortality or CHF ($P = 0.024$), whereas TIMI-flow grade assessment was not ($P = 0.693$). A subgroup of patients with TIMI-flow 0 to 1 after thrombolysis was identified by rapid ST-segment resolution of ≥50% with relatively benign outcomes [36]. In addition, data from the GUSTO-I study [37] revealed that patients with higher T-waves (>98% percentile of the upper limit of normal) had a lower 30-day mortality than those without high T waves (5.2% versus 8.6%, $P = 0.001$) and were less likely to develop CHF (15% versus 24%, $P < 0.001$) or cardiogenic shock (6.1% versus 8.6%, $P = 0.0023$). The study suggested that T-wave amplitude had prognostic significance after controlling the data for time to treatment in acute MI.

Table 1 provides a summary of the most significant ECG changes in CHF and their implications for clinical diagnosis of the patients.

Cardiac repolarization in heart failure

Cardiac repolarization may be disturbed in patients with CHF, and in principle, these alterations may be measured by QT- or QTc-duration, QT variability, QT-dispersion, and the detection of microvolt T-wave alternans. As CHF patients might have areas of fibrosis and scars the evaluation of changes in cardiac repolarization might be diagnostically and prognostically useful with respect to life-threatening ventricular tachyarrhythmias.

Table 1
Outline of significant parameters of indices of increased dispersion of ventricular repolarization and disturbed sympatho-vagal balance and their clinical significance for assessing patients with congestive heart failure

Method/Index	Definition	Pathophysiology	Advantage	Disadvantage	Clinical use
QT variability (QTV)	Beat-to-beat or diurnal variations of QT duration	Increased dispersion of repolarization (susceptibility to reentrant ventricular tachycardias)	Simple measured Parameter (QT duration)	Computer algorithm not generally available Criteria not standardized	Experimental
QT dispersion (QTd)	Difference between longest and shortest QT interval in 12-lead or 3-lead (Holter) ECG	Increased dispersion of repolarization (susceptibility to reentrant ventricular tachycardias)	Simple measured parameter	Too many technical problems and pitfalls Variable and Inconsistent results	Obsolete
T wave alternans (TWA)	Macro-TWA: beat-to-beat changes of T-wave polarity and/or shape Micro-TWA: beat-to-beat amplitude fluctuations of the T wave at the microvolt level	Increased dispersion of repolarization (susceptibility to reentrant ventricular tachycardias)	Macro: direct (eyball) detection from conventional ECG Strong parameter of ventricular vulnerability	Micro: complicated protocol Algorithm not generally available Ventricular premature beats may interfere with computer analysis Increased heart rate by exercise or emotion necessary for analysis	Experimental (near clinical)

Heart rate variability (HRV)	Beat-to-beat oscillations of relative risk-intervals	Disturbed sympathovagal balance (susceptibility to life-threatening ventricular tachyarrhythmias)	Computer algorithms widely available Relative simple automated measurement Well standardized technique and parameters	Many overlapping parameters (time/frequency domain) Not valid at periods of physical activity, postural changes or emotional stimuli Low sensitivity and positive predictive value (PPV)	Clinically useful
Heart rate turbulence (HRT)	Fluctuations of sinus rhythm cycles after a single VPB	Disturbed sympathovagal balance (susceptibility to life-threatening ventricular tachyarrhythmias)	Simple parameter of BRS Standardized (automated) measurement	Computer algorithm not generally available Requires single ventricular premature beats Not applicable in AF Low sensitivity and positive predictive value (PPV)	Experimental (near clinical)
Baroreflex sensitivity (BRS)	Reflex heart rate response to physiologic activation and deactivation of baroreceptors following IV—phenylephrine	Disturbed sympathovagal balance (susceptibility to life-threatening ventricular tachyarrhythmias)	Clear pathophysiologic concept Well standardized technique	Advanced and complicated technique Low sensitivity and positive predictive value (PPV)	Experimental

Ancillary parameters

Table 2 provides an overview of the most significant tests and indexes related to disturbed cardiac repolarization and sympathovagal balance, their pathophysiologic role in the initiation of malignant ventricular tachyarrhythmias, and clinical significance for investigating CHF patients.

QT interval duration

In the study of Harding and colleagues [38] significant changes of QRS- and both QT- and QTc-duration were observed in 23 patients who received an LV assist device (LVAD) for CHF. QRS duration decreased from 117 ± 6 to 103 ± 6 milliseconds ($P < 0.01$), the absolute QT-duration increased from 359 ± 6 to 378 ± 8 milliseconds ($P < 0.05$), and the QTc-interval increased from 379 ± 10 to 504 ± 11 milliseconds ($P < 0.01$). None of these immediate changes were observed among 22 patients undergoing routine coronary artery bypass grafting. The findings that QRS- and QT-duration were significantly influenced by the load on the failing heart and that the action potential shortened, may contribute to the improved cellular contractile performance after sustained LVAD support. Similar findings were noted by Gaudron and colleagues [39] in 134 patients after

Table 2
Summary of the most significant ECG alterations and their relation to pathophysiologic and clinical factors in congestive heart failure

Observation	Implication
Normal	• Left ventricular systolic dysfunction very unlikely
	• Negative predictive value for CHF >90%
ST-T wave changes	• Myocardial ischemia
	• Arrhythmogenic right ventricular cardiomyopathy
	• Hypertrophic cardiomyopathy
Left ventricular hypertrophy	• Arterial hypertension
	• Aortic stenosis
	• Hypertrophic cardiomyopathy
	• Early (subclinical) stages of dilated cardiomyopathy
Left bundle branch block (LBBB)	• Usually associated with structural heart disease
	• Indicates diffuse myocardial disease and fibrosis
	• Prevalence: about 25% in CHF
	• 5-year mortality about 35%
	• Only weak correlation between QRS duration and left ventricular mechanical dyssynchrony
LBBB and right axis deviation	• Prevalence: extremely rare (<1% of LBBB)
	• Relatively specific for diffuse disease like dilated congestive cardiomyopathy (DCM)
LBBB with left axis deviation	• Most common in diffuse structural heart disease
Right bundle branch block (RBBB)	• No clear association with heart failure except for cor pulmonale
	• Prevalence only about 6% in CHF
Small QRS complexes	• Pericardial effusion
	• Hypothyroidism
	• Amyloidosis
Is there a typical ECG pattern of CHF?	• left ventricular hypertrophy in percordial leads with small voltage in frontal leads (HT, AS)
	• left bundle branch block with left axis deviation atrial fibrillation (DCM, CHD)
	• LBBB with right axis deviation (DCM)
What ECG markers best correlate with low LVEF?	• Q waves in precordial leads or LBBB in patients with known CHD
	• Left atrial "enlargement" (P-wave) and/or LVH in (decompensated) diseases with pressure overload

Abbreviations: As, aortic stenosis; CHD, coronary heart cartery disease; CHF, congestive heart failure; DCM, dilated cardiomyopathy; HT, systemic (arterial) hypertension; LVH, left ventricular hypertrophy; LBBB, left bundle branch block.

acute MI, in whom LV dilatation was closely related to the end-diastolic LV volume index, Lown-ventricular premature beat (VPB) score ($r = 0.98$, $P < 0.01$), and the QTc-prolongation ($r = 0.998$, $P < 0.01$), respectively. Patients with progressive LV remodeling reflected by LV dilatation on echocardiography, and QTc prolongation may be more susceptible to enhanced electrical instability. LV remodeling after MI might serve as a link between dysfunction, electrical instability, and sudden cardiac death.

In a recent study Vrtovec and colleagues [40] measured corrected QT interval using Bazett formula from standard 12-lead ECGs in 241 patients with CHF and elevated BNP levels >400 pg/mL. QTc intervals were prolonged in 122 (52%) and normal in 119 (49%) patients, but BNP levels were comparable in both groups. After 6-month follow-up 46 patients died, 9 underwent transplantation, and another 17 underwent LV assist device implantation. The deaths were attributed to pump failure ($n = 24$), sudden cardiac death ($n = 18$), and noncardiac causes ($n = 4$). Kaplan-Meier survival rates were three times higher in the normal QTc group than in the prolonged QTc group, and on multivariate analysis prolonged QTc interval was an independent predictor of all-cause death ($P = 0.0001$), cardiac death ($P = 0.0006$), sudden cardiac death ($P = 0.004$), and pump failure death ($P = 0.0006$). A prolonged QTc interval is thus a strong, independent predictor of adverse outcome in CHF patients with BNP levels >400 pg/mL.

As a more recent parameter of increased dispersion of repolarization, QT variability was studied by Berger and colleagues [41]. In 83 patients with ischemic and nonischemic dilated cardiomyopathy and 60 control subjects QT variability index was calculated in each subject as the logarithm of the ratio of normalized QT variance to heart rate variance, and the coherence between heart rate and QT interval fluctuations was determined by spectral analysis. Patients with dilated cardiomyopathy had greater QT variance than control subjects (60.4 ± 63.1 versus 25.7 ± 24.8 ms^2, $P < 0.0001$) despite reduced heart rate variance (6.7 ± 7.8 versus 10.5 ± 10.4 bpm^2, $P = 0.01$). The QT variability index was higher in patients with dilated cardiomyopathy than in control subjects with a high degree of significance, and QT variability index did not correlate with LVEF but did depend on NYHY functional class. QT variability index did not differ between patients with ischemic and those with nonischemic

origin. Coherence between heart rate and QT interval fluctuations at physiologic frequencies was lower in patients with dilated cardiomyopathy compared with those without dilated cardiomyopathy and QT interval variability increased with worsening of functional class but was independent of LVEF, indicating that dilated cardiomyopathy leads to temporal lability in ventricular repolarization.

QT dispersion

QT dispersion (QTd) is simply measured as the difference between the longest and shortest QT interval within the normal 12-lead ECG. QTd is often increased in patients with idiopathic dilated cardiomyopathy and CHF, but it does not necessarily predict an increased risk of arrhythmic death [42,43]. Pinsky and colleagues [44] studied 108 consecutive patients referred for heart transplantation, 80 of whom were placed on the waiting list. During 25 months of follow-up comparison of QTd ≥ 140 milliseconds versus ≤ 140 milliseconds, and a QTc of $\geq 9\%$ of normal predicted a 4.1 increase of the risk of cardiac death. In a recent study of Brooksby and colleagues [45] in 554 ambulatory outpatients with CHF, the heart rate corrected QT-dispersion and maximum QT-interval were significant univariate predictors of all-cause mortality during a follow-up period of 471 ± 168 days ($P = 0.026$, and <0.0001, respectively), and of sudden death and progressive heart failure death. These indices were not related to outcome in the multivariate analysis, in which independent predictors of all-cause mortality consisted of cardiothoracic ratio ($P = 0.0003$), echocardiographically derived end-diastolic dimension ($P = 0.007$), and ventricular couplets on 24-hour ECG monitoring ($P = 0.015$).

These results could not be reproduced in the Evaluation of Losartan In the Elderly trial (Losartan Heart Failure Survival Study) [46], in which 986 high-uality ECGs were retained and analyzed for heart rate, QRS duration, maximum QT and JT intervals,and QT and JT dispersion from a pool of 3118 ECGs of 1804 patients. During a follow-up of 540 ± 153 days there were 140 (14%) deaths from all causes, including 119 cardiac (12%) and 59 (6%) sudden cardiac deaths. The mean heart rate was significantly faster in nonsurvivors than in survivors (77 ± 16 versus 74 ± 14 bpm, $P = 0.0006$) and in patients who died of cardiac causes (76 ± 16 bpm, $P = 0.04$

versus survivors). Mean QRS duration was significantly longer in nonsurvivors (107 ± 25 milliseconds), and in the subgroups who died of cardiac (107 ± 24 milliseconds) or sudden death (112 ± 23 milliseconds) than in survivors (99 ± 24 milliseconds, $P < 0.01$ for all). The maximum QTc and QT intervals were similar for nonsurvivors, regardless of cause of death and in survivors. There were no significant differences in QTd or JTd (JT dispersion from the end of the QRS to the end of the T wave) between patients with any mode of death and survivors ($P < 0.1$ for all). Neither losartan nor captopril significantly modified QTd or JTd. Therefore, the investigators concluded that increased QTd is not associated with increased mortality in CHF patients, and it is inappropriate to examine drug efficacy in such patients [47]. Although QTd might be easily measured from the 12-lead ECG, this parameter is virtually of no diagnostic and prognostic value in CHF patients.

ECG-derived parameters for assessing sympathetic nervous system activity–heart rate variability include: (1) time domain parameters: root-mean-square of successive differences, percent difference between adjacent normal to normal relative risk (RR) intervals >50 milliseconds computed over the entire 24-hour ECG recording (pNN50), percent difference between adjacent normal RR intervals >50 milliseconds computed over the entire 24-hour ECG recording (pNN50) for short term; standard deviation of the averages normal to normal RR intervals in all 5-minute segments of a 24-hour ECG recording, standard deviation of all normal to normal RR intervals (SDNN), and mean of standard deviation for all 5-minute segments of RR intervals in 24 hours for long-term heart rate variability. (2) Frequency domain parameters of heart rate variability: ultralow-frequency power, very low-frequency power, low-frequency power, high-frequency power, baroreflex sensitivity, and heart rate turbulence.

Activation of the sympathetic (adrenergic) nervous system is one of the hallmarks of chronic CHF. Adrenergic activation may be estimated by measuring norepinephrine (NE) concentration in the blood, determining heart rate variability, that is, RR interval fluctuations in short- and long-term ECG recordings, by studying baroreflex sensitivity (the control of vagal and sympathetic outflow to the heart and peripheral vessels), and by quantifying heart rate turbulence.

Heart rate variability may be measured in short 1- to 5- to 10-minute ECG strips or 24-hour long-term ECG recordings, both in time and the frequency domain. Baroreflex sensitivity assesses the reflex heart rate response to physiologic activation and deactivation of the baroreceptors secondary to drug-induced changes in arterial pressure. These are measured by correlating spontaneous fluctuations of systolic blood pressure with the corresponding heart rate (RR interval) both at rest and after administration of the pure alpha-adrenoreceptor stimulant phenylephrine.

The method of heart rate turbulence quantifies the fluctuations of sinus rhythm cycles after single ventricular premature complexes (VPCs). In normal or low-risk groups, sinus rhythm exhibits a characteristic biphasic pattern of early acceleration and subsequent deceleration after a VPC. However, in high-risk (mostly postinfarction) patients, hear rate turbulence is attenuated or missing.

Heart rate variability

Increased sympathetic tone in cardiovascular conditions was elegantly demonstrated by Grassi and colleagues [47] in 243 subjects: 38 normotensive healthy controls, 113 with untreated essential hypertension, 27 normotensive and obese, and 65 with CHF. Heart rate was correlated with venous plasma NE, and postganglionic muscle sympathetic nerve activity (microneurography at a peroneal nerve). In the whole group, the heart rate was correlated with both plasma NE (r = 0.32, $P < 0.0001$) and muscle sympathetic nerve activity (r = 0.38, $P < 0.0001$). Heart rate values were greater in the obese and CHF patients than in controls, as was plasma NE and muscle sympathetic nervous activity (all differences statistically significant). In the subjects with essential hypertension, no significant relationship was found between these three indices of sympathetic activity. The results suggested that supine heart rate can be regarded as a marker of intersubject differences in sympathetic tone in the general population and individuals with cardiovascular disease.

In patients with CHF, heart rate variability (HRV) is frequently decreased, with a significant increase in the low-frequency component of the frequency domain HRV measurements, together with high levels of catecholamines, BNP, and an altered baroreflex sensitivity. The prognostic significance of HRV in CHF patients remains unclear. In one of the first studies in 40 patients with CHF, comparing normal individuals and patients with a history of nonsustained ventricular tachycardia and normal cardiac function, there was no significant difference in the HRV parameters despite a significantly lowered HRV in CHF patients [48]. In a prospective study of 71 patients with idiopathic dilated cardiomyopathy and CHF, Hoffman and colleagues [49] studied HRV by time and frequency domain methods. After a follow-up period of 15 ± 5 months, there was no significant difference of time or frequency domain indices of HRV in patients with arrhythmic events compared with those without major arrhythmic events. In a further study of 159 patients with idiopathic dilated cardiomyopathy and CHF, 30 patients died during follow-up, and there was a significant correlation between LVEF, increased SDNN and the percentage of adjacent RR intervals that vary by more than 50 milliseconds (pNN50) and an increased risk of cardiac death. However, the risk of sudden cardiac death correlated only with LVEF. This was in contrast to an increased low-frequency power and impairment of pNN50 that strongly correlated with an increased risk of death from progressive pump failure [50]. Another two studies showed that HRV was reduced in patients with CHF with a strong correlation between HRV and LV function and peak oxygen consumption [51,52].

HRV may have prognostic impact in hospitalized patients for decompensated CHF, as shown by Aronson and colleagues [53] in 199 patients with NYHA class III or IV CHF using 24-hour Holter recordings, and time and frequency HRV parameters. During a mean follow-up of 312 ± 150 days after discharge from the hospital, 40 patients (21.1%) died. Kaplan-Meier analysis indicated that patients with abnormal values of standard deviation of the RR intervals over a 24-hour period ($P = 0.027$), of SD of all 5-minute mean RR intervals ($P = 0.043$), of total power ($P = 0.022$), and of ultralow-frequency power ($P = 0.008$) in the lower tertile were at higher risk of death. In a multivariate Cox regression model, the same indexes in the lower tertile were independent predictors of mortality (RR from 2.2 to 2.6). The severity of autonomic dysfunction during hospitalization for CHF can thus predict survival after hospital discharge using measurements of overall HRV.

The predictive power of HRV for cardiac as well as sudden cardiac death was shown in three recent studies. In the VA trial [54] of 179 patients with CHF, the lowest quartile of patients were compared with the remaining, using SDNN as the sole HRV parameter. Among 127 patients

meeting the inclusion criteria, SDNN <65.3 milliseconds (the lowest quartile) was the sole independent factor predictive of survival in a multivariate model ($P = 0.0001$). A Cox proportional-hazards model revealed that each increase in 10 milliseconds in SDNN conferred a 20% decrease in risk of mortality ($P = 0.0001$). Furthermore, patients with SDNN <65.3 milliseconds had a significantly increased risk of sudden death ($P = 0.016$). Thus, in this study HRV was the sole independent predictor of overall mortality, and was significantly associated with sudden death. La-Rovere and colleagues [55] developed a multivariate survival model for the identification of sudden (presumably arrhythmic) death from data of 202 consecutive patients with moderate to severe CHF. Time- and frequency-domain HRV parameters obtained from 8-minute ECG recordings at baseline and during controlled breathing were challenged against clinical and functional parameters. This model was then validated in 242 consecutive patients referred for CHF as the validation sample. Sudden death was independently predicted by a model that included low frequency power of HRV during controlled breathing ≤ 13 milliseconds^2 and left ventricular end-diastolic diameter ≥ 77 mm (RR 3.7, 95% CI, 1.5 to 9.3, and RR 2.6, 95% CI, 1.1 to 6.3, respectively). Low-frequency power ≤ 11 milliseconds^2 during controlled breathing and ≥ 83 VPCs/hr on Holter monitoring were both independent predictors of sudden death (RR 3.0, 95% CI, 1.2 to 7.6, and RR 3.7, 95% CI, 1.5 to 9.0, respectively). The results showed that reduced short-term low-frequency power during controlled breathing is a powerful and independent predictor of sudden death in CHF patients. Similar results by the same group were reported by Guzzetti and colleagues [56], who studied 330 consecutive CHF patients. Using time, frequency, and fractal analyses, the risk of pump failure and of sudden death could be differentiated as follows: depressed power of night time HRV (≤ 509 milliseconds^2) very low-frequency power (<0.04 Hz), high pulmonary wedge pressure (≥ 18 mmHg), and low LVEF ($\leq 24\%$) were independently related to pump failure, while reduction of low frequency power (≤ 20 milliseconds^2) and increased LV end-systolic diameter (≥ 61 mm) were linked to sudden (arrhythmic) mortality.

From a technical point of view it is interesting that HVR parameters may also be retrieved from implanted devices. In this respect Adamson and colleagues [57] studied 397 patients where continuous HRV was measured as the standard deviation of 5-minute median atrial–atrial intervals (SDAAM) sensed by the biventricular pacing device. SDAAM < 50 milliseconds when averaged over 4 weeks was associated with increased mortality risk (HR 3.2, $P = 0.02$), and SDAAM were persistently lower over the entire follow-up period in patients who required hospitalization or died. Automated detection of decreases in SDAAM was 70% sensitive in detecting cardiovascular hospitalisations, with 2.4 false-positives per patient-year follow-up.

Last, it should be mentioned that HRV may be improved by exercise training [58], by drugs like candesartan [59] or valsartan, whose effect was comparable with lisinopril [60], and by biventricular pacing for cardiac resynchronization [61]. Whether these effects influence the prognosis of CHF patients remains to be investigated in larger studies. In conclusion, based on present experience assessing HRV either by time or frequency domain parameters may be a valuable tool for predicting an adverse prognosis in CHF patients irrespective of the underlying heart disease.

References

[1] Lonn E, Mathew J, Pogue J, et al, and the Heart Outcomes Prevention Evaluation Study Investigators. Relationship of electrocardiographic left ventricular hypertrophy to mortality and cardiovascular morbidity in high-risk patients. Eur J Cardiovasc Prev Rehab 2003;10:420–8.

[2] Fonseca C, Oliveira AG, Mota T, et al. The value of the electrocardiogram and chest X-ray for confirming or refuting a suspected diagnosis of heart failure in the community. Eur J Heart Fail 2004;6:807–12.

[3] Sanders P, Morton JB, Davidson NC, et al. Electrical remodeling of the atria in congestive heart failure: electrophysiological and electroanatomical mapping in humans. Circulation 2003;108:1461–8.

[4] Song J, Kalus JS, Caron MF, et al. Effect of diuresis on P-wave duration and dispersion. Pharmacotherapy 2002;22:564–8.

[5] Camsari A, Pekdemir H, Akkus MN, et al. Long-term effects of beta blocker therapy on P-wave duration and dispersion in congestive heart failure patients: a new effect? J Electrocardiol 2003;36:111–6.

[6] Faggiano P, Dáloia A, Zanelli E, et al. Contribution of left atrial pressure and dimension to signal-averaged P-wave duration in patients with chronic congestive heart failure. Am J Cardiol 1997;179:219–22.

[7] Yamada T, Fukunami M, Shimonagata T, et al. Prediction of paroxysmal atrial fibrillation in patients with congestive heart failure: a prospective study. J Am Coll Cardiol 2000;35:405–13.

[8] Dixen U, Wallevik L, Hansen MS, et al. Prolonged signal-averaged P wave duration as a prognostic marker for morbidity and mortality in patients with congestive heart failure. Scan Cardiovasc J 2003;37:193–8.

[9] Shamim W, Yousufuddin M, Xiao HB, et al. Septal q waves as an indicator of risk of mortality in elderly patients with chronic heart failure. Am Heart J 2002;44:740–4.

[10] Krüger S, Filzmaier K, Graf J, et al. QRS prolongation on surface ECG and brain natriuretic peptide as indicators of left ventricular systolic dysfunction. J Intern Med 2004;255:206–12.

[11] Bode-Schnurbus L, Bocker D, Block M, et al. QRS duration: a simple marker for predicting cardiac mortality in ICD patients with heart failure. Heart 2003;89:1157–62.

[12] Iuliano S, Fisher SG, Karasik PE, et al. Department of Veterans Affairs Survival Trial of Antiarrhythmic Therapy in Congestive Heart Failure. QRS duration and mortality in patients with congestive heart failure. Am Heart J 2002;143:1085–91.

[13] Morgera T, Di Lenarda A, Sabbadini G, et al. Idiopathic dilated cardiomyopathy: prognostic significance of electrocardiographic and electrophysiological findings in the nineties. Ital Heart J 2004;5:593–603.

[14] Shenkman HJ, Pampati V, Khandelwal AK, et al. Congestive heart failure and QRS duration: establishing prognosis study. Chest 2002;122:528–34.

[15] Shamim W, Yousufuddin M, Cicoria M, et al. Incremental changes in QRS duration in serial ECGs over time identify high risk elderly patients with heart failure. Heart 2002;88:47–51.

[16] Bloomfield DM, Steinman RC, Namerow PB, et al. Microvolt T-wave alternans distinguishes between patients likely and patients not likely to benefit from implanted cardiac defibrillator therapy: a solution to the Multicenter Automatic Defibrillator Implantation Trial (MADIT) II conundrum. Circulation 2004;110:1885–9.

[17] Nicolic G, Marriott HJL. Left bundle branch block with right axis deviation: a marker of congestive cardiomyopathy. J Electrocardiol 1985;18:395–404.

[18] Childers R, Lupovich S, Sochanski M, et al. Left bundle branch block and right axis deviation: a report of 36 cases. J Electrocardiol 2000;33:93–102.

[19] Leclercq C, Kass DA. Retiming the failing heart: principles and current clinical status of cardiac resynchronization. J Am Coll Cardiol 2002;39:194–201.

[20] Leclercq C, Kass DA. Retiming the failing heart: principles and current clinical status of cardiac resynchronization. J Am Coll Cardiol 2002;39:194–201.

[21] Kass DA. Pathology of cardiac dyssynchrony and resynchronization. In: Ellenbogen KA, Kay GN,

Wilkoff BL, editors. Device therapy for congestive heart failure. Philadelphia (PA): WB Saunders; 2004. p. 27–46.

[22] Tedrow U, Sweeney MO, Stevenson WG. Physiology of cardiac resynchronization. Curr Cardiol Rep 2004;6:189–93.

[23] Vassallo JA, Cassidy DM, Miller JM, et al. Left ventricular endocardial activation during right ventricular pacing: effect of underlying heart disease. J Am Coll Cardiol 1986;7:1228–33.

[24] Cazeau S, Leclercq C, Lavergne T, et al, and the Multisite Stimulation in Cardiomyopathies (MUSTIC) Study Investigators. Effects of multisite biventricular pacing in patients with heart failure and intraventricular conduction delay. N Engl J Med 2001;344:873–80.

[25] Abraham WT, Fisher WG, Smith AL, et al, and the MIRACLE Study Group. Multicenter InSync Randomized Clinical Evaluation. Cardiac resynchronization in chronic heart failure. N Engl J Med 2002; 346:1845–53.

[26] Bristow MR, Saxon LA, Boehmer J, et al, and the Comparison of Medical Therapy, Pacing, and Defibrillation in Heart Failure (COMPANION) Investigators. Cardiac-resynchronization therapy with or without an implantable defibrillator in advanced chronic heart failure. N Engl J Med 2004;350: 2140–50.

[27] Cleland JG, Daubert JC, Erdmann E, et al, and the Cardiac Resynchronization-Heart Failure (CARE-HF) Study Investigators. The effect of cardiac resynchronization on morbidity and mortality in Heart failure. N Engl J Med 2005;352: 1539–49.

[28] Strickberger SA, Conti J, Daoud EG, et al. Patient selection for cardiac resynchronization therapy: from the Council on Clinical Cardiology Subcommittee on Electrocardiography and Arrhythmias and the Quality of Care and Outcomes Research Interdisciplinary Working Group, in collaboration with the Heart Rhythm Society. Circulation 2005; 111:2146–50.

[29] Sutton MG, Plappert T, Hilpisch KE, et al. Sustained reverse left ventricular structural remodeling with cardiac resynchronization at one year is a function of etiology: quantitative Doppler echocardiographic evidence from the Multicenter InSync Randomized Clinical Evaluation (MIRACLE). Circulation 2006;113:266–72.

[30] Knight BP, Desai A, Coman J, et al. Long-term retention of cardiac resynchronization therapy. J Am Coll Cardiol 2004;44:72–7.

[31] Kashani A, Barold SS. Significance of QRS complex duration in patients with heart failure. J Am Coll Cardiol 2005;46:2183–92.

[32] Yu CM, Wing-Hong Fung J, Zhang Q, et al. Understanding nonresponders of cardiac resynchronization therapy—current and future perspectives. J Cardiovasc Electrophysiol 2005;16:1117–24.

[33] Barrabes JA, Figuears J, Moure C, et al. Q-wave evolution of a first acute myocardial infarction without significant ST segment elevation. Int J Cardiol 2001;77:55–62.

[34] Mager A, Sclarovsky S, Herz I, et al. Value of the initial electrocardiogram in patients with inferior-wall acute myocardial infarction for prediction of multivessel coronary artery disease. Coron Artery Dis 2000;11:415–20.

[35] Barrabes JA, Figueras J, Moure C, et al. Prognostic value of lead aVR in patients with a first non-ST-segment elevation acute myocardial infarction. Circulation 2003;108:814–9.

[36] Shah A, Wagner GS, Granger CB, et al. Prognostic implications of TIMI flow grade in the infarct related artery compared with continuous 12-lead ST-segment resolution analysis: reexamining the "gold standard" for myocardial reperfusion assessment. J Am Coll Cardiol 2000;35:666–72.

[37] Hochrein J, Sun F, Pieper KS, et al. Higher T-wave amplitude associated with better prognosis in patients receiving thrombolytic therapy for acute myocardial infarction (a GUSTO-I substudy). Global Utilization of Streptokinase and Tissue plasminogen Activator for Occluded Coronary Arteries. Am J Cardiol 1998;81:1078–84.

[38] Harding JD, Piacentino V, Gaughan JP, et al. Electrophysiological alterations after mechanical circulatory support in patients with advanced cardiac failure. Circulation 2001;104:1241–7.

[39] Gaudron P, Kugler I, Hu K, et al. Time course of cardiac structural, functional and electrical changes in asymptomatic patients after myocardial infarction: their inter-relation and prognostic impact. J Am Coll Cardiol 2001;38:33–40.

[40] Vrtovec B, Delgado R, Zewail A, et al. Prolonged QTc interval and high B-type natriuretic peptide levels together predict mortality in patients with advanced heart failure. Circulation 2003;107: 1764–9.

[41] Berger RD, Kasper EK, Baughman KL, et al. Beat-to-beat QT interval variability: novel evidence for repolraization lability in ischemic and nonischemic dilated cardiomyopathy. Circulation 1997;96: 1557–65.

[42] Grimm W, Steder U, Menz V, et al. QT dispersion and arrhythmic events in idiopathic dilated cardiomyopathy. Am J Cardiol 1996;78:458–61.

[43] Bodi-Peris V, Monmeneu-Menadas JV, Marin-Ortuno F, et al. QT interval dispersion in hospital patients admitted with cardiac insufficiency. Determinants and prognostic value. Rev Esp Cardiol 1999;52:563–9.

[44] Pinsky DJ, Sciacca RR, Steinberg JS. QT dispersion as a marker of risk in patients awaiting heart transplantation. J Am Coll Cardiol 1997;29:1576–84.

[45] Brooksby P, Batin PD, Nolan J, et al. The relationship between QT intervals and mortality in ambulant patients with chronic heart failure. The United

Kingdom heart failure evaluation and assessment of risk trial (UK-HEART). Eur Heart J 1999;20: 1335–41.

[46] Gang Y, Ono T, Hnatkova K, et al. ELITE II investigators. QT dispersion has no prognostic value in patients with symptomatic heart failure: an ELITE II substudy. Pacing Clin Electrophysiol 2003;26: 394–400.

[47] Grassi G, Vailati S, Bertinieri G, et al. Heart rate as a marker of sympathetic activity. J Hypertens 1998; 16:1635–9.

[48] Fei L, Keeling PJ, Gill JS, et al. Heart rate variability and it's relation to ventricular arrhythmias in congestive heart failure. Br Heart J 1994;71:322–8.

[49] Hoffman J, Grimm W, Menz V, et al. Heart rate variability and major arrhythmias in patients with idiopathic dilated cardiomyopathy. Pacing Clin Electrophysiol 1996;19:1841–4.

[50] Szabo BM, van Veldhuisen DJ, van der Veer N, et al. Prognostic value of HRV in chronic congestive heart failure secondary to idiopathic or ischemic dilated cardiomyopathy. Am J Cardiol 1997;79:978–80.

[51] Yi G, Goldman JH, Keeling PJ, et al. Heart rate variability in idiopathic dilated cardiomyopathy: relation to disease severity and prognosis. Heart 1977; 77:108–14.

[52] Fauchier L, Babuty D, Cosnay P, et al. Heart rate variabilty in idiopathic dilated cardiomyopathy: characteristics and prognostic value. J Am Coll Cardiol 1997;30:1009–14.

[53] Aronson D, Mittleman MA, Burger AJ. Measures of heart period variability as predictors of mortality in hospitalized patients with decompensated congestive heart failure. Am J Cardiol 2004;93:59–63.

[54] Bilchick KC, Fetics B, Djoukeng R, et al. Prognostic value of heart rate variability in chronic congestive heart failure (Veterans Affairs Survival Trial of Antiarrhythmic Therapy in Congestive Heart Failure). Am J Cardiol 2002;90:24–8.

[55] La Rovere MT, Pinna GD, Maestri R, et al. Short-term heart rate variability strongly predicts sudden cardiac death in chronic heart failure patients. Circulation 2003;107:565–70.

[56] Guzzetti S, La Rovere MT, Pinna GD, et al. Different spectral components of 24 h heart rate variability are related to different modes of death in chronic heart failure. Eur Heart J 2005;26:357–62.

[57] Adamson PB, Smith AL, Abraham WT, et al, and the InSync III Model 8042 and Attain OTW Lead Model 4193 Clinical Trial Investigators. Continuous autonomic assessment in patients with symptomatic heart failure: prognostic value of heart rate variability measured by an implanted cardiac resynchronization device. Circulation 2004;110: 2389–94.

[58] Larsen AI, Gjesdal K, Hall C, et al. Effect of exercise training in patients with heart failure: a pilot study on autonomic balance assessed by heart rate variability. Eur J Cardiovasc Prev Rehab 2004;11:162–7.

[59] Tambara K, Fujita M, Sumita Y, et al. Beneficial effect of candesartan treatment on cardiac autonomic nervous system activityin patients with chronic heart failure: simultaneous recording of ambulatori electrocardiogram and posture. Clin Cardiol 2004;27: 300–3.

[60] De Tommasi E, Iacoviello M, Romito R, et al. Comparison of the effect of valsartan and lisinopril on autonomic nervous system activity in chronic heart failure. Am Heart J 2003;146:E17.

[61] Livanis EG, Flevari P, Theodorakis GN, et al. Effect of biventricular pacing on heart rate variability in patients with chronic heart failure. Eur J Heart Fail 2003;5:175–8.

ELSEVIER
SAUNDERS

CARDIOLOGY
CLINICS

Cardiol Clin 24 (2006) 427–437

The 12-Lead Electrocardiogram in Supraventricular Tachycardia

Uday N. Kumar, MD, Rajni K. Rao, MD, Melvin M. Scheinman, MD*

Division of Cardiology, Department of Medicine, 500 Parnassus Avenue, Box 1354, University of California, San Francisco, San Francisco, California 94143, USA

The term supraventricular tachycardia (SVT) encompasses a range of common arrhythmias in which the atrial or atrioventricular (AV) node is essential for the perpetuation of the tachyarrhythmia [1]. Because of misdiagnosis and inconsistent classification, the exact prevalence of SVT is not clear but may be as high as six to eight per 1000 people in the United States [2]. SVT affects patients of varied ages, often can lead to symptoms, and may occur in patients with or without structural heart disease.

The diagnosis of SVT is made primarily by using the 12-lead electrocardiogram (ECG). Correct ECG diagnosis of SVT is important for several reasons. First, because symptomatic patients who may have SVT often require rapid and accurate treatment, misidentification of the type of SVT can lead to inappropriate acute management. Second, making the correct ECG diagnosis of the type of SVT is important for long-term prognosis and treatment strategies, including the selection of effective medications or the decision to refer a patient for catheter ablation. Finally, for patients who do go on to catheter ablation, a correct ECG diagnosis of the type of SVT facilitates the appropriate choice of ablation strategy. The correct choice is essential because the risk, duration, complexity, and success rate of catheter ablation varies based on the type of SVT [3].

Despite its importance, making the correct ECG diagnosis of SVT type may be difficult for numerous reasons. First, during the acute care of highly symptomatic or unstable patients who have possible SVT, the health care provider may be pressed for time. Second, the correct diagnosis may also be elusive when only a rhythm strip (as opposed to a 12-lead ECG) is available. Similarly, SVT may be suspected in hospitalized patients who are monitored on telemetry, but such monitoring equipment may not be able to generate a true 12-lead ECG. Third, the ECG morphology may be more unusual in patients taking antiarrhythmic medications or in patients who have had prior ablation or surgical procedures. For instance, patients who have congenital heart disease and have undergone corrective surgeries frequently develop SVT as a late complication [4,5]. Fourth, variability in the placement of ECG electrodes may affect the ECG tracing. Finally, the ECG computer diagnosis of arrhythmias is unreliable. These potential difficulties represent just a few of the challenges to accurate ECG diagnosis of SVT.

General points

This article provides a stepwise approach to the 12-lead ECG diagnosis of SVT. It first presents an initial approach to categorization and diagnosis. Then, the common ECG manifestations of each type of SVT are discussed individually. Finally, it presents a systematic algorithm for diagnosing suspected SVT based on the ECG.

The various forms of SVT include sinus tachycardia (ST), focal atrial tachycardia (AT), multifocal atrial tachycardia (MAT), atrial fibrillation (AF), atrial flutter (AFl), AV node reentrant

---

* Corresponding author.
  E-mail address: scheinman@medicine.ucsf.edu (M.M. Scheinman).

tachycardia (AVNRT), AV reentrant tachycardia (AVRT), junctional tachycardia (JT), and permanent junctional reciprocating tachycardia (PJRT).

The first step in diagnosing SVT is to categorize the rhythm as narrow complex (QRS < 120 milliseconds) or wide complex (QRS ≥ 120 milliseconds) and as regular (fixed R-R cycle lengths) or irregular (variable R-R cycle lengths) (Table 1). Some tachycardias are represented in more than one category. The next step is to look for evidence of atrial activity. If a discrete P wave is visible, the relationship of the P wave to the QRS complex should be evaluated. This relationship is characterized as either a "short-RP tachycardia" or a "long-RP tachycardia." In short-RP tachycardia, the time from the P wave to the preceding R wave is less than the time from the P wave to the following R wave (RP < PR). In long-RP tachycardia, the opposite is true (RP > PR) (see Table 1).

In addition to cycle regularity and QRS width, the following ECG criteria may help differentiate the various types of SVT: heart rate during tachycardia; mechanism of initiation/termination; P wave/QRS/ST morphology; changes in cycle length with the appearance of bundle-branch block; and ECG changes in response to maneuvers such as carotid sinus massage or adenosine administration. One study reports that viewing the ECG at both normal (25 mm/s) and faster (50 mm/s) paper speeds may improve diagnostic accuracy [6]. The findings and criteria helpful in the diagnosis of each particular SVT are discussed in greater detail later.

Sinus tachycardia

ST is a long-RP tachycardia that presents with a heart rate over 100 beats/min (bpm). The P wave morphology is identical to that of normal sinus rhythm. There usually is a gradual onset and termination that often can be appreciated on Holter or telemetry monitoring. A variant of ST, sinus node reentrant tachycardia, comprises a reentrant loop originating in the sinus node, behaves clinically like an SVT, and has a sudden onset and abrupt termination. In sinus node reentry tachycardia, the PR interval during tachycardia may differ from normal sinus rhythm, although the P wave morphology is identical. True sinus node reentrant tachycardia seems to be uncommon, with most of the reported cases originating from high in the crista terminalis [7]. Patients who have another variant of ST, termed "inappropriate sinus tachycardia," show persistent tachycardia during the day with marked increases in heart rate in response to exercise. This diagnosis is made from the 24-hour Holter recording, and beta-blockers are the drugs of choice.

Table 1
Initial categorization of tachycardic rhythms using the 12-lead electrocardiogram

Rhythm	Narrow	Wide

Regular	Short-RP
	  Typical (slow-fast) AVNRT
	  Atypical (slow-slow) AVNRT (usually)
	  Orthodromic AVRT
	  JT
	  AT (less commonly)
	Long-RP
	  Atypical (fast-slow) AVNRT
	  Orthodromic AVRT (slowly conducting
	    accessory pathway)
	  ST
	  AT (more commonly)
	  PJRT
	Flutter waves
	  AFl (fixed AV block)
		ST, JT, AT, AVNRT, orthodromic AVRT,
		  or AFl with aberrancy
		Antidromic AVRT
		Monomorphic ventricular tachycardia

Irregular	AF AFl (variable AV block) MAT	AF, AFl, or MAT with aberrancy AF, AFl with pre-excitation Polymorphic ventricular tachycardia

Abbreviations: AF, atrial fibrillation; AFl, atrial flutter; AT, atrial tachycardia; AVNRT, atrioventricular node reentrant tachycardia; AVRT, atrioventricular reentrant tachycardia; JT, junctional tachycardia; MAT, multifocal atrial tachycardia; PJRT, permanent junctional reciprocating tachycardia; ST, sinus tachycardia.

Focal atrial tachycardia

AT is initiated and sustained within the atria and is manifested by a single P wave morphology. The P wave morphology depends of the site of origin of the tachycardia. AT may be caused by automaticity, triggered activity, or microreentry [8–10]. Rarely, digitalis toxicity can result in AT, usually with accompanying AV nodal block [11]. AT is usually a long-RP tachycardia with an atrial rate usually less than 250 bpm and a ventricular rate dependent on the presence or absence of AV nodal block [1]. A classic example of focal AT is shown in Fig. 1.

AT caused by abnormal automaticity often exhibits a "warm-up" phenomenon in which the heart rate gradually speeds up before reaching a fixed peak. The diagnosis of AT caused by triggered activity is often made in the electrophysiology laboratory when the AT can be initiated by pacing the atrium at a critical rate. AT caused by microreentry is often seen in patients who have structural heart disease, usually is initiated by a premature atrial beat, and typically is paroxysmal. It often is impossible to distinguish triggered from reentrant AT. For AT caused by abnormal automaticity, adenosine usually results in AV nodal block without terminating the AT. On the ECG, this AT is manifested as discernible P waves continuing at the AT rate with occasionally conducted QRS complexes. In contrast, triggered ATs usually are terminated with adenosine. Although these general aspects of the different types of AT can be useful in diagnosis, significant overlap of these properties exists.

To help localize the origin of the AT, one can begin by analyzing the P wave polarity. To distinguish a right atrial from a left atrial location, aVL and V1 are the essential leads. P waves that are positive in V1 usually arise from the left atrium, whereas P waves that are positive in aVL usually arise from the right atrium or occasionally from the right pulmonary vein [12–15]. Positive P wave polarity in leads II, III, and aVF predicts a superior origin; negative P wave polarity in these leads predicts an inferior origin. The polarity of the P wave may be difficult to interpret if the P wave is inscribed upon the ST segment or T wave. Thus, the P wave morphology is interpreted best when the heart rate or ventricular rate is slowed, such as after adenosine administration. The finer points of P wave polarity during AT that are most relevant for the site of ablation are described in Table 2.

Multifocal atrial tachycardia

MAT is thought to be caused by enhanced automaticity of multiple competing atrial foci. MAT is almost always associated with pulmonary disease and rarely, if ever, is seen in the setting of digitalis toxicity. To make the diagnosis of MAT, at least three different P wave morphologies must be observed, which typically do not have a fixed relationship to one another. The heart rate is greater than 100 bpm and usually is irregular (varying R-R intervals); the PR intervals may vary; and AV nodal block may be present.

Atrial flutter

AFl is caused by a rapid macroreentrant circuit occurring in the atria. The atrial rate is usually 240 to 340 bpm; the ventricular rate varies,

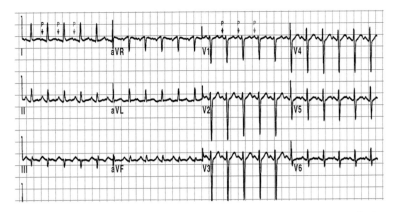

Fig. 1. Focal atrial tachycardia with 1:1 conduction. Note the narrow, regular tachycardia. The P waves are marked with arrows (long-RP interval), and the P wave morphology differs from that of sinus rhythm.

Table 2
P wave morphology in atrial tachycardia—general principles

Location			P wave polarity during atrial tachycardia
Right atrium	+ or ± in aVL and − in V1	Crista terminalis (CT)	May be +, ±, or − in II, II, aVF in the high, mid, and inferior CT, respectively; − or ± in V1; − in aVR
		Tricuspid annulus	− in V1-V2; + in aVL and frequently in I
		Right atrial appendage	Insufficient data
Left atrium	− in aVL and + in V1	Right pulmonary veins	+ in V1–V6; + in I; narrow P wave in V1
		Left pulmonary veins	+ in V1–V6; −/isoelectric in aVL; broad or notched P wave in V1
		Mitral annulus	± with initially narrow negative deflection in V1; −/isoelectric in I, aVL; slightly +/isoelectric in II, III, aVF
		Left atrial appendage	Broadly + in V1–V6; − in I, aVL; + in II, III, aVF
Interatrial septum and adjacent structures	Specific to location	Coronary sinus ostium	+ in V1; isoelectric in I; − in II, III, aVF; + in aVL, aVR
		Anteroseptum	−/± in V1; +/± in II, III, aVF
		Mid septum	−/± in V1; − in two of three inferior leads (II, III, aVF)
		Left septum	Uncommon; variable findings

Abbreviations: +, positive; −, negative; ±, biphasic.
From Refs. [12,15,42].

depending on the degree of AV nodal block. Of note, chronic antiarrhythmic therapy may prolong atrial refractoriness and slow the AFl rate [16]. The atrial-to-ventricular ratio can be regular (eg, 2:1, 4:1) or irregular if the degree of AV nodal block is variable. Unless the atrial rate is relatively slow, 1:1 conduction is unusual unless it occurs by an accessory pathway, which can result in wide pre-excited QRS complexes.

The nomenclature of AFl is based on electro-anatomic relationships observed during electrophysiology studies; if the circuit is dependent upon the cavotricuspid isthmus, it is defined as typical AFl [17–20]. The reentrant circuit in typical AFl traverses the musculature around the tricuspid valve. If this circuit activates the lateral right atrium from superior to inferior and the septum from inferior to superior, it is termed counterclockwise typical AFl. If the lateral and septal activations occur in reverse, while still being dependent on the cavotricuspid isthmus, it is termed clockwise typical AFl. In contrast to discrete P waves, typical AFl usually results in flutter waves having a saw-tooth pattern. An analysis of their polarity demonstrates that counterclockwise typical flutter waves are positive in V1 and negative in leads II, III, and aVF

(Fig. 2). Clockwise typical flutter waves are negative in V1 and positive in leads II, III, and aVF. Of note, although the macroreentrant circuit is located in the right atrium, the saw-tooth pattern and its polarity primarily reflect the axis and sequence of left atrial activation.

In contrast to typical AFl, atypical AFl is any other AFl that does not display a typical activation sequence. On the ECG, the saw-tooth flutter waves may be absent, and the flutter wave polarity differs from typical AFl. The flutter waves may be quite varied in appearance and may appear similar to discrete P waves. For example, in atypical AFl arising from the left atrial septum, the flutter waves are prominent in V1 but are flat in the other leads and may appear similar to AT [21,22]. The atrial rate of atypical AFl may also be quite varied, depending on the location and spatial extent of the macroreentrant circuit. Atypical AFl can originate in the left or right atrium, around a scar or surgical site, or around other structures, which partly explains the variability in its morphology and rate. The administration of adenosine can be important in the diagnosis of any type of AFl by virtue of its effect on the AV node: the slowing of the ventricular rate can make flutter waves more readily discernible.

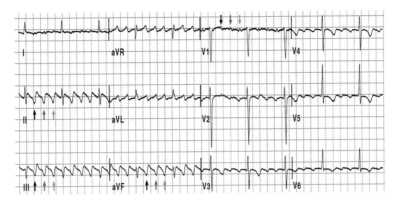

Fig. 2. Typical, counterclockwise atrial flutter. The flutter waves are marked with arrows. Four-to-one atrioventricular block is present, which facilitates examination of the flutter wave morphology. Note the characteristic saw-tooth appearance in the inferior leads (II, III, aVF) and the positive flutter wave polarity in lead V1.

ECG diagnosis of typical versus atypical flutter is clinically relevant, because the approach and success rate of catheter ablation differ [3,23,24].

Atrial fibrillation

The ECG hallmarks of AF include an irregularly irregular variation in R-R interval and the absence of organized atrial activity. Underlying AF may still be present even if the R-R intervals are regular when concomitant complete AV nodal block with a junctional or subjunctional escape rhythm is present (occasionally seen with digitalis toxicity). Coarse AF may be confused with AFl; very fine AF may be confused with atrial paralysis. In addition to AF, irregular junctional rhythms, MAT, and AFl with variable block are also in the differential diagnosis for irregularly irregular rhythms (see Table 1). The atrial rates in AF are variable but are usually greater than 350 bpm. The ventricular rate is usually significantly slower and varies depending on AV nodal function, unless an accessory pathway capable of antegrade conduction is present.

Atrioventricular node reentrant tachycardia

Initiation of AVNRT is dependent on the presence of dual AV node physiology, with two pathways having differing conduction and refractory times. AVNRT can be divided into typical and atypical forms, with the typical form being more common [2,25]. Typical AVNRT, also known as slow-fast AVNRT, uses a slow AV nodal pathway for antegrade conduction and a fast pathway for retrograde conduction

(Fig. 3). Atypical AVNRT can be slow-slow AVNRT, using a slow antegrade and another slow retrograde pathway (with different properties), or fast-slow, using a fast antegrade and a slow retrograde pathway. The heart rate in AVNRT can vary from 118 to 264 bpm (mean, 181 ± 35) and is similar to the rates seen in AVRT [26]. There typically is a 1:1 AV relationship in AVNRT, but because the reentrant circuit resides within the area of the AV node, 2:1 AV block can be seen. Retrograde AV nodal atrial block can occur also, although less commonly. Typical AVNRT is initiated with an atrial premature beat and terminates with a P wave (antegrade slow pathway). AVNRT is terminated by adenosine (>90% of the time) or vagal maneuvers, which can be useful in making a diagnosis [27].

Typical AVNRT is a short-RP tachycardia in which the earliest retrograde atrial activity is detected on the septum, near the AV node. The RP interval is usually less than 70 milliseconds [28]. Because retrograde atrial activation occurs over a fast pathway, the retrograde P wave is superimposed on the QRS and appears as a pseudo S wave (present during AVNRT but not during normal sinus rhythm) that is best seen in leads II, III, and aVF. Similarly, a pseudo R′ may also be present in lead V1. These ECG findings are important because they are infrequently seen in AVRT [29,30]. Having a pseudo S, a pseudo R′, or both is 90% to 100% specific for typical AVNRT and has an 81% positive predictive value for typical AVNRT [29,30]. These criteria are only 42% sensitive for typical AVNRT, however [29]. Occasionally in typical AVNRT (20% of the time), the P wave is buried

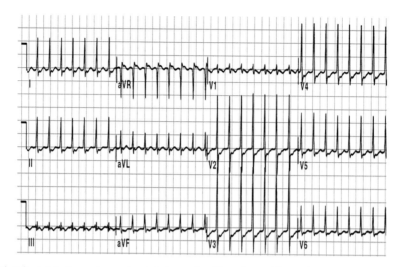

Fig. 3. Typical atrioventricular node reentrant tachycardia. Note the rapid, regular, narrow complexes, the pseudo S wave in leads I, II, and aVF, and the small pseudo R′ wave in lead V1.

within the QRS and is invisible [26]. Additionally, ST segment depression of ≥2 mm is less common in AVNRT and is seen to a lesser extent and in fewer leads than in AVRT [29]. In contrast to AVRT, QRS alternans is an uncommon finding in AVNRT and may be related more to the rapidity of the heart rate than to the underlying SVT mechanism [29,31]. Taking into account the pseudo S/R′ waves, the RP interval, and the lack of significant ST depression in multiple leads (the Jaeggi algorithm), a correct diagnosis of typical AVNRT can be made by ECG analysis 76% of the time [28,29].

In atypical (slow-slow) AVNRT, the retrograde atrial activation usually is seen first near the coronary sinus ostium. The P wave may be distinct from the QRS and appears negative in leads II, III, and aVF and positive in leads V1, V2, aVR, and aVL [32]. Atypical (slow-slow) AVNRT is usually a short-RP tachycardia and often cannot be distinguished from orthodromic AVRT, as discussed later [31,33].

Atypical (fast-slow) AVNRT is a long-RP tachycardia in which the earliest retrograde atrial activity is seen in the posteroseptal right atrium or in the coronary sinus. This form of AVNRT is thought to use the same pathways as in typical AVNRT, but in reverse [34]. The P wave precedes the QRS and is negative in leads II, III, and aVF and is positive in leads V1, V2, aVR, and aVL. Atypical (fast-slow) AVNRT may be indistinguishable from a low AT or orthodromic AVRT with a posteroseptal pathway.

Orthodromic atrioventricular reentrant tachycardia

The reentrant loop in AVRT is comprised of the atria, AV node, ventricle, and accessory pathway. In orthodromic AVRT, conduction occurs antegrade through the AV node and retrograde through an accessory pathway. Orthodromic AVRT is usually a short-RP tachycardia with an RP interval greater than 100 milliseconds [28,29]. If the accessory pathway has slow retrograde conduction, however, the RP is significantly longer, consistent with a long-RP tachycardia. Orthodromic AVRT also is a narrow complex tachycardia, unless bundle-branch block or aberrancy is present (Fig. 4). The heart rate in AVRT ranges from 124 to 256 bpm (mean, 183 ± 32 bpm) [32]. AVRT usually is initiated with one or more ventricular premature beats and usually terminates with a QRS complex. AVRT can be terminated by adenosine (>90% of the time) or vagal maneuvers [27].

In normal sinus rhythm, antegrade conduction over an accessory pathway resulting in a short PR interval and a delta wave on the surface ECG is the hallmark of the Wolff-Parkinson-White ECG pattern (Fig. 5). The delta wave is the ECG manifestation of ventricular pre-excitation. If no antegrade conduction is evident, but the pathway is capable of retrograde conduction, the pathway is defined as concealed. In Wolff-Parkinson-White, the disappearance of the delta wave during tachycardia is caused by orthodromic AVRT. The loss

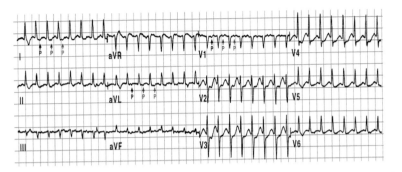

Fig. 4. Orthodromic atrioventricular reentrant tachycardia. Note the narrow, regular, rapid tachycardia. The P waves buried in the ST segment (short-RP interval) are marked with an arrow. No pseudo S/R' waves are seen.

of the delta wave during sinus rhythm results from the loss of pre-excitation caused by a poorly conducting accessory pathway incapable of conducting at higher rates.

Most patients who have orthodromic AVRT (81%–87%) have visible retrograde P waves that are best seen in leads I, II, III, aVF, and V1 [29,32]. QRS alternans (alternating QRS amplitude) is common (45% of cases), unlike AVNRT [29]. Also unlike AVNRT, ST segment depression of ≥2 mm is common in AVRT, particularly in patients who have no visible P wave or who have an RP interval less than 100 milliseconds; the ST depressions also are seen in several leads (mean, 4.4 ± 1.4 leads) [29]. By using the Jaeggi algorithm, which takes into account the absence of pseudo S/R' waves, an RP interval greater than 100 milliseconds, and the presence of ST depression of ≥2 mm, a correct diagnosis of AVRT can be made using the surface ECG 88% of the time [28,29].

After diagnosing AVRT, it is helpful to localize the pathway because the feasibility, approach, and success of catheter ablation depend on the pathway site. In Wolff-Parkinson-White syndrome, the polarity of the delta wave during normal sinus rhythm often predicts accessory pathway location unless multiple accessory pathways are present (an occasional finding) [36,37]. Accessory pathway localization based on the delta wave during normal sinus rhythm has been described in detail previously [38,39]. The polarity and morphology of the retrograde P wave during orthodromic AVRT also may assist in pathway localization [14,32,35]. In general, a positive P wave in leads II, III, and aVF suggests an anterior accessory pathway; a negative P wave in leads II, III, and aVF suggests an inferior accessory pathway; a positive P wave in lead V1 or a negative P wave in lead I suggests a left-sided accessory pathway; and a negative P wave in lead V1 or a positive P wave in lead I suggests a right-sided accessory pathway.

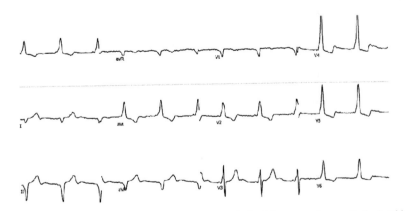

Fig. 5. Wolff-Parkinson-White pattern. Note the short PR interval, the delta waves (pre-excitation), which are positive in leads I and aVL and negative in leads II, III, and aVF, and the transition of the delta wave axis from lead V1 to V2 (consistent with a right posteroseptal accessory pathway).

The development of bundle-branch block aberrancy during SVT also can be a helpful clue. If the tachycardia cycle length slows when bundle-branch block appears, then the SVT is an AVRT and not AVNRT or AT, because the ventricle is not an integral component of the circuit in these latter two arrhythmias. More importantly, the slowing of the tachycardia cycle length in with the appearance of bundle branch block proves that this AVRT uses an accessory pathway with the pathway on the same side as the blocked bundle branch. The increase in cycle length can be explained by the additional conduction time required for the depolarization wave front to go from the normally conducting bundle branch (on the contralateral side) across the ventricular septum and into the accessory pathway and atrium.

Focal junctional tachycardia

JT is uncommon in adults and often is a diagnosis of exclusion. This arrhythmia is more common in children and often is irregular. In adults, JT manifests as a regular, short-RP tachycardia (if ventriculo-atrial [VA] conduction is present) with a narrow QRS complex, unless bundle-branch aberrancy is present. It can be caused by enhanced automaticity or triggered activity. The VA relationship may be dissociated, associated with 1:1 retrograde conduction, or associated with various degrees of VA retrograde block [36]. When dissociation is present, the P waves seen on the ECG are most likely caused by sinus rhythm. If the P waves appear associated with the QRS rhythm, they typically are negative in leads II, III, and aVF because of retrograde atrial activation. The diagnosis of JT is based primarily on tachycardia initiation without the need for a critical AV nodal delay. Beta-blockers are

the initial drug of choice, and ablation may be recommended for drug-refractory cases.

Permanent junctional reciprocating tachycardia

PJRT is an incessant long-RP tachycardia, typically seen in children but occasionally seen in adults, which may lead to tachycardia cardiomyopathy [37]. The cardiomyopathy frequently abates after successful treatment of the arrhythmia. In PJRT the heart rate is usually between 100 and 200 bpm but can vary significantly because of autonomic influences [37]. The arrhythmia uses the atria, AV node, the ventricle, and an accessory pathway and is similar to orthodromic AVRT. PJRT enters into the differential diagnosis of atypical AVNRT or AT originating from the inferior atrium. The accessory pathway usually is concealed and possesses decremental conduction properties. In most cases, the accessory pathway is within or near the coronary sinus ostium. PJRT usually starts spontaneously after a sinus beat and does not require a premature beat or a change in the PR interval for initiation. On the ECG, the QRS complexes usually are narrow and have a 1:1 AV relationship. The P waves usually are broad and negative in leads II, III, and aVF [38]. The RP interval is much longer in PJRT than in most orthodromic AVRTs. PJRT usually terminates in the retrograde limb, which is sensitive to vagal maneuvers [38,39].

Wide-complex supraventricular tachycardias caused by pre-excitation

It is important to differentiate patients who have pre-excited wide-complex tachycardia (WCT) from those who have SVT with aberrancy or ventricular tachycardia. Of particular concern are patients who have AF and AFl with antegrade

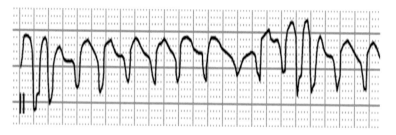

Fig. 6. Wide-complex tachycardia caused by atrial fibrillation in a different patient who had Wolff-Parkinson-White syndrome. Note the very rapid rate, the irregularity, and the wide, bizarre, varying QRS morphology caused by varying degrees of fusion from AV node conduction and antegrade accessory pathway conduction. The negative delta wave in lead II suggests a posterior (inferior) accessory pathway location.

conduction through an accessory pathway. Because the accessory pathway does not possess the same decremental conduction properties as the AV node, AF or AFl with antegrade conduction through an accessory pathway may conduct rapidly, often with ventricular rates greater than 280 to 300 bpm, and may degenerate into ventricular fibrillation. An irregular, rapid WCT should raise suspicion for AF with pre-excitation (Fig. 6). Similarly, AFl or AT with very rapid or 1:1 AV conduction should raise concern for pre-excitation. In all cases, delta waves should be present during tachycardia but may be overshadowed by the wide-complex morphology. In AF, AFl, or AT, varying degrees of fusion through the pathway and through the AV node may produce beat-to-beat variation in the QRS morphology. If the rhythm is maximally pre-excited, the QRS morphology may appear similar to that of patients who have ventricular tachycardia, but conversion to sinus rhythm will produce the pre-excitation pattern in patients who have Wolff-Parkinson-White syndrome.

Antidromic AVRT is a WCT that exhibits maximal pre-excitation (Fig. 7). In antidromic AVRT, conduction occurs antegrade through an accessory pathway and retrograde through the AV node. Delta waves should be evident both during normal sinus rhythm and during tachycardia. The retrograde P waves in antidromic AVRT are frequently seen in a 1:1 VA relationship preceding the QRS [40]. Because dual AV node physiology (having both fast and slow pathways) is common in patients who have accessory pathways, retrograde conduction may occur during antidromic AVRT by a slow AV nodal pathway,

a fast AV nodal pathway, or alternate between fast and slow AV nodal pathways [41]. Thus, the characteristics of the P wave and PR interval may vary during tachycardia.

Summary of steps required for ECG diagnosis of SVT

1. Assess QRS width and regularity.
2. Look for evidence of atrial activity.
3. If distinct P waves are seen
   - Determine the RP relationship
   - Evaluate the P wave morphology during SVT and, if possible, during normal sinus rhythm
   - Evaluate the AV relationship (eg, 1:1, 2:1, dissociated)
4. If flutter waves are seen or suspected
   - Evaluate their morphology, preferably if the ventricular rate can be slowed
5. If no P waves are seen
   - Look for irregularity or the absence of an isoelectric baseline, both suggesting AF
   - Look for a pseudo S/R′ to suggest AVNRT
6. Assess the underlying atrial and ventricular rates.
7. Examine the initiation (atrial premature beat, ventricular premature beat, warm-up, no initiating factors) and termination. (Does the SVT terminate with a P wave or a QRS; does it cool down slowly?)
8. Examine the response to adenosine. (Does it terminate the tachycardia, and, if so, how? Does it cause AV block, and, if so, what happens to the underlying atrial rhythm?)

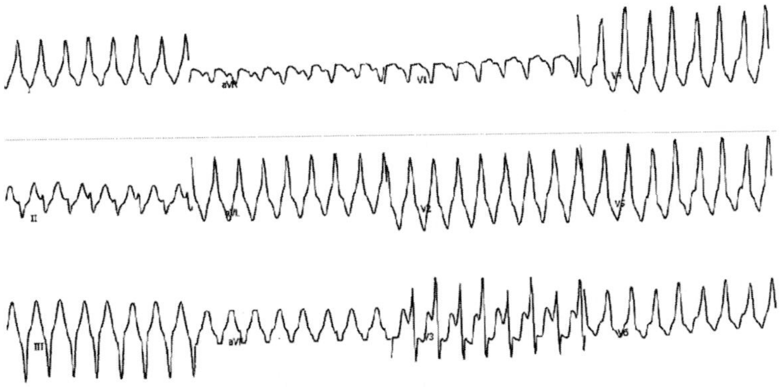

Fig. 7. Antidromic atrioventricular reentrant tachycardia in the same patient as in Fig. 5, using a right posteroseptal accessory pathway. Note the wide-complex, regular rhythm. The delta waves are more prominent because of maximal pre-excitation.

References

[1] Ganz LI, Friedman PL. Supraventricular tachycardia. N Engl J Med 1995;332:162–73.

[2] Blomstrom-Lundqvist C, Scheinman MM, Aliot EM, et al. ACC/AHA/ESC guidelines for the management of patients with supraventricular arrhythmias—executive summary. A report of the American College of Cardiology/American Heart Association Task Force on Practice Guidelines and the European Society of Cardiology Committee for Practice Guidelines (Writing Committee to Develop Guidelines for the Management of Patients with Supraventricular Arrhythmias) developed in collaboration with NASPE-Heart Rhythm Society. J Am Coll Cardiol 2003;42:1493–531.

[3] Scheinman MM, Huang S. The 1998 NASPE prospective catheter ablation registry. Pacing Clin Electrophysiol 2000;23:1020–8.

[4] van den Bosch AE, Roos-Hesselink JW, Van Domburg R, et al. Long-term outcome and quality of life in adult patients after the Fontan operation. Am J Cardiol 2004;93:1141–5.

[5] Weipert J, Noebauer C, Schreiber C, et al. Occurrence and management of atrial arrhythmia after long-term Fontan circulation. J Thorac Cardiovasc Surg 2004;127:457–64.

[6] Accardi AJ, Miller R, Holmes JF. Enhanced diagnosis of narrow complex tachycardias with increased electrocardiograph speed. J Emerg Med 2002;22:123–6.

[7] Marrouche NF, Beheiry S, Tomassoni G, et al. Three-dimensional nonfluoroscopic mapping and ablation of inappropriate sinus tachycardia. Procedural strategies and long-term outcome. J Am Coll Cardiol 2002;39:1046–54.

[8] Chen SA, Chiang CE, Yang CJ, et al. Sustained atrial tachycardia in adult patients. Electrophysiological characteristics, pharmacological response, possible mechanisms, and effects of radiofrequency ablation. Circulation 1994;90:1262–78.

[9] Haines DE, DiMarco JP. Sustained intraatrial reentrant tachycardia: clinical, electrocardiographic and electrophysiologic characteristics and long-term follow-up. J Am Coll Cardiol 1990;15:1345–54.

[10] Wu D, Amat-y-leon F, Denes P, et al. Demonstration of sustained sinus and atrial re-entry as a mechanism of paroxysmal supraventricular tachycardia. Circulation 1975;51:234–43.

[11] Smith TW, Antman EM, Friedman PL, et al. Digitalis glycosides: mechanisms and manifestations of toxicity. Part II. Prog Cardiovasc Dis 1984;26: 495–540.

[12] Kistler PM, Kalman JM. Locating focal atrial tachycardias from P-wave morphology. Heart Rhythm 2005;2:561–4.

[13] Tang CW, Scheinman MM, Van Hare GF, et al. Use of P wave configuration during atrial tachycardia to predict site of origin. J Am Coll Cardiol 1995;26: 1315–24.

[14] Waldo AL, Maclean AH, Karp RB, et al. Sequence of retrograde atrial activation of the human heart. Correlation with P wave polarity. Br Heart J 1977; 39:634–40.

[15] Yamane T, Shah DC, Peng JT, et al. Morphological characteristics of P waves during selective pulmonary vein pacing. J Am Coll Cardiol 2001;38: 1505–10.

[16] Tai CT, Chen SA. Mechanisms of antiarrhythmic drug action on termination of atrial flutter. Pacing Clin Electrophysiol 2001;24:824–34.

[17] Lee KW, Yang Y, Scheinman MM. Atrial flutter: a review of its history, mechanisms, clinical features, and current therapy. Curr Probl Cardiol 2005;30: 121–67.

[18] Yang Y, Varma N, Keung EC, et al. Reentry within the cavotricuspid isthmus: an isthmus dependent circuit. Pacing Clin Electrophysiol 2005;28:808–18.

[19] Scheinman MM, Yang Y, Cheng J. Atrial flutter: part II nomenclature. Pacing Clin Electrophysiol 2004;27:504–6.

[20] Olgin JE, Kalman JM, Fitzpatrick AP, et al. Role of right atrial endocardial structures as barriers to conduction during human type I atrial flutter. Activation and entrainment mapping guided by intracardiac echocardiography. Circulation 1995; 92:1839–48.

[21] Bochoeyer A, Yang Y, Cheng J, et al. Surface electrocardiographic characteristics of right and left atrial flutter. Circulation 2003;108:60–6.

[22] Goya M, Takahashi A, Nuruki N, et al. A peculiar form of focal atrial tachycardia mimicking atypical atrial flutter. Jpn Circ J 2000;64:886–9.

[23] Della BP, Fraticelli A, Tondo C, et al. Atypical atrial flutter: clinical features, electrophysiological characteristics and response to radiofrequency catheter ablation. Europace 2002;4:241–53.

[24] Marrouche NF, Natale A, Wazni OM, et al. Left septal atrial flutter: electrophysiology, anatomy, and results of ablation. Circulation 2004;109: 2440–7.

[25] Sung RJ, Styperek JL, Myerburg RJ, et al. Initiation of two distinct forms of atrioventricular nodal reentrant tachycardia during programmed ventricular stimulation in man. Am J Cardiol 1978;42:404–15.

[26] Tai CT, Chen SA, Chiang CE, et al. A new electrocardiographic algorithm using retrograde P waves for differentiating atrioventricular node reentrant tachycardia from atrioventricular reciprocating tachycardia mediated by concealed accessory pathway. J Am Coll Cardiol 1997;29:394–402.

[27] DiMarco JP, Miles W, Akhtar M, et al. Adenosine for paroxysmal supraventricular tachycardia: dose ranging and comparison with verapamil. Assessment in placebo-controlled, multicenter trials. The Adenosine for PSVT Study Group. Ann Intern Med 1990;113:104–10.

[28] Jaeggi ET, Gilljam T, Bauersfeld U, et al. Electrocardiographic differentiation of typical atrioventricular

node reentrant tachycardia from atrioventricular reciprocating tachycardia mediated by concealed accessory pathway in children. Am J Cardiol 2003; 91:1084–9.

[29] Arya A, Kottkamp H, Piorkowski C, et al. Differentiating atrioventricular nodal reentrant tachycardia from tachycardia via concealed accessory pathway. Am J Cardiol 2005;95:875–8.

[30] Kalbfleisch SJ, el-Atassi R, Calkins H, et al. Differentiation of paroxysmal narrow QRS complex tachycardias using the 12-lead electrocardiogram. J Am Coll Cardiol 1993;21:85–9.

[31] Kay GN, Pressley JC, Packer DL, et al. Value of the 12-lead electrocardiogram in discriminating atrioventricular nodal reciprocating tachycardia from circus movement atrioventricular tachycardia utilizing a retrograde accessory pathway. Am J Cardiol 1987;59:296–300.

[32] Chen SA, Tai CT, Chiang CE, et al. Electrophysiologic characteristics, electropharmacologic responses and radiofrequency ablation in patients with decremental accessory pathway. J Am Coll Cardiol 1996;28:732–7.

[33] Oh S, Choi YS, Sohn DW, et al. Differential diagnosis of slow/slow atrioventricular nodal reentrant tachycardia from atrioventricular reentrant tachycardia using concealed posteroseptal accessory pathway by 12-lead electrocardiography. Pacing Clin Electrophysiol 2003;26:2296–300.

[34] Yamabe H, Shimasaki Y, Honda O, et al. Demonstration of the exact anatomic tachycardia circuit in the fast-slow form of atrioventricular nodal reentrant tachycardia. Circulation 2001;104:1268–73.

[35] Chen SA, Tai CT, Chiang CE, et al. Role of the surface electrocardiogram in the diagnosis of patients with supraventricular tachycardia. Cardiol Clin 1997;15:539–65.

[36] Scheinman MM, Gonzalez RP, Cooper MW, et al. Clinical and electrophysiologic features and role of catheter ablation techniques in adult patients with automatic atrioventricular junctional tachycardia. Am J Cardiol 1994;74:565–72.

[37] Lindinger A, Heisel A, von Bernuth G, et al. Permanent junctional re-entry tachycardia. A multicentre long-term follow-up study in infants, children and young adults. Eur Heart J 1998;19:936–42.

[38] Gaita F, Haissaguerre M, Giustetto C, et al. Catheter ablation of permanent junctional reciprocating tachycardia with radiofrequency current. J Am Coll Cardiol 1995;25:648–54.

[39] Prystowsky EN, Yee R, Klein GJ. Wolff-Parkinson-White syndrome. In: Zipes DP, Jalife J, editors. Cardiac electrophysiology: from cell to bedside. 4th edition. Philadelphia: Saunders; 2004. p. 874.

[40] Packer DL, Gallagher JJ, Prystowsky EN. Physiological substrate for antidromic reciprocating tachycardia. Prerequisite characteristics of the accessory pathway and atrioventricular conduction system. Circulation 1992;85:574–88.

[41] Chen YJ, Chen SA, Chiang CE, et al. Dual AV node pathway physiology in patients with Wolff-Parkinson-White syndrome. Int J Cardiol 1996;56:275–81.

[42] Marrouche NF, SippensGroenewegen A, Yang Y, et al. Clinical and electrophysiologic characteristics of left septal atrial tachycardia. J Am Coll Cardiol 2002;40:1133–9.

ELSEVIER
SAUNDERS

CARDIOLOGY
CLINICS

Cardiol Clin 24 (2006) 439–451

Value of the 12-Lead ECG in Wide QRS Tachycardia

John M. Miller, MD*, Mithilesh K. Das, MD, Anil V. Yadav, MD,
Deepak Bhakta, MD, Girish Nair, MD, Cesar Alberte, MD

*Indiana University School of Medicine, Krannert Institute of Cardiology, 1801 N. Capitol Avenue,
Indianapolis, IN 46202, USA*

Mr. V., A 64-year-old man, came to the emergency room because of sudden onset of palpitations 2 hours earlier. He was mildly short of breath but had no chest pain; there was neither history of prior episodes nor even any cardiovascular illness aside from hypertension. On examination, he appeared somewhat anxious but comfortable, had blood pressure 110/70 and a regular heart rate at 155 beats per minute (bpm); he had no evidence of heart failure except for "occasional elevation in jugular venous pressure." ECG showed a regular rhythm at 145 bpm with a QRS duration of 160 milliseconds (Fig. 1); he had no prior ECGs. The staff doctors argued among themselves whether this was supraventricular tachycardia (SVT) or ventricular tachycardia (VT), eventually reasoning that with his normal blood pressure and mentation, it must be SVT. Just as he was about to receive an injection of adenosine, the tachycardia reverted to sinus rhythm at 75 bpm. After another hour's observation to ensure he was stable, Mr. V. was sent home with a diagnosis of SVT and told to make an appointment with a cardiologist. Two weeks later, he had another episode of palpitations but suddenly became very short of breath and passed out. His wife called 911, but when rescue workers arrived, refractory ventricular fibrillation was present and sinus rhythm could not be restored.

This story illustrates several of the difficulties encountered when a patient develops a wide QRS tachycardia (WQRST). A fundamental error—assuming that with a normal blood pressure and mental status, the rhythm must be SVT—led to an incorrect diagnosis with a relatively benign prognosis, whereas Mr. V. actually had VT (his peculiar neck vein pattern was cannon A waves) that put him at risk of sudden cardiac death—which, sadly, occurred 2 weeks later. In fact, his ECG in the emergency room (Fig. 1) clearly demonstrated most of the criteria that strongly favor a diagnosis of VT.

Few clinical situations cause more anxiety among physicians than caring for a patient with an ongoing episode of WQRST; one must act quickly and decisively (but often without the confidence that the action is correct), and the consequences of making an incorrect diagnosis are potentially disastrous. Because optimal long-term management depends on a correct initial diagnosis, the importance of correctly identifying the nature of the WQRST is obvious. In this article, we will review the ECG criteria that can help the clinician distinguish among the possible diagnoses. Most of these criteria have been in the literature for more than 15 years, but are still poorly recognized or applied by clinicians [1–8]. Clinical history [9] as well as nonelectrocardiographic methods, such as evaluation of neck veins for cannon A waves, variable intensity of S1, and use of carotid sinus massage, are also valuable in the differential diagnosis of WQRST and should not be ignored; however, a detailed discussion of these is beyond the scope of this article.

Definitions

In the following discussion, we will use these definitions:

> *Wide QRS complex tachycardia:* rhythm with QRS duration ≥120 milliseconds and rate ≥100 bpm

* Corresponding author.
E-mail address: jmiller6@iupui.edu (J.M. Miller).

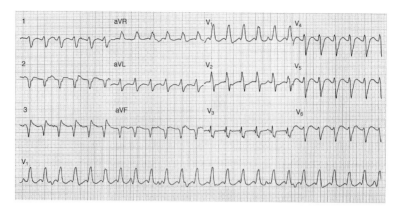

Fig. 1. ECG of patient in emergency room diagnosed as supraventricular tachycardia because of stable blood pressure. Correct diagnosis is ventricular tachycardia, by virtue of QRS duration, rightward superior axis, monophasic R in V1, R/S ratio <1 in V6, and atrioventricular dissociation.

Ventricular tachycardia: tachycardia requiring participation of structures below the bundle of His

Supraventricular tachycardia: tachycardia requiring participation of structures above bundle of His

Left bundle branch block (LBBB) configuration: QRS duration ≥120 milliseconds with predominantly negative terminal portion of lead V1

Right bundle branch block (RBBB) configuration: QRS duration ≥120 milliseconds with predominantly positive terminal portion of lead V1

Diagnostic possibilities

Possible causes of WQRST include the following (examples of leads V1 and V6 shown in Fig. 2):

1) Ventricular tachycardia—This is the most common cause of WQRST in all published series, accounting for 70% to 80% of cases depending on the population studied. Most cases occur in the setting of significant structural heart disease, and many patients are quite ill at the time of the rhythm. These features and the implications of the diagnosis of VT are in part responsible for the anxiety

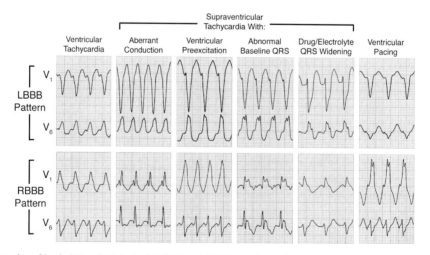

Fig. 2. Examples of leads V1 and V6 in both **LBBB** and **RBBB** configurations in each cause of WQRST. See text for further clarification.

provoked by seeing a patient with WQRST. Because ventricular activation is not mediated to any significant extent by the normal His-Purkinje system (HPS; His bundle, bundle branches, and fascicles), but is instead dependent on muscle–muscle conduction, the QRS complex during VT generally does not resemble true LBBB or RBBB.

2) Supraventricular tachycardia with:

a. Aberrant interventricular conduction (SVT-A)—BBB may be present at all times, including during the resting rhythm ("permanent"), or only during some episodes of WQRST due to refractoriness of one of the bundle branches. This may be purely due to the rapid rate or the suddenness of rate increase ("rate-related") from the baseline rhythm ("functional"). Because ventricular activation is mediated by the nonblocked portion of the HPS, the QRS complex in SVT resembles known patterns of BBB and fascicular block. In most WQRST series, SVT-A accounts for the second largest group after VT.

b. Abnormal ventricular activation using an atrioventricular (AV) accessory pathway (AP), such as with Wolff-Parkinson-White syndrome. In these so-called preexcited tachycardias, ventricular activation proceeds, at least in part, over an AP that bypasses the AV node. These pathways almost always insert into the epicardial aspect of ventricular muscle near the AV groove, remote from the HPS; muscle–muscle conduction is responsible for ventricular activation, as is the case with VT. Preexcited SVT is a relatively uncommon cause of WQRST among adults.

c. Abnormal baseline QRS configuration—Patients with a variety of disorders that alter the QRS complex during resting rhythm may have episodes of SVT conducted to the ventricles with the same abnormal QRS pattern. Disorders that produce bizarre QRS patterns include dilated and hypertrophic cardiomyopathy and repaired congenital heart disease. This group currently accounts for a small portion of all WQRSTs, but will probably increase in prevalence as more patients with repaired congenital heart disease reach adulthood, and patients with severe cardiomyopathies have improved longevity.

d. Nonspecific QRS widening due to electrolyte or drug effects—Transient metabolic abnormalities such as hyperkalemia and acidosis, as well as drug effects (procainamide and other Type IA or IC antirrhythmic drugs, amiodarone, and so on) can diffusely widen the QRS complex and transform an otherwise narrow complex SVT into one with a wide QRS. This is an uncommon but important group of WQRSTs; correct diagnosis relies on a good history and strong clinical suspicion of specific disorders. One clue to the presence of hyperkalemia is a normal or even short QT interval (usually with characteristic peaked T waves) during WQRST, in contrast to the slight prolongation of QT in the presence of a wide QRS complex.

3) Ventricular pacing—Although patients with ventricular pacemakers can certainly have ventricular rates > 100 bpm with a wide QRS, pacemaker stimulus artifacts ("spikes") are usually easily visible, and the nature of the rhythm is evident. However, in some cases pacemaker artifacts may be very small, such that the rhythm is not clearly recognized as paced. This relatively uncommon cause of WQRST is likely to become somewhat more prevalent with continuing advances in pacemaker technology (voltage regulation to pace just above threshold, and so on).

In all large series concerned with the differential diagnosis of WQRST, the overwhelming majority of cases are VT (up to 80%); the next largest group is SVT-A, with other diagnoses contributing a small fraction of cases. From a practical standpoint, it is thus clear that the major differential diagnosis of WQRST is between VT and SVT-A. In most other diagnoses, the QRS complex does not resemble any typical form of aberration. Thus, one approach to establishing the correct diagnosis for WQRST is to pose the question, "is the QRS complex compatible with some form of aberration?" If it is, the rhythm is likely SVT; if it is not, the rhythm is more than likely VT, with other possible diagnoses depending on clinical circumstances (pacemaker present, suspicion of hyperkalemia or drug effect, and so on).

ECG criteria

Many ECG criteria have been proposed to distinguish VT from SVT-A. These may be difficult to remember in the urgency of a clinical setting; however, if one recalls their basis—is the QRS compatible with aberration, or not?—it is easier to "reconstruct" the criteria and apply them correctly. These criteria have had variable sensitivity and specificity in prior studies, many of which contained relatively few cases. We therefore examined a series of 650 WQRSTs and evaluated the accuracy of the established criteria. In each case, the correct diagnosis was confirmed by electrophysiology study; ECGs were obtained from 385 individuals (279 [73%] men), aged 9–89 years (mean 53 ± 19 years) among whom structural heart disease was present in 54% (prior myocardial infarction in 38%, cardiomyopathy in 13%, and repaired congenital heart disease in 2%). Within this series, 473 (73%) WQRSTs were VT, 132 (20%) were SVT-A, 37 (6%) were preexcited SVT, 6 (<1%) were SVT with abnormal baseline QRS complex, 2 (<1%) were ventricular pacing with poorly evident stimulus artifacts; none in this series of WQRST evaluated at electrophysiology study were SVT with drug/electrolyte-based QRS widening. The proportion of preexcited SVT is probably higher than one would expect in a consecutive series of adult patients presenting to the health care system with WQRST, due to the selected nature of the population (referred for electrophysiology study).

The following paragraphs discuss the established criteria for the diagnosis of WQRST and particularly their ability to distinguish VT from SVT-A (Table 1).

1) *QRS duration*. It has been noted that in most cases of SVT-A, the QRS duration is ≤140 milliseconds in RBBB aberration, and up to 160 milliseconds in LBBB aberration [1]. Therefore, QRS complexes wider than this are less likely to be aberration, and thus VT is the more probable diagnosis. As noted above, influences that nonspecifically widen the QRS such as drug effects can decrease the value of this rule. In patients with VT occurring in the absence of structural heart disease, or in VTs with earliest activation in the septum in patients with structural heart disease, the QRS complex can be relatively narrow (sometimes even <120 milliseconds). Among SVT-A cases in our series, the mean (±SD) QRS duration was 136 ± 18 milliseconds (for VT, 166 ± 38 milliseconds, $P < 0.001$ compared with SVT-A); 77/132 (58%) of SVT-As had QRS duration ≤140 milliseconds versus 125/473 (26%) VTs

(sensitivity 0.58, specificity 0.73, negative predictive accuracy 0.86); thus, 348/473 (74%) of VTs had QRS duration >140 milliseconds. Further, only 28 (21%) of SVT-As in our series had a QRS duration in excess of 160 milliseconds, compared with 302 (64%) VTs ($P < 0.001$; sensitivity 0.64, specificity 0.79).

2) *QRS axis*. In most cases of SVT-A, the QRS axis is either normal (0° to +90°) or shows left anterior fascicular block (0° to −90°) or left posterior fascicular block (+90° to 180°). In our series, 124/132 (94%) of SVT-A ECGs had a frontal plane axis within these bounds versus 378/473 (80%) of VTs. However, an axis between −90° and 180° (rightward superior) is not readily achieved with any combination of BBB or fascicular block, and is thus unlikely to be SVT-A (therefore, VT). This is easily recognized on the standard 12-lead ECG, because leads 1, 2, and 3 are all predominantly negative (Fig. 1) [3]. In our series, 93/473 (20%) of VTs had an axis between −90° and 180° versus 5/132 (4%) of SVT-As ($P < 0.001$; sensitivity 0.20, specificity 0.96). Thus, although this is a highly specific criterion, preexisting QRS abnormalities can produce a rightward superior axis; a previous resting ECG, if available, can aid the analysis.

3) *QRS concordance*. A concordant pattern is one in which the predominant QRS deflection is either all positive or all negative across the precordial leads. This is a relatively uncommon pattern in SVT-A because with LBBB aberration, the negative QRS complex in V1 and V2 becomes positive in V4-6, and in RBBB aberration, tall terminal R waves in V1 and V2 diminish by V3 and V4 before increasing again in V5 and V6. In our series, 72/81 (88%) of ECGs with a concordant pattern were VT (Fig. 3). Although relatively specific for VT, only 15% of VTs demonstrated this finding. We found this to be more useful in RBBB-type QRS complexes ("positive" concordance): concordance was present in 46/254 (18%) of VTs with RBBB-type pattern, only 5/93 (5%) RBBB-type SVT-As showed concordance ($P < 0.005$, sensitivity 0.18, specificity 0.95). On the other hand, a negative concordant pattern discriminated poorly: only 26/219 (12%) of LBBB-type VTs showed negative concordance while 4/39 (10%) of SVT-As

Table 1
Summary of electrocardiographic criteria to distinguish VT from SVT-A

Criterion	VT	SVT-A	P value	Sensitivity	Specificity	PPA	NPA
QRS duration							
Mean ± SD	166 ± 38 ms	136 ± 18 ms	<0.001	—	—	—	—
≤140 ms	125/473 (26%)	77/132 (58%)	<0.001	0.58	0.73	0.38	0.86
≤160 ms	171/473 (36%)	104/132 (79%)	<0.001	0.64	0.79	0.38	0.92
QRS Axis							
Right superior (−90° to 180°)	93/473 (20%)	5/132 (4%)	<0.001	0.20	0.96	0.95	0.25
Right inferior (90° to 180°) w/LBBB	44/219 (20%)	1/39 (3%)	<0.01	0.20	0.97	0.98	0.18
Normal (0° to + 90°) w/RBBB	7/254 (3%)	21/93 (23%)	<0.001	0.23	0.97	0.75	0.77
QRS concordance							
Positive (RBBB-type)	46/254 (18%)	5/93 (5%)	<0.005	0.18	0.95	0.90	0.30
Negative (LBBB-type)	26/219 (12%)	4/39 (10%)	NS	0.12	0.90	0.87	0.15
Atrioventricular relationship							
AV dissociation	145/473 (31%)	0/132 (0%)	<0.001	0.31	1.00	1.00	0.29
1:1 AV relationship	38/473 (8%)	69/132 (52%)	<0.001	0.08	0.48	0.36	0.13
2:1 VA conduction	19/473 (4%)	0/132 (0%)	<0.02	0.04	1.00	1.00	0.22
VA Wenckebach	4/473 (1%)	0/132 (0%)	NS	0.01	1.00	1.00	0.22
Atrial fibrillation/flutter	20/473 (4%)	6/132 (5%)	NS	0.04	0.95	0.77	0.22
Indeterminate	247/473 (52%)	57/132 (43%)	NS	0.52	0.57	0.81	0.25
Dissociated, 2:1 or wenckebach	168/473 (36%)	0/132 (0%)	<0.001	0.36	1.00	1.00	0.30
QRS configuration in V1							
VT criteria[a]	460/473 (97%)	16/132 (12%)	<0.001	0.97	0.88	0.97	0.90
Onset-S Nadir >60 ms w/LBBB	170/219 (77%)	6/39 (15%)	<0.001	0.78	0.85	0.97	0.40
"Rs" complex	26/473 (5%)	0/132 (0%)	<0.01	0.05	1.00	1.00	0.23
"W" complex	26/473 (5%)	0/132 (0%)	<0.01	0.05	1.00	1.00	0.23
SVT-A criteria[a]	13/473 (3%)	116/132 (88%)	<0.001	0.97	0.88	0.97	0.90
QRS configuration in V6 in RBBB-type							
R/S ratio <1	188/254 (74%)	20/94 (24%)	<0.001	0.73	0.79	0.90	0.52
RS complex in precordial leads							
RS absent	139/473 (29%)	16/132 (12%)	<0.001	0.29	0.88	0.90	0.26
RS present, R-S interval >100 ms	241/334 (75%)	9/116 (8%)	<0.001	0.72	0.92	0.96	0.54
QRS alternans							
Present	7/473 (2%)	6/132 (5%)	<0.05	0.1	0.95	.054	0.21

Abbreviations: LBBB, left bundle branch block-type tachycardia; NPA, negative predictive accuracy; PPA, positive predictive accuracy; RBBB, right bundle branch block-type tachycardia; SVT-A, supraventricular tachycardia with aberration; VT, ventricular tachycardia.

[a] See text for details.

with LBBB pattern did so (P = NS; sensitivity 0.12, specificity 0.90). Of note, positive concordance can be observed in preexcited SVT because APs activate the ventricles from base to apex (positive complexes in precordial leads); right ventricular apical pacing can sometimes produce a negative concordant pattern.

4) *Atrioventricular relationship.* In SVT-A, with extremely rare exceptions, one must have at least as many atrial complexes as ventricular; in VT, atrial activation is not necessary for continuation of the rhythm, and thus one may observe a variety of non-1:1 AV relationships in VT. These include complete dissociation (generally sinus rhythm in the

A. Positive Concordance

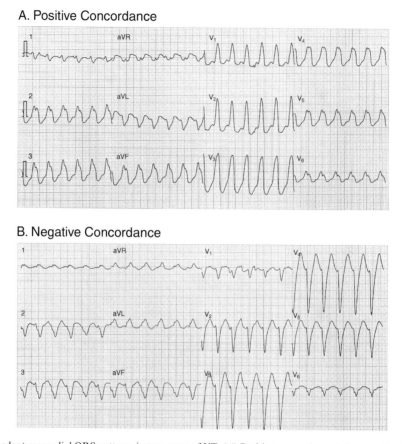

B. Negative Concordance

Fig. 3. Concordant precordial QRS patterns in two cases of VT. (*A*) Positive concordance (all precordial leads positive). (*B*) Negative concordance (all precordial leads negative). Note dissociated atrial activity in V1 of each ECG.

atria; Figs. 1 and 3), 2:1 retrograde (VA) conduction, and retrograde Wenckebach block. All of these are best discerned on a long rhythm strip rather than analyzing individual ECG leads (2–3 seconds' worth). ECG leads of greatest value in finding P waves are 2, 3, aVF, V1, and aVR. It is important to note that VT can have 1:1 retrograde conduction, mimicking SVT-A; this is especially problematic in young patients with VT in the absence of structural heart disease. Of equal importance is realizing that atrial activation may be unrelated to that of the ventricles, but one cannot discern this on the ECG either because of a rapid ventricular rate resulting in too much QRS complex, ST segment, and T wave to be able to see distinct P waves, the presence of atrial activation "buried" in a wide QRS complex, or the presence of atrial fibrillation or flutter. In our series, 145/473 (31%) of VTs

showed AV dissociation, 19 (4%) showed 2:1 retrograde conduction, and 4 (1%) had retrograde Wenckebach; thus, in 36%, the AV relationship was diagnostically helpful. On the other hand, 38 (8%) of VTs showed 1:1 retrograde conduction, atrial fibrillation was evident in 20 (4%), and in 247 (52%), the AV relationship could not be determined. Thus, in over half of VT cases, this criterion was not helpful. However, among available criteria for distinguishing SVT-A from VT, all but the AV relationship depend on having a relatively normal baseline ECG (which is not available for comparison in the vast majority of cases). Of note, not all cases of SVT-A show 1:1 conduction: surprisingly, this was clearly present in only 69/132 (52%) of SVT-A cases. In 6 (5%), atrial flutter was evident, while in 57 (47%), atrial activity could not clearly be discerned (occurring simultaneously with the wide QRS or otherwise obscured).

5) *Fusion and capture complexes.* Fused QRS complexes are those in which the QRS is a blend of two sources of activation (Fig. 4). This is typically seen in VT when an atrial complex encounters an AV node and HPS that have recovered from refractoriness related to the prior QRS and can activate some of the ventricular muscle over a portion of the HPS, while the next VT complex is also occurring. Rarely, a complete supraventricular capture complex occurs (all ventricular muscle activated from HPS). Understandably, these phenomena depend on (1) a non-1:1 AV relationship during VT and (2) a relatively slow VT rate; in the absence of these, the AV node would be maintained in refractoriness, and no atrial activations could penetrate the AV conduction system. Fusion complexes can occur during SVT-A (a premature ventricular complex occurring during SVT), but this is exceedingly rare. Although fusion/capture complexes are practically diagnostic of VT, they are very uncommon; only two VTs in our series showed this phenomenon (0.5%).

6) *Specific patterns in leads V1 and V6.* Configurations of the QRS in V1 and V6 can aid in distinguishing VT from SVT-A (also based on the principle that only certain patterns are compatible with aberration); examples of leads V1 and V6 from each diagnostic category are shown in Fig. 2 and more extensively in Fig. 5. These morphologic criteria are as follows:

a. *V1 in RBBB-type QRS.* Normally, initial ventricular activation occurs independent of the right bundle branch; thus, RBBB aberration should only affect the latter portion of the QRS, not its onset. In accordance with this principle, several patterns have been recognized as consistent with aberration (rR', rsR', rSr', rSR') [1], and others inconsistent therewith, indicating VT instead (qR, Rsr', monophasic R wave). Within our series, 116/132 (88%) SVT-As had a V1 configuration consistent with one of the listed aberration patterns compared with 13/473 (3%) VTs ($P < 0.001$; sensitivity 0.97, specificity 0.88). However, this criterion can occasionally be difficult to apply because the end of the T wave may distort the onset of the QRS in V1, simulating or obscuring a Q wave. Similarly, atrial activity (especially atrial flutter or fibrillation) may distort the initial portion of V1.

b. *V1 in LBBB-type QRS.* In true LBBB aberration, the initial portion of the QRS in V1 shows rapid activation, with an R wave duration (if present) ≤30 milliseconds and interval from QRS onset to S-wave nadir ≤70 milliseconds [4]. This pattern was observed in 33/39 (85%) of LBBB-type SVT-A ECGs, but only 49/219 (22%) 170/176 of LBBB-type VT ECGs. In contrast, a broad initial R wave (>30 milliseconds) or longer interval from QRS onset to S-nadir (>70 milliseconds) is not compatible with typical aberration, and thus WQRST with this pattern is more likely VT; 170/176 (97%) of ECGs with such a pattern were VT ($P < 0.001$; sensitivity 0.78, specificity 0.85, positive predictive accuracy 0.97). In addition, notching or slurring off the QRS complex suggests myocardial disease, the presence of which suggests a higher likelihood of VT.

c. *Other specific patterns in V1.* In cases of a tall R/small S ("Rs") as well as so-called

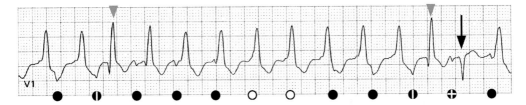

Fig. 4. Fusion and capture complexes. A rhythm strip of lead V1 is shown in a patient with RBBB-type VT; *black dots* indicated dissociated atrial activity (*white circle in center of dots* indicates a probable P wave hidden within a QRS complex). A fortuitously timed P wave (*black dot with vertical line*) can conduct and depolarize some of the ventricles (*arrowheads*), or rarely (*black dot with white cross*), completely capture the ventricles (*arrow*).

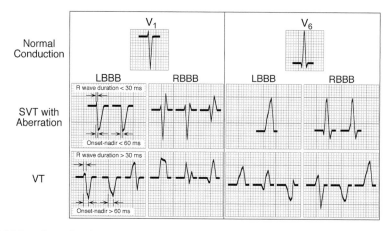

Fig. 5. Typical QRS configurations in SVT with aberration and VT in both LBBB and RBBB-type complexes. Note that with LBBB aberration, initial deflections are relatively rapid, whereas they occur much more slowly in VT. See text for further clarification.

"W" configuration in V1 (examples in Fig. 6), VT is the overwhelming diagnosis; in our series, all cases (26 [5%] "Rs," 26 [5%] "W") with either of these patterns were VT (specificity 1.0). It is difficult to achieve either of these patterns with any type of aberration.

d. *V6 in RBBB-type QRS.* Normally, the right ventricle's relatively small muscle mass contributes a small deflection in its direction, toward V1 and away from V6.

With RBBB aberration, this small contribution to the QRS is shifted later to appear as a small S wave. QRS patterns consistent with aberration are thus qRs or Rs. In contrast, because practically all RBBB-type VTs arise in the left ventricle, all of the right ventricular voltage plus some left ventricular voltage travels away from V6, yielding a different set of QRS patterns (qRS, qrS, rS, QS). This is the origin of the familiar R/S <1 rule (suggests

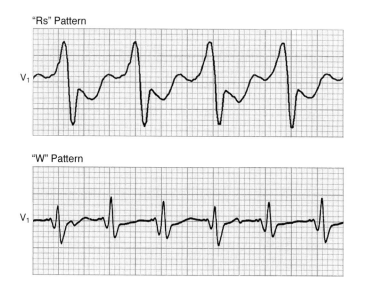

Fig. 6. Uncommon but highly specific configurations of lead V1 found only in VT. (*Top*) The "Rs" configuration; (*bottom*) the "W" configuration. Neither is compatible with standard aberration.

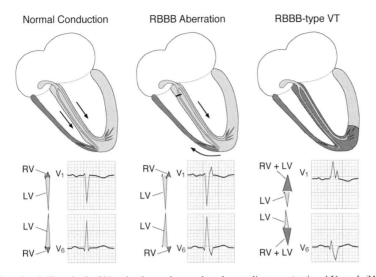

Fig. 7. Explanation for R/S ratio in V6 rule. In each panel, a heart diagram (atria, AV node/His bundle/bundle branches) and right (RV) and left ventricles (LV) is shown above representative ECGs of V1 and V6 in normal conduction, RBBB aberration, and RBBB-type VT. At the left of each ECG panel, the relative contribution of each ventricle to the ECG complex is depicted. The normal RV has a smaller mass and contributes less voltage than the LV. In normal conduction, the RV and LV components occur simultaneously, resulting in a narrow QRS. In RBBB aberration, the RV component is shifted later, resulting in the standard small terminal R in V1 and small terminal S in V6. In RBBB-type VT, all of the RV plus some of the LV voltage proceeds toward V1 and away from V6, resulting in a tall R wave in V1 and large S wave in V6 (R/S ratio <1).

VT; see Fig. 7). Among cases in our series showing RBBB-type QRS in which an RS complex was present in V6, 188/254 (74%) of VT ECGs had an R/S ratio <1, whereas 20/94 (24%) of SVT-A ECGs showed this. In 188/208 (90%) of ECGs with an R/S ratio <1, the correct diagnosis was VT ($P < 0.001$; sensitivity 0.73, specificity 0.79, positive predictive accuracy 0.9).

e. *V6 in LBBB-type QRS.* In typical LBBB aberration, V6 usually shows a monophasic R wave with a slow upstroke. This is, unfortunately, quite common in VT as well; however, a qR or QS should not be seen in V6 with true LBBB aberration and these strongly suggest VT when present.

7) *Absent RS in precordial leads* [10]. In most cases of either RBBB or LBBB aberration, at least one precordial lead has an "RS" configuration, and the interval from R wave onset to S wave nadir is ≤100 milliseconds; in a WQRST in which none of the precordial leads has an RS complex, or in which the R–S interval exceeds 100 milliseconds, aberration is unlikely to be the cause, and

therefore, VT is the likely diagnosis (Fig. 3A and Fig. 8). In the original series incorporating these criteria, the "absent RS" feature was not frequently present (only 15% of VTs, but no SVTs); adding the R–S interval >100 milliseconds criterion allowed a diagnosis in almost half of their cases (AV dissociation and traditional patterns in V1 and V6 were also used in the algorithm). In our series, an RS complex was absent in 140/473 (30%) VT ECGs as opposed to 9/132 (8%) SVT-A ECGs. Thus, 140/156 (90%) ECGs in our series showed no RS complex in the precordial leads (positive predictive accuracy 0.9). The utility of the R-S interval was somewhat less than the originators or the criterion found (sensitivity 0.99, specificity 0.97). As with the criteria for lead V1 noted above, other features of the ECG (particularly T waves) can distort the QRS complex to either simulated or obscure a small Q wave, the presence of which would make the criterion "negative."

8) *Miscellaneous features.* Rightward inferior axis deviation in LBBB SVT-A is extremely rare (1/39 LBBB SVTs [3%] in our series);

A. Ventricular Tachycardia

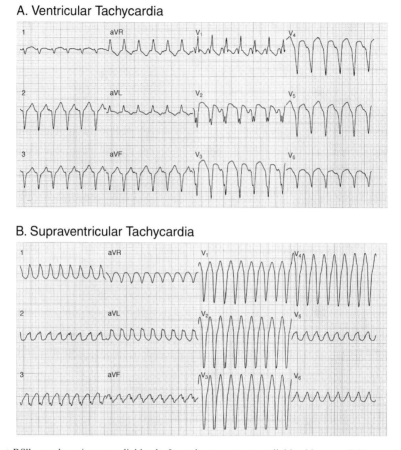

B. Supraventricular Tachycardia

Fig. 8. "Absent RS" complexes in precordial leads. In each case, no precordial lead has an "RS" complex (hence, "absent RS"). Although considered to be highly suggestive of VT, the *bottom* panel shows a LBBB SVT tachycardia with no RS complexes in precordial leads.

this combination should suggest VT as the WQRST diagnosis (present in 44/219 [20%] of LBBB-type VTs in our series [$P < 0.01$, specificity 0.97]). In addition, RBBB-type VT rarely has a normal axis (0° to +90°); this combination should likewise suggest SVT-A (combination was present in 21/93 [23%] of RBBB-type SVT-As in our series versus 7/254 [3%] RBBB-type VTs; [$P < 0.01$, specificity 0.97]).

9) *QRS alternans* (Fig. 9). Beat-to-beat alternation of the QRS amplitude is often associated with narrow-complex orthodromic SVT incorporating an accessory AV pathway; alternans of ≥ 0.1 mV can also be seen in WQRST, whether SVT-A or VT. In one study of WQRST, alternans was present in about equal frequency in SVT-A and VT

(35%) but more leads showed alternans in SVT-A (mean seven leads) than in VT (mean three leads) [11]. In our series, alternans was far less common; only 15 cases showed this feature, with a disproportionate number in the SVT-A group (6/132 [5%]) as opposed to the VT group (7/473 [2%]; $P < 0.05$, sensitivity 0.05, specificity 0.99). It is not clear why the findings in the current series differ so greatly from the prior one. The presence of alternans did not appear to have any relationship to tachycardia cycle length, and of interest, patients with multiple WQRSTs typically showed alternans in only one. Further, two episodes of the same tachycardia did not necessarily both show alternans. Reasons for these peculiar features are not known.

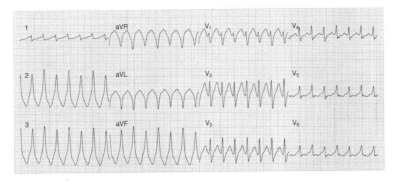

Fig. 9. QRS alternans during VT. Voltage changes in alternate complexes are noted in all limb leads as well as V1 and to a lesser extent, all other leads except V3 and V4 (alternans is also noted in Fig. 8A).

The preceding criteria can be applied when only the WQRST ECG is available; as health information systems become more integrated, it should be possible to readily access a WQRST patient's prior ECGs for comparison. In such cases, the following additional criteria can be applied [2,5]:

1) *Identical QRS configuration between baseline and WQRST* [2,12,13]. In cases in which the WQRST complexes are identical to those of the baseline ECG, it is very likely that the WQRST is SVT. Only very rare cases of VT show this similarity; the one important exception is bundle branch reentrant VT, in which both the resting ECG and VT have a LBBB pattern [14,15].

2) *Contralateral BBB patterns in baseline versus WQRST ECGs.* If a patient has resting RBBB in sinus rhythm and has an episode of LBBB-type tachycardia, the tachycardia is very unlikely to be SVT with LBBB aberration, because (at least in principle) both conduction pathways would be blocked and one should see only P waves. However, it is clear that some cases of apparent BBB are instead bundle branch delay (especially in a diseased left bundle branch), and thus, it is not uniformly true that contralateral BBB in resting rhythm versus WQRST is diagnostic of VT.

3) *WQRST complexes narrower than baseline ECG* [14]. In this situation, the baseline ECG must have a very wide BBB pattern, with a narrower QRS complex during tachycardia caused by a septal tachycardia origin (activating both ventricles nearly simultaneously) or early engagement of the HPS. Because of these considerations, this unusual

phenomenon suggests VT as the cause of the WQRST.

It is worth noting in passing that rate and regularity of the rhythm are not helpful discriminators between SVT-A and VT. A ventricular rate of 150 bpm should prompt one to think of atrial flutter, but otherwise, the degree of overlap in ventricular rate among WQRSTs is such that it has no differential diagnostic value. An irregular WQRST is almost always atrial fibrillation; other SVTs and VT are only rarely irregular (enough R-R variation to be evident on the surface ECG—usually >40 milliseconds).

Some authors have attempted to use combinations of ECG criteria to yield a higher proportion of correct diagnoses. In one such effort, Griffith and colleagues [16] found that a history of myocardial infarction, QRS morphology in aVF and V1, and frontal plane axis deviation >40° different from the baseline ECG correctly identified 90% of WQRSTs. This algorithm relies on clinical history and prior ECG, one or both of which may not be available.

Application of criteria

Correct application of established diagnostic criteria remains a significant problem in management of patients with WQRST. As an example of this, two cardiologists and two emergency physicians were asked to apply the algorithm by Brugada and colleagues [17] to 157 WQRSTs; the sensitivity and specificity of diagnoses were 0.85–0.91 and 0.55–0.60, respectively, for the cardiologists, while the emergency physicians' numbers were 0.79–0.83 and 0.43–0.70, respectively.

These contrast to the sensitivity (0.987) and specificity (0.965) in the original paper by the algorithm's developers. This disparity does not call into question either the validity of the algorithm or its designers' honesty; expert ECG interpreters who are focused on the task of carefully applying an algorithm would naturally be expected to yield better results than those who are less practiced in this exercise. These results do illustrate that even relatively simple and straightforward criteria for differentiating among causes of WQRST often fall short in their "real world" application.

Time and again, instead of intelligently applying valid ECG criteria to a WQRST patient (perhaps because of the difficulty in either recalling or correctly applying them), clinicians fall back on the appearance of the patient to make their diagnosis: if he has a good blood pressure and mental status, the WQRST must be SVT. Inappropriate treatment based on incorrect diagnoses has led to disastrous results [18,19]. However, if one recalls nothing else about diagnosing the cause of WQRST, in most clinical settings a simple guess of VT will be correct >70% of the time [20]. A corollary to this is that if there is doubt as to the diagnosis of WQRST, it is safest to treat as VT.

Summary

A wealth of useful diagnostic criteria is available to assist the health care worker in arriving at the correct diagnosis in cases of WQRST. Despite the abundance of good criteria for determining the diagnosis in cases of WQRST, they are of no use if they cannot be readily applied in an urgent clinical situation because they cannot be easily recalled or are too complex and cumbersome to use. It may be that refresher courses in the differential diagnosis of WQRST, especially for emergency physicians who are often the "first responders" to patients with WQRST, can improve physicians' diagnostic accuracy in this important disorder.

References

[1] Wellens HJ, Bär FW, Lie KI. The value of the electrocardiogram in the differential diagnosis of a tachycardia with a widened QRS complex. Am J Med 1978;64:27–33.

[2] Dongas J, Lehmann MH, Mahmud R, et al. Value of preexisting bundle branch block in the electrocardiographic differentiation of supraventricular from ventricular origin of wide QRS tachycardia. Am J Cardiol 1985;55(6):717–21.

[3] Reddy GV, Leghari RU. Standard limb lead QRS concordance during wide QRS tachycardia. A new surface ECG sign of ventricular tachycardia. Chest 1987;92(4):763–5.

[4] Kindwall KE, Brown J, Josephson ME. Electrocardiographic criteria for ventricular tachycardia in wide complex left bundle branch morphology tachycardias. Am J Cardiol 1988;61(15): 1279–83.

[5] Kremers MS, Black WH, Wells PJ, et al. Effect of preexisting bundle branch block on the electrocardiographic diagnosis of ventricular tachycardia. Am J Cardiol 1988;62(17):1208–12.

[6] Marriott HJ. Differential diagnosis of supraventricular and ventricular tachycardia. Cardiology 1990; 77(3):209–20.

[7] Antunes E, Brugada J, Steurer G, et al. The differential diagnosis of a regular tachycardia with a wide QRS complex on the 12-lead ECG: ventricular tachycardia, supraventricular tachycardia with aberrant intraventricular conduction, and supraventricular tachycardia with anterograde conduction over an accessory pathway. Pacing Clin Electrophysiol 1994; 17(9):1515–24.

[8] Alberca T, Almendral J, Sanz P, et al. Evaluation of the specificity of morphological electrocardiographic criteria for the differential diagnosis of wide QRS complex tachycardia in patients with intraventricular conduction defects. Circulation 1997;96(10):3527–33.

[9] Baerman JM, Morady F, DiCarlo LA Jr, et al. Differentiation of ventricular tachycardia from supraventricular tachycardia with aberration: value of the clinical history. Ann Emerg Med 1987;16(1): 40–3.

[10] Brugada P, Brugada J, Mont L, et al. A new approach to the differential diagnosis of a regular tachycardia with a wide QRS complex. Circulation 1991;83(5):1649–59.

[11] Kremers MS, Miller JM, Josephson ME. Electrical alternans in wide complex tachycardias. Am J Cardiol 1985;56(4):305–8.

[12] Halperin BD, Kron J, Cutler JE, et al. Misdiagnosing ventricular tachycardia in patients with underlying conduction disease and similar sinus and tachycardia morphologies. West J Med 1990; 152(6):677–82.

[13] Olshansky B. Ventricular tachycardia masquerading as supraventricular tachycardia: a wolf in sheep's clothing. J Electrocardiol 1988;21(4):377–84.

[14] Miller JM. The many manifestations of ventricular tachycardia. J Cardiovasc Electrophys 1992;3:88–107.

[15] Oreto G, Smeets JL, Rodriguez LM, et al. Wide complex tachycardia with atrioventricular dissociation and QRS morphology identical to that of sinus rhythm: a manifestation of bundle branch reentry. Heart 1996;76(6):541–7.

[16] Griffith MJ, De Belder MA, Linker NJ, et al. Multivariate analysis to simplify the differential diagnosis of broad complex tachycardia. Br Heart J 1991; 66(2):166–74.

[17] Isenhour JL, Craig S, Gibbs M, et al. Wide-complex tachycardia: continued evaluation of diagnostic criteria. Acad Emerg Med 2000;7(7):769–73.

[18] Stewart RB, Bardy GH, Greene HL. Wide complex tachycardia: misdiagnosis and outcome after emergent therapy. Ann Intern Med 1986;104(6): 766–71.

[19] Buxton AE, Marchlinski FE, Doherty JU, et al. Hazards of intravenous verapamil for sustained ventricular tachycardia. Am J Cardiol 1987;59(12):1107–10.

[20] Steinman RT, Herrera C, Schuger CD, et al. Wide QRS tachycardia in the conscious adult. Ventricular tachycardia is the most frequent cause. JAMA 1989; 261(7):1013–6.

CARDIOLOGY
CLINICS

Cardiol Clin 24 (2006) 453–469

Electrocardiographic Markers of Sudden Death

Peter Ott, MD*, Frank I. Marcus, MD

*Sarver Heart Center, University of Arizona Health Sciences Center, 1501 N. Campbell Avenue,
Tucson, AZ 85724, USA*

Sudden cardiac death (SCD) is defined as abrupt loss of consciousness due to cardiac arrest in a person who was previously in a stable condition. That most of these events are due to ventricular arrhythmias is supported by data from (a) fortuitous Holter ECG recordings of patients at the time of sudden death, (b) electrocardiographic recordings at the scene of a patient in cardiac arrest, and (c) stored electrogram data from patients with an implantable cardioverter defibrillator (ICD). However, it can be difficult to know the actual cause of death even in patients who die suddenly. For example, autopsy studies in patients with known heart disease and at high risk for ventricular arrhythmias showed that sudden death events were due to nonarrhythmic or noncardiac death mechanisms in 7 of 17 sudden death victims [1].

Sudden death accounts for >60% of all cardiac deaths, and remains a significant public health problem. The SCD rates range from 270/100,000 in female to 410/100,000 in male adults >35 years of age. For each gender group the rate is higher in African Americans than in the White population. Each year, approximately 400,000 to 450,000 patients die form this condition in the United States alone [2]. Citing retrospective data, Myerberg and colleagues [3] have drawn attention to the fact that, although the risk for SCD is greatest in those patients with significant structural heart disease, these high-risk patients contribute a relatively low number of total SCD victims. The greatest number of SCD occurs in a population with minimal or no prior history of heart disease. In those patients, SCD is the first presentation of heart disease.

A prospective study in The Netherlands [4] collected clinical data in patients suffering sudden death over a 3-year period. A total of 2030 deaths occurred in inhabitants age 25 to 75; of those, 375 (18%) were sudden deaths. A history of prior heart disease was absent in half of all sudden death victims, and less the half of those with a prior myocardial infarction (MI) had significant left ventricular (LV) dysfunction (ejection fraction [EF] <30%). These prospective data confirm that the majority of sudden death victims cannot be identified before the event.

During the last 10 years, the ICD has been shown to be effective in terminating sustained ventricular arrhythmias, thus aborting sudden arrhythmic death. Several clinical trials [5,6] have shown that ICD therapy, when added to optimal medical therapy, significantly improves survival in selected patients with decreased LV function. To significantly decrease the total number of SCD events, risk stratification is needed to identify patients at risk from a large pool of adults with no or minimal overt symptoms of heart disease, because it is this group that contributes the largest number of SCD victims.

Sudden death in the general population

Autopsy studies of victims of SCD show a healed MI in more than one half of these cases, even if there is no prior history of coronary artery disease. Significant coronary artery disease is present in 70% to 80% of SCD victims, while 10% to 15% have a dilated cardiomyopathy (CMP) [7,8]. Other abnormalities seen are ventricular hypertrophy, inflammation, and infiltration. In clinical reports structural abnormalities were absent in up to 10% of SCD survivors [9,10].

---

* Corresponding author.
E-mail address: ottp@email.arizona.edu (P. Ott).

454   OTT & MARCUS

A routine 12-lead ECG may identify a prior MI by showing typical Q-wave infarct pattern, or it may show increased R-wave voltage, suggesting primary or secondary ventricular hypertrophy. Nonspecific ST/T wave changes with intraventricular conduction delay may suggest the presence of a possible CMP. These ECG abnormalities raise the clinical suspicion of structural heart disease, but they are not specific predictors for sudden death, because the incidence of SCD is relatively low even in the presence of such structural heart disease.

Sudden cardiac death in patients with coronary artery disease

Acute ischemia, during an MI, leads to major metabolic and cellular abnormalities, which may result in ventricular fibrillation (VF) and SCD (Fig. 1). This can be the first manifestation of coronary artery disease (CAD); VF due to acute ischemia is a major cause of SCD in the general population [11].

The typical Q-wave infarct pattern on the 12-lead ECG persists indefinitely in >80% of patients but disappears after months to years in approximately 15% of patients. In 15% to 40% of infarcts the classical Q-wave pattern does not develop (non-Q-wave infarction).

The presence of a remote or recent MI is not specific for predicting future SCD events. In the era of aggressive reperfusion therapy for MI, the incidence of sudden death early after MI is low. In the GISSI-2 trial [12], 8600 patients were followed after thrombolytic therapy for acute MI. During a 6-month follow-up, the total mortality rate was only 3%, with one third of these deaths being classified as SCD. Although the presence of ventricular arrhythmias was a predictor of both sudden death (relative risk [RR] 2.2) and total mortality (RR 1.4), the absolute risk of SCD was low. In another trial [13], in which 1400 MI survivors with frequent nonsustained ventricular arrhythmias were randomized to placebo or amiodarone therapy, the annual sudden death rate was only 3.5% over a 2-year follow-up in either group, and was unaffected by amiodarone therapy. Thus, given the low absolute risk for SCD in most patients post-MI, it remains difficult to attempt to reliably identify those at high risk for SCD.

In a recent ICD trial [5], the benefit for ICD therapy seemed to be greatest in those patients with a prolonged QRS duration (>120 milliseconds) on the baseline 12-lead ECG. This raised the question as to the predictive value of QRS duration with regard to arrhythmic death. Zimetbaum and colleagues [14] reviewed electrocardiographic data of patients from the MUSTT trial. In this trial, 1638 patients with chronic ischemic heart disease, who had a reduced LVEF (<40%) and nonsustained V, and who were not inducible during electrophysiologic study, were

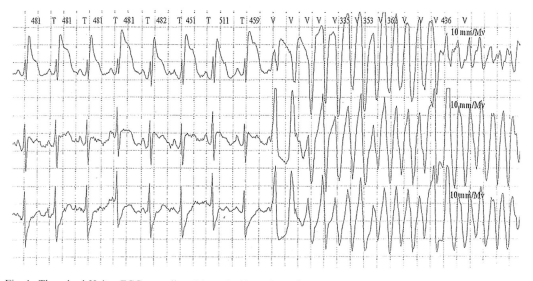

Fig. 1. Three-lead Holter ECG recording (25 mm/s, 10 mm/mV) from a 65-year-old male with CAD and normal LV function. He died suddenly while wearing the Holter recorder. Note the ST segment elevation, indicating myocardial ischemia, preceding the onset of VF.

followed in a registry for 5 years. Indeed, electrocardiographic findings of left bundle branch block (LBBB) (but not right bundle branch block [RBBB]) or LV hypertrophy (LVH) were associated with increased risk (hazard ratio of 1.49 and 1.35) for arrhythmic death.

There is no reliable ECG marker that is both sensitive and specific to predict SCD in patients with CAD. The combination of prior MI and reduced LVEF identified patients that benefit form an ICD as primary prophylaxis for SCD.

Sudden cardiac death and congestive heart failure

Despite optimal medical therapy, the mortality rates are high (15–35% at 2 years) for patients with symptomatic heart failure, and one third to two thirds of these deaths are sudden [15,16]. Although clinical data show that most of these events are due to ventricular arrhythmias, a subset of these patients with severe heart failure have sudden death due to bradyarrhythmias and electromechanical dissociation [17]. In patients with chronic systolic LV dysfunction, the 12-lead ECG may show evidence of a prior MI or nonspecific changes: 25% to 50% have an intraventricular conduction delay or BBB pattern, and many show nonspecific ST/T wave changes [18]. Atrial and ventricular arrhythmias are frequently seen. However, there are no specific 12-lead ECG markers that would predict the risk for sudden death. In particular, patients with chronic heart failure frequently have premature ventricular beats (PVCs) and/or nonsustained ventricular tachycardia (VT), which may be seen on routine ECG. However, while asymptomatic nonsustained ventricular arrhythmias predict total mortality, they have not been shown to be an independent specific predictor of SCD [19].

There is no reliable ECG marker that is both sensitive and specific to predict SCD in patients with congestive heart failure (CHF). The combination of prior CHF and impaired LV systolic function identified patients that benefit form an ICD as primary prophylaxis for SCD [6].

Sudden cardiac death in hypertrophic cardiomyopathy

This is an autosomal dominant disease with variable penetrance, affecting specific proteins of the cardiac myocyte contractile apparatus [20]. Over one half of genotyped patients show mutations in genes encoding for proteins of the beta-myosin heavy chain, myosin binding protein C and cardiac troponin-T.

Patients may present with dyspnea due to diastolic LV dysfunction, palpitations due to atrial dysrhythmias or syncope, and sudden death due to ventricular arrhythmias. A hallmark of this disease is ventricular hypertrophy, which may be regionally pronounced such as in the septum or at the LV apex. The main role of the 12-lead ECG is to provide a clue for the presence of this condition by showing clinically unexpected signs of LVH with or without precordial voltage and ST/T wave changes (Fig. 2). These abnormalities can be very striking [21]. Up to one third of patients may have abnormal Q waves, mostly in the anterolateral leads (I, aVL, V4–V6), often mimicking MI. These Q waves are thought to be related to septal hypertrophy and abnormal septal forces at the onset of ventricular depolarization. Left atrial enlargement and atrial arrhythmias are common [22]. The association of hypertrophic CMP (HCMP) and accessory pathways remains poorly defined, and atrioventricular (AV) conduction disturbances are uncommon.

Based on data from tertiary centers, the annual mortality rate is 3% to 6% [23]. However, recent data from nontertiary centers, representing community cohorts of patients, not influenced by referral bias, report a 1% annual mortality rate [24]. Except for accidental death, HCMP is the most common cause of SCD in young people including athletes [25]. VF is the mechanism of sudden death that has been supported by stored electrogram data from ICDs. Several clinical markers have been found to identify high-risk patients: history of prior cardiac arrest or sustained VT, family history of sudden death, unexplained syncope, decreased blood pressure response to exercise, severe LVH (>30 mm). Of note, the QRS voltage on a 12-lead ECG correlates poorly with echocardiographic LVH [26]. Electrocardiographic evidence of progressive LVH, however, portends a poor overall prognosis [27]. The apical form of HCMP [28], which may show impressive T-wave inversions in the precordial leads, has a low risk for sudden death.

Sudden cardiac death and arrhythmogenic right ventricular dysplasia/cardiomyopathy

The pathologic hallmark of arrhythmogenic right ventricular dysplasia/cardiopmyopathy

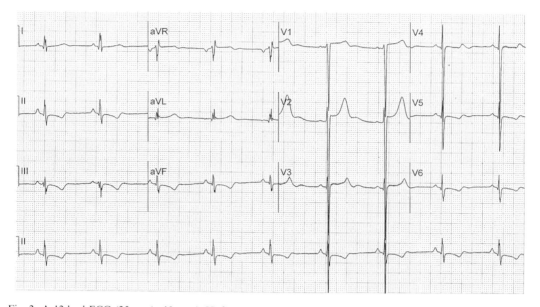

Fig. 2. A 12-lead ECG (25 mm/s; 10 mm/mV) from a 19-year-old male with HCMP and a family history of sudden death. Note the increased S-wave voltage in leads V1 to V5 consistent with LVH. Diffuse ST/T wave changes are also present. This patient's LV wall thickness measured 28 mm on echocardiography.

(ARVD/C) is patchy, fibrofatty replacement of myocytes altering myocardial depolarization and repolarization. Patients may present with PVCs or nonsustained or sustained VT, which may result in syncope. These arrhythmias typically have a LBBB morphology [29]. Some individuals may have cardiac arrest as a result of ventricular arrhythmias. In endemic areas for ARVD/C, autopsy studies suggest that up to 20% of unexpected deaths in individuals younger than 35 years may be due to ARVD/C [30]. This condition is genetically determined, and a familial history of syncope premature sudden death can be found in a sizeable minority of patients. Genetic studies have revealed both autosomal dominant and autosomal recessive transmission patterns. Eight genetic loci have been identified that primarily affect genes encoding for cell junction proteins such as desmosomes as well as the gene encoding the cardiac ryanodine receptor, suggesting altered intracellular myocyte calcium handling [31,32].

Important clinical clues for the diagnosis are abnormal findings in the 12-lead ECG in individuals with apparently normal hearts: (1) T-wave inversion in V1 to V3, (2) QRS duration ≥110 milliseconds in V1 to V3, (3) presence of epsilon waves. These ECG findings are included as diagnostic criteria [33].

Repolarization abnormalities, such as precordial T-wave inversion in leads V1 to V3 can be seen frequently in normal children. Although T-wave inversion in V1 is also seen frequently in young adults of both genders, T-wave inversion in leads V2 and V3 is not seen in healthy male adults and only rarely seen in female adults [34]. Thus, in a young adult, presenting with PVCs or VT of LBBB pattern, precordial T-wave inversion in V1 to V3 should raise the suspicion for ARVD/C (Fig. 3). At least one half of ARVD/C patients presenting with VT will have precordial T-wave inversion, and the extent of T-wave inversion correlates with the degree of RV dysplasia.

Abnormalities in depolarization are common in patients with ARVD/C. Fontaine [35] reported that a prolonged QRS duration (>110 milliseconds) in lead V1 had a sensitivity of 55% and specificity of 100% for ARVD/C. About one third of patients show an epsilon wave: a discrete late potential after the end of the QRS (Fig. 4). Its recognition is enhanced by recording the ECG at double speed (50 mm/s), double scale (20 mm/mV), and altered filter settings (40 Hz) [36]. A prolonged S wave upstroke in V1 to V3 (S wave nadir to isoelectric baseline: ≥55 milliseconds) was identified in 37 of 39 (95%) patients with ARVD/C. Other ECG features relate to the delay in RV depolarization—the so-called parietal

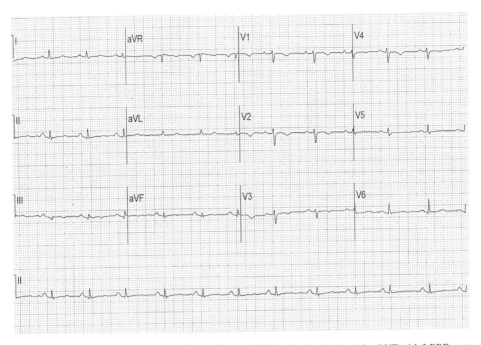

Fig. 3. A 12-lead ECG (25 mm/s; 10 mm/mV) from a 39-year old female, who had sustained VT with LBBB pattern. She was diagnosed with ARVD/C. Note the T-wave inversion in leads V1 to V4.

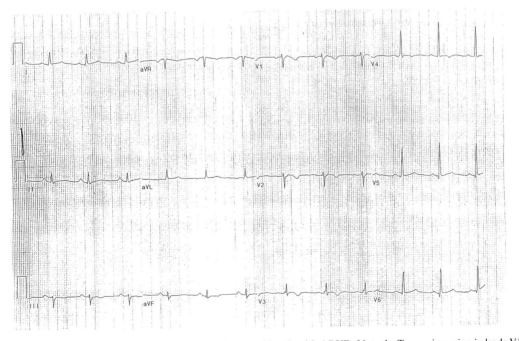

Fig. 4. A 12-lead ECG (25 mm/s; 10 mm/mV) in a 47-year-old male with ARVD. Note the T-wave inversion in leads V1 and V2 and low-amplitude, low-frequency "epsilon waves" following the QRS in leads V1 and V2.

block: these include a QRS duration in lead V1 to V3 exceeding QRS duration in V6 and the ratio of QRS duration V1 to V3/V4 to V6 ≥1.2.

When evaluating young adults with LBBB/inferior axis PVCs or VT, the challenge is to determine the etiology of the arrhythmia. The differential diagnosis is: RV outflow tract (RVOT) PVC/VT or ARVD/C. The former tends to be benign, and is not genetically determined; the latter may be associated with SCD, and may be genetically determined. In a recent study [36] evaluating ECG features in both clinical conditions, precordial T-wave inversion in V1 to V3 was present in 33 of 39 (85%) patients with ARVD/C but in none of 28 patients with RVOT PVC/VT. Similarly, delayed S-wave upstroke in V1 to V3 was present in 37 or 39 (95%) of ARVD/C patients and only in 1 of 28 (7%) RVOT PVC patients. This suggests that these two ECG markers could be useful in determine the etiology of the arrhythmia and clinical decision making.

These ECG findings, together with morphologic evaluation of RV, structure and function aid in the clinical diagnosis of ARVD/C. Risk stratification for sudden death has been evaluated by two groups [37,38]. In general, low-risk patients have the following characteristics: (1) upright T waves in V1 to V6, (2) less QRS and QT dispersion, (3) no history of syncope, (4) no LV involvement, or (5) normal or minimal RV involvement. However, prospective evaluation of these risk factors alone or in combination has not been done.

Sudden cardiac death and long QT syndrome

In the mid-1950s, Jervell and Lange-Nielson [39] described the association of an abnormally long QT interval on the 12-lead ECG and sudden death in individuals with congenital hearing loss. This was found to be an autosomal recessive condition. Later, a familial long QT syndrome (LQTS) was also recognized in those with normal hearing and found to be an autosomal dominant disorder. The disease prevalence is estimated at 1:7000. Patients, often with familial clustering, show QT interval prolongation on the 12-lead ECG, and are prone to polymorphic VT, which may result in syncope or SCD. Structural heart disease is absent. The normal corrected QT interval (QTc; QT interval corrected for heart rate, Bazett formula) in 578 adults is <430 milliseconds in men and <450 milliseconds in women. A prolonged QTc interval, seen in only 1% of

individuals is ≥460 milliseconds for men and ≥480 milliseconds for woman [40]. QT interval prolongation, in the absence of structural heart disease, electrolyte abnormalities, and drugs that prolong the QT interval is suggestive of LQTS (for a list see www.QTdrug.org). However, the measurement of the QTc interval to diagnose the LQTS reveals overlap with normal values. A recent study [41] examined the QTc intervals of 83 genotyped carriers and 119 noncarriers. The QTc ranged from 410 to 590 milliseconds (mean 490 milliseconds) for gene carriers and 380 to 470 milliseconds (mean 420 millseconds) for noncarriers. A diagnostic QTc cutoff of >440 milliseconds would have misdiagnosed 22 of 199 (11%) noncarrier individuals, whereas a diagnostic cutoff of >470 milliseconds would have resulted in a false negative diagnosis in 40% of male and 20% of female gene carriers. Thus, a diagnostic scoring system [42] using clinical factors and ECG features, including QTc interval and T-wave abnormalities, has been proposed to estimate the likelihood of LQTS.

Although originally attributed to an "imbalance" in sympathetic cardiac innervations, it is now established that mutations of genes coding for various cardiac ion channels are responsible for this disease. These genetic defects result in prolongation of the action potential repolarization and thus an increase in the QT interval on the 12-lead ECG. Genetic analyses have identified defects in six genes of genotyped patients; 90% have defects in the genes coding for ion channels carrying repolarizing potassium currents: the I-Ks ion channel (LQT1, chromosome 11) (Fig. 5) and the I-Kr ion channel (LQT2, chromosome 7). A smaller proportion of patients carry genetic mutations in the gene coding for the sodium channel (LQT3, chromosome 5). The T-wave morphology on the 12-lead ECG can provide clues to the underlying genetic defect: broad-based prolonged T-wave in LQT1, low-amplitude T wave in LQT2 and late onset T wave in LQT 3 [43] (Fig. 6). Clinical data has shown gene specific risk [44] and triggers [45] for arrhythmias.

Cardiac potassium channels are sensitive to catecholamines, and cardiac events frequently occur during stress or exertion particular in LQT1. Thus, several groups have evaluated infusion of epinephrine on the QT interval and T waves in patients with LQTS. In one study [46], the infusion of low-dose epinephrine (0.5 μg/kg/min) resulted in an increase in the QT interval (+82 ± 34 milliseconds) in 19 patients with LQT1 syndrome,

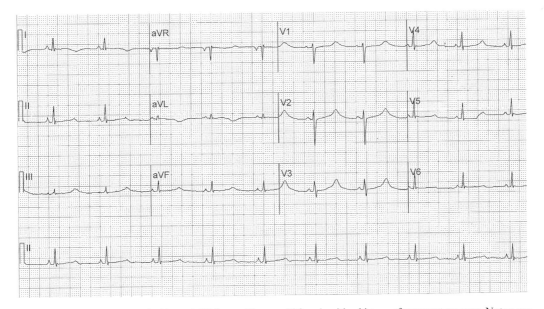

Fig. 5. A 12-lead ECG (25 mm/s; 10 mm/mV) from a 35-year-old female with a history of recurrent syncope. Note a pro-longed QT interval (QTc = 540 milliseconds) with a broad-based T wave. Genotype testing in this patient documented a defect in the I-Ks ion channel gene (LQT1 syndrome). The patient later had syncope while swimming due to docu-mented VF and survived due to successful ICD therapy.

compared to no change (-7 ± 13 milliseconds) in 27 control patients. The same group [47] also de-scribed epinephrine-induced qualitative T-wave changes during infusion of low-dose epinephrine; notched T waves appeared in 75% of LQT2 pa-tients, but were also seen in 26% and 34% of LQT1 and controls, respectively. T-wave notching beyond the peak of the T wave, however, was seen exclusively in patients with LQT2 syndrome. These data suggest a role of epinephrine infusion in diag-nosing LQTS, especially in patients with borderline electrocardiographic findings.

Risk stratification in patients with suspected LQTS relies on clinical and family history: syn-cope, sudden death, and documented torsade de pointes. Electrocardiographic parameters such as

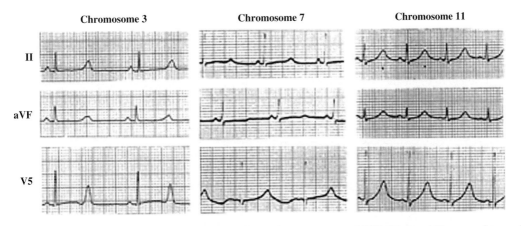

Fig. 6. ECG tracings in patients with different long QT syndrome genotype. LQT3: late-onset T waves of normal duration; LQT2: flat low-amplitude T waves; LQT1: early-onset of broad-based T waves. (*From* Moss AJ, Zareba W, Benhorin J, et al. ECG T-wave patterns in genetically distinct forms of the hereditary long QT syndrome. Circulation 1995;92:2929–34, with permission.)

QT duration and T-wave morphology also appear to be useful. A recent report [48] on data form 647 genotyped patients, of whom 90% were LQT1 and LQT2, correlate the risk for arrhythmic events with sex, QTc duration, and genotype. In a multivariate analysis, a QTc > 500 milliseconds was highly predictive of arrhythmic events in patients with LQT1 and LQT2. The presence of T-wave alternans on an ECG has long been recognized as a predictor for arrhythmic events. A recent study [49] from the LQT registry confirmed a high risk of clinical events in 30 patients with T-wave alternans (Fig. 7). However, the presence of T-wave alternans was strongly related to QTc prolongation, and after adjustment for this, it was no longer an independent marker for arrhythmic events. T-wave notching [50], independent of QT duration, may be a predictor for arrhythmic events. In a small study, T-wave notching, present in 33 of 53 (62%) LQTS patients was more prevalent in 30 of 37 (81%) patients with a history of syncope or cardiac arrest versus 3 of 16 (195) patients those without symptoms (P < 0.001).

Sudden cardiac death and short QT syndrome

Since its original description in 2000 [51], a small number of cases with familial sudden death and strikingly short QT interval (220–290

milliseconds) have been reported. The QRS complex is normal, and the ST segment is virtually nonexistent. The T waves are narrow based, tall, and symmetric (Fig. 8). The clinical spectrum ranges from aborted sudden death due to VF in an infant, to recurrent syncope in otherwise healthy adults [52]. Structural heart disease was absent, and secondary causes for QT interval shortening (hyperkalemia, hypercalcemia, and digitalis therapy) were carefully excluded. Some patients also had atrial fibrillation. During electrophysiologic evaluation, short atrial and ventricular refractory periods were noted and VF was easily induced with programmed ventricular stimulation. Recent genetic studies revealed mutations in genes coding for subunits of cardiac potassium channels, resulting in "gain of function" and thus an enhanced action potential repolarization [53]. A clear diagnostic cutoff for the QT interval has not yet been established. In a clinical series of 27 patients [54] the QT interval ranged from 210 to 320 milliseconds (mean 267 ± 33 milliseconds) and the QTc interval ranged from 250 to 340 milliseconds (mean 298 ± 21 milliseconds). Recent data [55] suggests that therapy with quinidine (but not sotalol or ibutilide) can prolong the abnormally short QT and render VF noninducible. It is not known if this will be a successful long-term therapy.

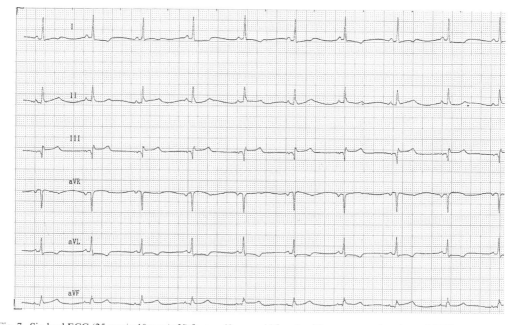

Fig. 7. Six-lead ECG (25 mm/s; 10 mm/mV) from a 40-year-old female with syncope and prolonged QT interval. T-wave alternans is present, best seen in lead I and lead II.

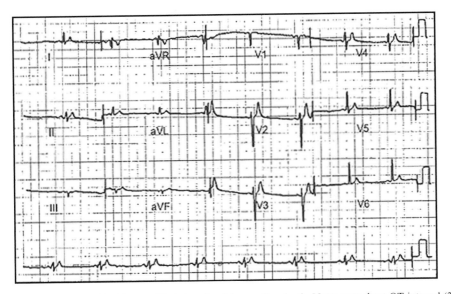

Fig. 8. Twelve-12 lead ECG of a 37-year-old victim of sudden cardiac death. Note: very short QT interval (266 milliseconds), normal QRS duration, and absence of ST segment. (*From* Gussak I. Brugada P, Brugada J, et al. Idiopathic short QT interval: a new clinical syndrome? Cardiology 2000;94:99–102; with permission.)

Sudden cardiac death and Brugada syndrome

In 1992, Brugada and colleagues [56] described a clinical syndrome consisting of apparently healthy adults presenting with syncope or sudden death. Their ECGs showed coved ST segment elevation and negative T waves in leads V1 and V2 (V3) in the absence of RBBB pattern (Fig. 9). This ECG pattern has become to be known as the "Brugada-ECG." These patients were thought to have no evidence of structural heart disease, and were at high risk for recurrent syncope or sudden death. In 15% to 20% of patients a genetic defect in the cardiac sodium channel was found [57]. It has been proposed that there is a premature termination of the epicardial action potential with loss of the phase-2 dome pattern. The ECG changes are believed to be due to regional epicardial–endocardial voltage gradient during the plateau phase of the action potential. This voltage gradient may give rise to VT due to phase-2 reentry caused by inhomogeneity of the voltage in adjacent areas of the myocardium [58]. In patients with the Brugada syndrome, syncope and sudden death are due to polymorphic VT. Since the original description, it has been observed that the "Brugada-ECG"-type ST segment elevation in the right precordial leads can be (1) cove shaped, (2) saddle shaped, (3) transient, and (4) be present in a multitude of clinical conditions. There has

been a recent attempt to standardize this diagnostic ECG feature as follows: type I; coved-shaped right precordial ST elevation, in more than one right precordial lead (V1–V3), of ≥2 mm followed by a negative T wave: type II: saddle-shaped ST elevation: and type III: ST elevation of <2 mm (Fig. 9). Only type I is said to be diagnostic of Brugada syndrome [59]. These ST elevations are sensitive to heart rate and the effects of autonomic stimulation [60]. Furthermore, sodium channel-blocking antiarrhythmic drugs such as procainamide or flecainide have been shown to "provoke" these ECG changes in patients with otherwise normal baseline ECG, and have been proposed as a screening tool in patients suspected to have the Brugada syndrome [61,62]. However, the sensitive, specificity and reproducibility of this drug provocation are not well established. Of interest, certain gene mutations are sensitive to temperature with regard to their phenotypic expression [63]. Indeed, Brugada-type ECG changes have been seen in patients only during febrile illness (Fig. 10). Some speculate that seizures during febrile illness may be related to self-terminating ventricular arrhythmias due to a temperature sensitive mutation in the sodium channel, giving rise to the "Brugada syndrome."

Patients with resuscitated sudden death or syncope or with a family history of premature sudden death and typical type I Brudaga ECG

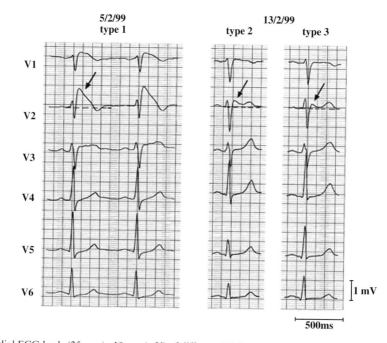

Fig. 9. Precordial ECG leads (25 mm/s; 10 mm/mV) of different ECG patterns in Brugada syndrome. Type I: coved ST segment elevation in leads V1 and V2 (and V3) followed by a negative T wave. Type II: saddleback-type ST segment elevation ≥2 mm. Type III: saddleback-type ST segment elevation <2 mm. (*From* Wilde AA, Antzelevitch C, Borggrefe M, et al. Proposed diagnostic criteria for the Brugada syndrome: consensus report. Circulation 2002;106: 2514–8; with permission.)

changes are at increased risk of recurrent events, and should be considered for ICD therapy. Asymptomatic patients who have an unprovoked typical Brudaga ECG (type I) are also at increased risk for arrhythmic events, but the magnitude of the risk is unclear. In one study the event rate over a mean of 24 months follow-up was 8% in these patients. Those presenting with typical Brugada ECG (type I) only after drug exposure or those presenting with nondiagnostic right precordial ECG abnormalities (type II, type III) are believed to be at low risk [59]. The role of electrophysiologic study and prognostic value of inducible VF remain controversial [64–66].

Sudden cardiac death and idiopathic ventricular fibrillation

A small group of patients with may have VF but have no demonstrable heart disease and have a normal 12-lead ECG. In particular, the QT interval will be normal, there are no changes suggestive of Brugada syndrome, and there is no family history of either condition. Minor structural and electrocardiographic abnormalities are

permitted [67]. This category is likely a heterogeneous group of patients, and further clinical and genetic studies may be able to focus on specific disorders within this group.

Based on careful analysis of clinical data, Coumel and his group described two distinct entities:

(1) Short coupled variant of torsade de pointes [68]: in this description, 14 patients (mean age 34 ± 10 years) of either sex, presented with syncope (one with resuscitated sudden death) and one third had a family history of sudden death. Structural heart disease was absent and the 12-lead ECG was normal. In particular, the QT interval was normal. Close coupled PVCs (coupling interval to preceding QRS: 245 ± 25 milliseconds) were noted and observed to degenerate into torsade de pointes (Fig. 11). Over a 7-year follow-up, five patients died (four suddenly) and nine were alive, three of whom had an ICD.

(2) Cathecholaminergic polymorphic VT [69]: in this series, 21 children (mean age 10 ± 4 years) of either sex presented with exertional

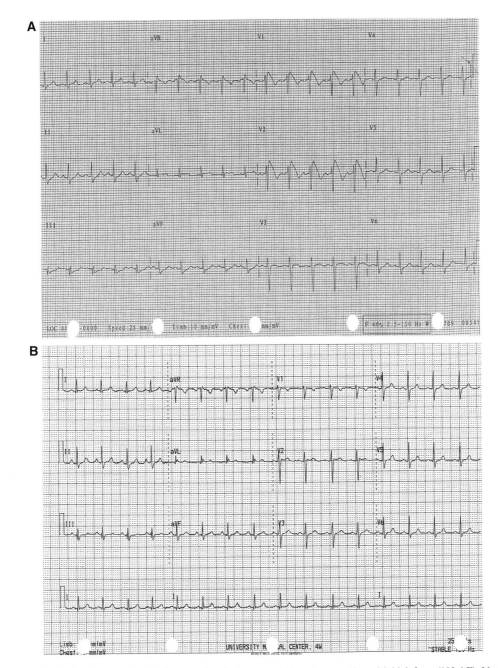

Fig. 10. (*A*) A12-lead ECG (25 mm/s; 10 mm/mV) of a 34-year-old female presenting with high fever (103.4 F). Note the coved ST elevation (3 mm) in leads V1 and V2, followed by a negative T wave – consistent with type I Brugada ECG pattern. (*B*) The ECG completely normalized once the fever resolved. Neither the patient nor her family had any history of syncope or sudden death.

syncope. Again, there was no structural heart disease and the QT interval was normal. One third of patients had a family history of syncope or sudden death. Adrenergic stimulation reproducibly resulted in a progressive pattern of polymorphic extrasystole, bidirectional tachycardia, and polymorphic VT degenerating into VF (Fig. 12). A recent

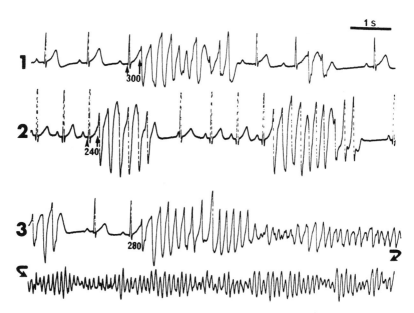

Fig. 11. Single-lead ECG strip from a 15-year-old male with syncope. Note: frequent close coupled PVCs, initiating non-sustained polymorphic VT degenerating into VF. (*From* Leenhardt A, Glaser E, Burguera M, et al. Short coupled variant of Torsade de Pointes. A new electrocradiographic entity in the spectrum of idiopathic ventricular fribrillation. Circulation 1994;89:206–15; with permission.)

study [70] in three affected families revealed mutations of the ryanodine receptor, indicating abnormalities in intracellular calcium handling as the mechanism of ventricular arrhythmias.

In a recent study [71], 18 patients with unexplained cardiac arrest and no evident cardiac disease (normal LV function, coronary arteries, and resting corrected QTc) underwent pharmacologic challenges with adrenaline and procainamide

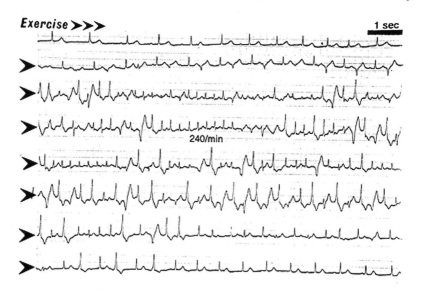

Fig. 12. Single-lead ECG strip during stress testing in a 7-year-old male with a history of exertional syncope. Note the progressive appearance of ventricular ectopy and bidirectional ventricular tachycardia. These arrhythmias disappeared with termination of exercise. (*From* Leenhardt A, Lucet V, Denjoy I, et al. Catecholaminergic polymorphic ventricular tachycardia in children. A 7-year follow-up of 21 patients. Circulation 1995;91:1512–9; with permission.)

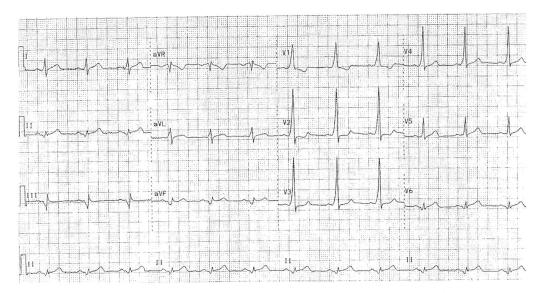

Fig. 13. Twelve-lead ECG (25 mm/s; 10 mm/mV) from a 35-year-old man with recurrent palpitations and documented SVT. The ECG shows a classic preexcitation pattern: short PR interval, slurred onset of QRS (delta wave), and increased QRS duration. Note: pseudo-Q waves in the inferior leads due to negative delta waves.

infusion to unmask subclinical primary electrical disease. The final diagnose was catecholaminergic VT in 10 patients (56%), Brugada syndrome in two patients (11%), and unexplained VF in six patients (33%).

Sudden cardiac death and Wolff-Parkinson-White syndrome

The presence of one or more accessory pathways spanning the AV groove gives rise to the typical preexcited pattern of the QRS complex on

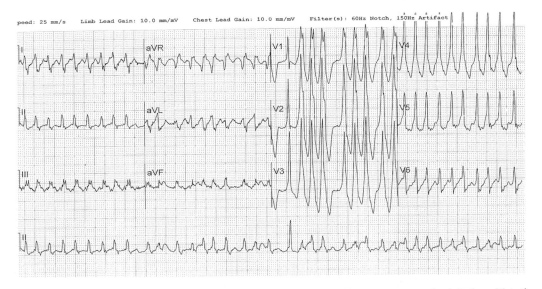

Fig. 14. A 12-lead ECG (25 mm/s; 10 mm/mV) from a 17-year-old male with near syncope and palpitations. Note the fast, irregularly irregular wide and narrow QRS complexes, typical for atrial fibrillation with fast AV conduction via the accessory pathway. The shortest preexcited RR interval is 200 milliseconds.

the 12-lead ECG: (a) short PR interval, (b) slurred onset of QRS complex (delta wave), and (c) prolonged QRS duration (Fig. 13). The prevalence of preexcitation on routine ECG is variably reported between approximately 3/1000 [72] to 5/10,000 [73]. Several algorithms, primarily using the delta wave polarity on the 12-lead ECG, allow accurate prediction the location of the accessory pathway [74]. This is quite useful when planning radiofrequency catheter ablation to treat patients with Wolff-Parkinson-White (WPW) syndrome. The need for possible transseptal puncture (left-sided accessory pathways) or the risk for AV block (anteroseptal pathway) can be anticipated.

Although orthodromic AV reentry tachycardia is the most common tachycardia in patients with WPW syndrome, these patients may also develop atrial fibrillation. In atrial fibrillation, the accessory pathway may allow rapid conduction to the ventricles, which can result in VF and sudden death. The risk for sudden death in patients with WPW sysdrome is estimated at 1 per 1000 patient-year follow-up [75]. The conduction properties of the accessory pathway are believed to be the prime determinant of VF induction during atrial fibrillation (Fig. 14). When compared to WPW patients with atrial fibrillation but with out sudden death, WPW with atrial fibrillation and survived sudden death have been found to have shorter minimum preexcited RR intervals (180 $\pm$ 30 milliseconds versus 240 $\pm$ 60 milliseconds) and shorter mean RR intervals (270 $\pm$ 60 milliseconds versus 340 $\pm$ 80 milliseconds) during induced atrial fibrillation [76]. However, a large overlap between these groups exists and a short ($<$250 millisecond) preexcited RR interval during induced atrial fibrillation was observed in approximately 17% of clinically asymptomatic WPW, resulting in a high false positive rate. Patients with VF are more likely to have multiple accessory pathways [77]. Thus, close attention to the preexcitation pattern at rest or during atrial fibrillation might provide a clue to the presence of more than one pathway. A clinically useful observation, although seen in only 5% to 15% of patients, is the loss of antegrade pathway conduction (loss of preexcitation) on a resting 12-lead ECG or during exercise stress testing [78]. This finding correlates well with an accessory pathway refractory period of $>$300 milliseconds and a mean RR interval (during atrial fibrillation) of $>$300 milliseconds. The loss of preexcitation has to be abrupt, and be associated with an increase in the PR interval to rule out enhanced AV nodal conduction. Such findings

characterize a pathway with poor antegrade conduction properties, which does not allow rapid AV conduction during atrial fibrillation; thus, there is a very low risk for VF and sudden death.

References

[1] Pratt CM, Grennway PS, Schoenfield MH, et al. Exploration of the precision of classifying sudden cardiac death. Implications for the interpretation of clinical trials. Circulation 1996;93:519–24.

[2] Zheng ZJ, Croft JB, Giles WH, et al. Sudden death in the United States 1989–1998. Circulation 2001; 104:2158–63.

[3] Myerburg RJ, Kessler KM, Castellanos A. Sudden death: epidemiology, transient risk and intervention assessment. Ann Intern Med 1993;119:1187–97.

[4] de Vreede-Swagemakers JJ, Gorgels APM, Dubois-Arbouw WI, et al. Out-of hospital cardiac arrest in the 1990s: a population based study in the Maastricht area on incidence, characteristics and survival. J Am Coll Cardiol 1997;30:1500–5.

[5] Moss AJ, Zareba W, Hall J, et al. Prophylactic implantation of a defibrillator in patients with myocardial infarction and reduced ejection fraction. N Engl J Med 2002;346:877–83.

[6] Bardy GH, Lee KL, Mark DB, et al. Amiodarone or an implantable cardioverter-defibrillator for congestive heart failure. N Engl J Med 2005;352:225–37.

[7] Kuller L, Cooper M, Perper J. Epidemiology of sudden death. Arch Intern Med 1972;129:714–9.

[8] Newman WP, Strong JP, Johnson WD. Community pathology of atherosclerosis and coronary artery disease in New Orleans. Morphologic findings in young black and white men. Lab Invest 1981;44: 496–501.

[9] Kudenchuck PJ, Cobb LA, Greene HL, et al. Late outcome of survivors of out of hospital cardiac arrest with left ventricular functions $>$50% and without significant coronary arterial narrowing. Am J Cardiol 1991;67:704–8.

[10] Freedman RA, Swerdlow CD, Soderholm-Difatte V, et al. Prognostic significance of arrhythmia inducibility or noninducibility at initial electrophysiologic study in survivors of cardiac arrest. Am J Cardiol 1988;61:578–82.

[11] Gorgeles APM, Gijsbers C, de Vreede-Swagemakers J, et al. Out of hospital cardiac arrest—the relevance of heart failure: the Maastricht Circulatory Arrest Registry. Eur Heart J 2003;24:1204–9.

[12] Maggioni AP, Zuanetti G, Franzosi MG, et al. Prevalence and prognostic significance of ventricular arrhythmias after acute myocardial infarction in the fibrinolytic era. GISSI-2 results. Circulation 1993; 87:312–22.

[13] Cairns JA, Connolly SJ, Roberts R, et al. Randomized trial of outcome after myocardial infarction in patients with frequent or repetitive ventricular

premature depolarizations: CAMIAT. Lancet 1997; 349:675–82.

[14] Zimetbaum PJ, Buxton AE, Batsford W, et al. Electrocardiographic predictors of arrhythmic death and total mortality in the Multicenter Unsustained Tachycardia Trial. Circulation 2004;110:766–9.

[15] Pitt B, Zannad F, Remme WJ, et al. The effect of spironolocatone on morbidity and mortality in patients with severe heart failure. N Engl J Med 1999;341: 709–17.

[16] MERIT-HF study group. Effect of metoprolol CR/XL in chronic heart failure: metoprolol CR/XL randomized intervention trial in congestive heart failure. Lancet 1999;353:2001–7.

[17] Luu M, Stevenson WG, Stevenson LW, et al. Diverse mechanisms of unexpected cardiac arrest in advanced heart failure. Circulation 1989;80:1675–80.

[18] Dec GW, Fuster V. Medical progress: idiopathic dilated cardiomyopathy. N Engl J Med 1993;331:1564.

[19] Teerlink JR, Jalaluddin M, Anderson S, et al. Ambulatory ventricular arrhythmias in patients with heart failure do not specifically predict in increased risk of sudden death. Circulation 2000;101:40–6.

[20] Schwartz K, Carrier L, Guicheney P, et al. Molecular basis for familial cardiomyopathies. Circulation 1995;91:532–40.

[21] Yamaguchi H, Ishimura T, Nishiyama S, et al. Hypertrophic non-obstructive cardiomyopathy with giant negative T waves (apical hypertrophy): ventriculographic and echocardiographic features in 30 patients. Am J Cardiol 1979;44:401–12.

[22] Frank S, Braunwald E. Idiopathic subaortic stenosis: clinical analysis of 126 patients with emphasis on the natural history. Circulation 1968; 37:759.

[23] Maron BJ. Hypertrophic cardiomyopathy: a systematic review. JAMA 2002;287:1308–20.

[24] Maron BJ, Casey SA, Poliac LC, et al. Clinical course of hypertrophic cardiomyopathy in a regional United States cohort. JAMA 1999;281:650–5.

[25] Maron BJ, Shirani J, Poliac LC, et al. Sudden death in young competitive athletes. Clinical, demographic and pathological profiles. JAMA 1996;276:199–204.

[26] Montgomery JV, Harris KM, Casey SA, et al. Relation of electrocardiographic patterns to phenotypic expression and clinical outcome in hypertrophic cardiomyopathy. Am J Cardiol 2005;96:270–5.

[27] McKenna WJ, Borggrefe M, England D, et al. The natural history of left ventricular hypertrophy in hypertrophic cardiomyopathy: an electrocardiographic study. Circulation 1982;66:1233.

[28] Erickson MJ, Sonnenberg B, Woo A, et al. Long term outcome in patients with apical hypertrophic cardiomyopathy. J Am Coll Cardiol 2002;39: 638–45.

[29] Marcus FI, Fontaine G. Arrhythmogenic right ventricular dysplasia/cardiomyopathy: a review. PACE 1995;18:1298–314.

[30] Thienne G, Nava A, Corrado D, et al. Right ventricular cardiomyopathy and sudden death in young people. N Engl J Med 1988;318:129–33.

[31] Rampazzo N, Nava A, Malacrida S, et al. Mutation in human desmoplakin domain binding to plakoglobin causes a dominant form of arrhythmogenic right ventricular cardiomyopathy. Am J Hum Genet 2002;71:1200–6.

[32] Tiso N, Stephan DA, Nava A, et al. Identification of mutation in the cardiac ryanodine receptor gene in families affected with arrhythmogenic right ventricular cardiomyopathy type 2 (ARVD2). Hum Mol Genet 2001;10:189–94.

[33] McKenna WJ, Thienne G, Nava A, et al. Diagnosis of arrhythmogenic right ventricular dysplasia/cardiomyopathy: task force of the working group myocardial and pericardial disease of the European Society of Cardiology and the Scientific Council on Cardiomyopathies of the international society and federation of cardiology. Br Heart J 1994;71:215–8.

[34] Marcus FI. Prevalence of T wave inversion beyond V1 in young normal individuals and usefulness for the diagnosis of arrhythmogenic right ventricular dysplasia/cardiomyopathy. Am J Cardiol 2005;95: 1070–1.

[35] Fontaine G, Umemura J, DiDonna P, et al. La duree des complexes QRS dans la dysplasie ventriculaire droite arythmogene. Un noveau marqueur diagnostique non-invasif. Ann Cardiol Angeiol (Paris) 1993; 42:399–405.

[36] Nasir K, Bomma C, Tandri H, et al. Electrocardiographic features of arrhythmogenic right ventricular dysplasia/cardiomyopathy according to disease severity. A need to broaden diagnostic criteria. Circulation 2004;110:1527–34.

[37] Turrini P, Corrado D, Basso C, et al. Noninvasive risk stratification in arrhythmogenic right ventricular cardiomyopathy. Ann Noninvasive Electrocardiol 2003;8:161–9.

[38] Peters S, Peters H, Thierfelder L. Risk stratification of sudden cardiac death and malignant ventricular arrhythmias in right ventricular dysplasia-cardiomyopathy. Int J Cardiol 1999;71:243–50.

[39] Jervell A, Lange-Nielsen F. Congenital deaf mutism, functional heart disease with prolonged QT interval and sudden death. Am Heart J 1957;54:59–68.

[40] Moss AJ, Robinson J. Clincial features of idiopathic long QT syndrome. Circulation 1992;85(suppl I): II40–4.

[41] Vincent GM, Timothy KW, Leppert M, et al. The spectrum of symptoms and QT intervals in carriers of the gene for the long-QT syndrome. N Engl J Med 1992;327:846–52.

[42] Schwartz PJ, Moss AJ, Vincent GM, et al. Diagnostic criteria for the long QT syndrome: an update. Circulation 1993;88:782–4.

[43] Moss AJ, Zareba W, Benhorin J, et al. ECG T-wave patterns in genetically distinct forms of the

hereditary long QT syndrome. Circulation 1995;92: 2929–34.

[44] Zareba W, Moss AJ, Schwartz PJ, et al. Influence of the genotype on the clinical course of the long QT syndrome. N Engl J Med 1998;339:960–5.

[45] Schwartz PJ, Priori SG, Spazzolini C, et al. Genotype-phenotype correlation in the long QT syndrome. Gene specific triggers for life-threatening arrhythmias. Circulation 2001;103:89–95.

[46] Ackerman MJ, Khositseth A, Tester D, et al. Epinephrine induced QT interval prolongation: a gene specific paradoxical response in congenital long QT syndrome. Majo Clin Proc 2002;77: 413–21.

[47] Khosiseth A, Hejlik J, Shen WK, et al. Epinephrine induced T wave notching in congenital long QT syndrome. Heart Rhythm 2005;2:141–6.

[48] Priori SG, Schwartz PJ, Napolitano C, et al. Risk stratification in the long-QT syndrome. N Engl J Med 2003;348:1866–74.

[49] Zareba W, Moss AJ, Vessie C, et al. T wave alternans in idiopathic long QT syndrome. J Am Coll Cardiol 1994;23:1541–6.

[50] Malfatto G, Beria G, Sala S, Bonazzi O, et al. Quantitative analysis of T wave abnormalities and their prognostic implications in the long QT syndrome. J Am Coll Cardiol 1994;23:296–301.

[51] Gussak I, Brugada P, Brugada J, et al. Idiopathic short QT interval: a new clinical syndrome? Cardiology 2000;94:99–102.

[52] Gaita F, Giustetto C, Bianchi F, et al. Short QT syndrome. A familial cause of sudden death. Circulation 2003;108:965–70.

[53] Bellocq C, Ginneken GC, Bezzina C, et al. Mutation in the KCNQ1 Gene leading to the short QT interval syndrome. Circulation 2004;109:2394–7.

[54] Giusetto C, Wolpert C, Anttonnen OM, et al. Clinical presentation of the patients with short QT syndrome. Heart Rhythm 2005;2(II):S61.

[55] Gaita F, Giustetto C, Bianchi F, et al. Short QT syndrome: pharmacological treatment. J Am Coll Cardiol 2004;43:1494–9.

[56] Brugada P, Brugada J. Right bundle branch block persistent ST segment elevation and sudden death: a distinct clinical and electrocardiographic syndrome. A multicenter report. J Am Coll Cardiol 1992;20:1391–6.

[57] Chen Q, Kirsch GE, Zhang D, et al. Genetic basis and molecular mechanism for idiopathic ventricular fibrillation. Nature 1998;392:293–5.

[58] Antzelevitch C. The Brugada syndrome: ionic basis and arrhythmia mechanisms. J Cardiovasc Electrophysiol 2001;12:268–72.

[59] Antzelevitch C, Brugada P, Borggrefe M, et al. Brugada syndrome. Report of the second consensus conference. Heart Rhyhtm 2005;2:429–40.

[60] Miyazaki T, Mitamura H, Miyoshi S, et al. Autonomic and antiarrhythmic drug modulation of ST

segment elevation in patients with Brugada syndrome. J Am Coll Cardiol 1996;27:1061–70.

[61] Fujiki A, Usui M, Nagasawa H, et al. ST segment elevation in the right precordial leads induced with class Ic antiarrhythmic drugs: insight into the mechanism of Brugada syndrome. J Cardiovasc Electrophysiol 1999;10:214–8.

[62] Gasparini M, Priori S, Mantica M, et al. Flecainide test in Brugada syndrome: a reproducible but risky tool. PACE 2003;26(pt II):338–41.

[63] Dumaine R, Towbin JA, Brugada P, et al. Ionic mechanism responsible for the electrocardiographic phenotype of the Brugada syndrome are temperature dependent. Circ Res 1999;85:803–9.

[64] Priori SG, Napolitano C, Gasparini M, et al. Natural history of Brugada syndrome. Insights for risk stratification and management. Circulation 2002; 105:1342–7.

[65] Brugada P, Brugada R, Mont L, et al. Natural history of Brugada syndrome: the prognostic value of programmed electrical stimulation of the heart. J Cardiovasc Electrophysiol 2003;14:455–7.

[66] Sarkozy A, Brugada P. Sudden cardiac death and inherited arrhythmia syndromes. J Cardiovasc Electrophysiol 2005;16(suppl):S8–20.

[67] Consensus Statement of the Joint Steering Committees of UCARE and of IVF-US. Survivors of out-of-hospital cardiac arrest with apparently normal heart: Need for definition and standardized clinical evaluation. Circulation 1997;95: 265–72.

[68] Leenhardt A, Glaser E, Burguera M, et al. Short coupled variant of torsade de pointes. A new electrocardiographic entity in the spectrum of idiopathic ventricular fibrillation. Circulation 1994; 89:206–15.

[69] Leenhardt A, Lucet V, Denjoy I, et al. Catecholaminergic polymorphic ventricular tachycardia in children. A 7 year follow-up of 21 patients. Circulation 1995;91:1512–9.

[70] Priori SG, Napolitano C, Natascia T, et al. Mutations of the cardiac ryanodine receptor gene (hRyR2) underlie catecholaminergic polymorphic ventricular tachycardia. Circulation 2001;103: 196–200.

[71] Krahn AD, Gollob M, Yee R, et al. Diagnosis of unexplained cardiac arrest: role of adrenaline and procainamide infusion. Circulation 2005;112: 2228–34.

[72] Krahn AD, Manfreda J, Tate RB. The natural history of electrocardiographic preexcitation in men. The Manitoba follow-up study. Ann Intern Med 1992;116:456–60.

[73] Orejerana LA, Vidaillet HJ, DeStefano F. Population prevalence of Wolff-Parkinson-White syndrome. J Am Coll Cardiol 1995; abstr 327A.

[74] Fitzpatrick AP, Gonzales RP, Lesh MD, et al. New algorithm for the localization of accessory

atrioventricular connections using a baseline electro-cardiogram. J Am Coll Cardiol 1994;23:107–16.

[75] Klein GJ, Prystowsky EN, Yee R, et al. Asymptom-atic Wolff-Parkinson-White. Should we intervene? Circulation 1989;80:1902–5.

[76] Klein GJ, Bashore TM, Sellers TD, et al. Ventricular fibrillation in the Wolff-Parkinson-White syndrome. N Engl J Med 1979;301:1080–5.

[77] Pappone C, Santinelli V, Rosanio S, et al. Usefulness of invasive electrophysiologic testing to stratify the risk of arrhythmic events in asymptomatic patients with Wolff-Parkinson-White syndrome. J Am Coll Cardiol 2003;41:239–44.

[78] Levy S, Broustedt JP. Exercise testing in the Wolff-Parkinson-White syndrome. Am J Cardiol 1981;48: 976–9.

ELSEVIER
SAUNDERS

Cardiol Clin 24 (2006) 471–490

CARDIOLOGY
CLINICS

Diagnostic Value of the 12-Lead Electrocardiogram during Conventional and Biventricular Pacing for Cardiac Resynchronization

S. Serge Barold, MD[a],*, Michael C. Giudici, MD[b],
Bengt Herweg, MD[a], Anne B. Curtis, MD[a]

[a]Division of Cardiology, University of South Florida College of Medicine and Tampa General Hospital,
Tampa, FL 33615, USA
[b]Division of Cardiology, Genesis Heart Institute, Davenport, IA, USA

The "low-tech" paced 12-lead surface ECG has fallen into disuse for routine pacemaker evaluation because it adds expense that is not usually reimbursed, and requires an additional piece of hardware. It is widely believed that the majority of pacemaker evaluation can be appropriately performed with a single-channel rhythm strip in conjunction with "high-tech" ECG/marker systems of pacemaker programmers. Intellectually, a 12-lead ECG would be ideal for all pacemaker evaluations, but most physicians do not have adequate support staff, time, and resources to do this when it will not be reimbursed by third-party payers. It is, however, important for the physician to recognize when a single-lead evaluation is inadequate and when a 12-lead ECG is essential to perform a proper evaluation [1]. This is especially important to evaluate patients with biventricular devices for cardiac resynchronization [2–7].

The pacemaker stimulus

Digital recorders distort pacemaker stimuli and produce striking changes in amplitude and polarity. Digital recorders can also miss some or all the of the pacemaker stimulus because of sampling characteristics involving a relatively narrow window. Some digital recorders process stimuli into an artifactual standard-size ECG deflection. Diagnostic evaluation of the pacemaker stimulus was possible with old analog-writing systems but no longer with modern digital technology.

Normal QRS patterns during right ventricular pacing

Pacing from the right ventricle (RV), regardless of site, virtually always produces a left bundle branch block (LBBB) pattern in the precordial leads (defined as the absence of a positive complex in lead V_1 recorded in the fourth or fifth intercostal space) [2,8,9]. Pacing from the RV apex produces negative paced QRS complexes in the inferior leads (II, III, and aVF) because depolarization begins in the inferior part of the heart and travels superiorly away from the inferior leads (Fig. 1). The mean paced QRS frontal plane axis is always superior, usually in the left, or less commonly in the right, superior quadrant.

Pacing from the right ventricular outflow tract

Primary lead placement in the right ventricular outflow tract (RVOT), septum, or lead displacement from the RV apex toward the RVOT shifts the frontal plane paced QRS axis to the left inferior quadrant, a site considered normal for spontaneous QRS complexes [8]. The inferior leads become positive. The axis then shifts to the right inferior quadrant as the stimulation site moves more superiorly toward the pulmonary

* Corresponding author.
E-mail address: ssbarold@aol.com (S.S. Barold).

cardiology.theclinics.com

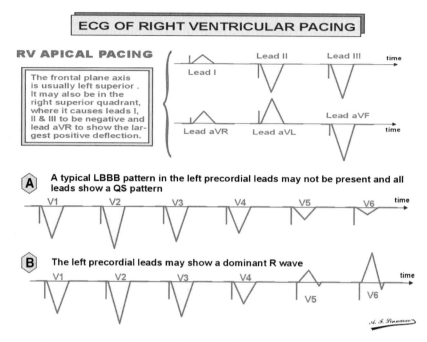

Fig. 1. Diagrammatic representation of the 12-lead ECG during apical RV pacing. (*Reproduced from* Barold SS, Stroobandt RX, Sinnaeve AF. Cardiac pacemakers step by step. An illustrated guide. Malden [MA]: Blackwell-Futura; 2004, with permission.)

valve (Fig. 2). With the backdrop of dominant R waves in the inferior leads, RVOT pacing may generate qR, QR, or Qr complexes in leads I and aVL (Fig. 3) [8]. Occasionally with slight displacement of the pacing lead from RV apex to the RV outflow tract, leads I and aVL may register a qR complex in conjunction with the typical negative complexes of RV apical stimulation in the inferior leads (Figs. 4 and 5). This qR pattern in

leads I and aVL must not be interpreted as a sign of myocardial infarction [10].

qR and Qr complexes in inferior and precordial leads

RV pacing from any site never produces qR complexes in V5 and V6 in the absence of myocardial infarction or ventricular fusion with

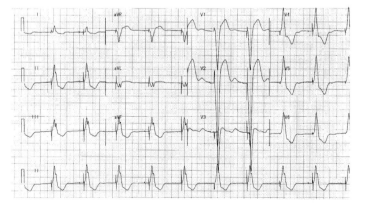

Fig. 2. Twelve-lead ECG during pacing the RV outflow tract. The frontal plane axis points to the left inferior quadrant, and there is a LBBB pattern in the precordial leads because there is no dominant R wave in lead V_1.

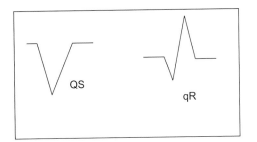

Fig. 3. Diagram showing the difference between a QS complex and a qR complex.

a spontaneous conducted QRS complex. A qR or Qr (but not QS, as shown in Fig. 3) complex in the precordial or inferior leads is always abnormal during RV pacing from any site in the absence of ventricular fusion (Fig. 6). In contrast, a q wave is common in the lateral leads (I, aVL, V_5, and V_6) during uncomplicated biventricular pacing (using the RV apex), and should not be interpreted as representing myocardial infarction or RVOT displacement of an RV apical lead. On the other hand, uncomplicated RV apical pacing rarely displays a qR complex in lead I (but not aVL) [2,8].

Dominant R wave of the paced QRS complex in lead V_1 during conventional right ventricular apical pacing

A dominant R wave in V_1 during RV pacing has been called a right bundle branch block (RBBB) pattern of depolarization, but this terminology is potentially misleading because this pattern may not be related to RV activation delay (Box 1). In our experience, a dominant R wave of a paced ventricular beat in the right precordial leads (V_1 and V_2 recorded in the fourth intercostal space) occurs in approximately 8% to 10% of patients with uncomplicated RV apical pacing [8,9,11,12]. The position of precordial leads V_1 and V_2 should be checked, because a dominant R wave can sometimes be recorded at the level of the third or second intercostal space during uncomplicated RV apical pacing (Figs. 7 and 8). The pacing lead is almost certainly in the RV (apex or distal septal site) if leads V_1 and V_2 show a negative QRS complex when recorded one space lower (fifth intercostal space). However, a dominant R wave may not be always eliminated at the level of the fifth intercostal space if RV pacing originates from the midseptal region [13].

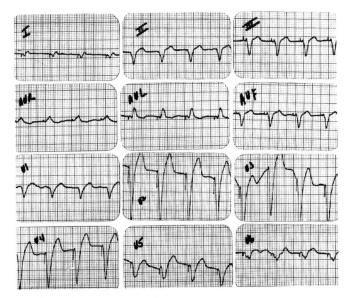

Fig. 4. Lead displacement from RV apex to mid-septal pacing simulating anterior myocardial infarction. ECG during VVI pacing in a patient with idiopathic cardiomyopathy, atrial fibrillation, complete heart block, and normal coronary arteries. After implantation of a pacemaker lead at the RV apex, the ECG showed a dominant QRS complex in leads I and aVL without a q wave. Three days after implantation this ECG shows qR complexes only in leads I and aVL, with major negativity in the inferior leads. The pacing lead was slightly displaced upwards toward the outflow tract as shown in Fig. 5. (*Reproduced from* Barold SS. Complications and follow-up of cardiac pacemakers. In: Singer I, Kupersmith, editors. Clinical manual of electrophysiology. Baltimore [MD]: Williams & Wilkins; 1993, with permission.)

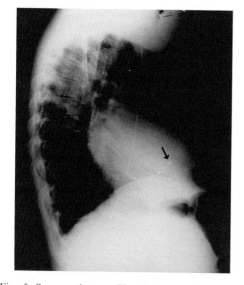

Fig. 5. Same patient as Fig. 4. Lateral chest X-ray showing displacement of the pacing lead toward the RV outflow tract.

Furthermore, in the normal situation with the ventricular lead in the RV, the "RBBB" pattern from pacing RV sites results in a vector change from positive to negative by lead V_3 in the precordial sequence. Therefore, a tall R wave in V_3 and V_4 signifies that a pacemaker lead is most probably not in the RV after excluding ventricular fusion from spontaneous atrioventricular conduction. However, left ventricular (LV) pacing generating a positive complex in lead V_1 may not necessarily be accompanied by a positive complex in leads V_2 and V_3. The ECG pattern with a truly posterior RV lead has not been systematically investigated as a potential cause of a tall R wave in V_1 during RV pacing.

We have never seen a so-called RBBB pattern in lead V_1 during uncomplicated RV outflow tract pacing, and it has never been reported so far. Right axis deviation of the ventricular paced beats in the frontal plane with a deep S wave in leads I and aVL does not constitute a RBBB pattern without looking at lead V_1.

Significance of a small r wave in lead V_1 during uncomplicated right ventricular pacing

A small early (r) wave (sometimes wide) may occasionally occur in lead V_1 during uncomplicated RV apical or outflow tract pacing. There is no evidence that this r wave represents a conduction abnormality at the RV exit site. Furthermore, an initial r wave during biventricular pacing does not predict initial LV activation [1].

Left ventricular endocardial pacing

Passage of a pacing lead into the LV rather than the RV occurs usually via an atrial septal defect (patent foramen ovale) or less commonly

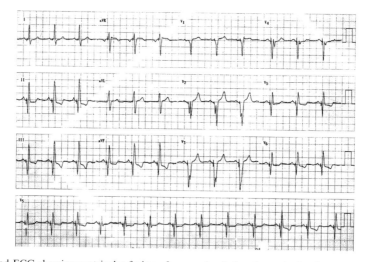

Fig. 6. Twelve-lead ECG showing ventricular fusion of pacemaker-induced ventricular depolarization with the native QRS complex generated by spontaneous atrioventricular conduction. The fusion QRS complex is narrow. Note the QR complexes in leads II, III, aVF, V_5, and V_6. The pattern simulates myocardial infarction during DDD pacing (AS-VP) in a patient with sick sinus syndrome, relatively normal AV conduction, and no evidence of coronary artery disease. The spontaneous ECG showed a normal QRS pattern.

Box 1. Causes of a dominant R wave in lead V1 during conventional ventricular pacing

- Ventricular fusion.
- Pacing in the myocardial relative refractory period.
- Left ventricular pacing from the coronary venous system.
- Left ventricular endocardial or epicardial pacing.
- Lead perforation of the right ventricle or ventricular septum with left ventricular stimulation.
- Uncomplicated right ventricular pacing (Lead V_1 recorded too high or in the correct place)

via the subclavian artery [13–28]. The diagnosis of a malpositioned endocardial LV lead will be missed in a single-lead ECG. The problem may be compounded if the radiographic malposition of the lead is not obvious or insufficient

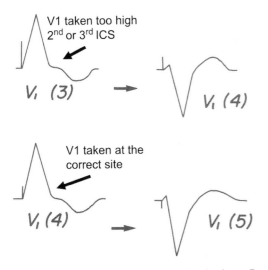

Fig. 7. Diagram showing evaluation of a dominant R wave in lead V_1 during uncomplicated RV pacing. When a dominant R wave occurs when V_1 is recorded one or two ICS too high, a negative QRS complex will often be recorded in the fourth ICS which is the correct site for V_1. If the dominant R wave persists or is initially recorded in the fourth ICS, a negative QRS complex will be recorded one ICS lower in the fifth ICS. (*Reproduced from* Barold SS. Complications and follow-up of cardiac pacemakers. In: Singer I, Kupersmith J, editors. Clinical manual of electrophysiology. Baltimore [MD]: Williams & Wilkins; 1993, with permission.)

projections are taken. A 12-lead paced ECG will show an RBBB pattern of paced ventricular depolarization, commonly with preserved QRS positivity in the right precordial leads or at least V_1 (Fig. 9). The positive QRS complexes are unaltered when leads V_1 and V_2 are recorded one intercostal space lower. During LV pacing, the frontal plane axis of paced beats can indicate the site of LV pacing, but as a rule, with a RBBB configuration the frontal plane axis cannot differentiate precisely an endocardial LV site from one in the coronary venous system. The diagnosis of an endocardial LV lead is easy with transesophageal echocardiography. In the usual situation, it will show the lead crossing the atrial septum then passing through the mitral valve into the LV. An endocardial LV lead is a potential source of cerebral emboli. Most patients with neurologic manifestations do not exhibit echocardiographic evidence of thrombus on the pacing lead. In symptomatic patients, removal of the lead after a period of anticoagulation should be considered. A chronic LV lead in asymptomatic or frail elderly patients is sometimes best treated with long-term anticoagulant therapy.

A Medline search from the years 2000 to 2005 revealed a substantial number of reports documenting inadvertent endocardial LV lead placement (pacing and implantable cardioverter-defibrillator leads). The true incidence of this problem is unknown, but the Medline data suggest that there are probably many unreported cases. It is disturbing that this serious but avoidable complication (simply by looking at a 12-lead ECG at the time of implantation) is still being recognized at late follow-up when lead extraction can be problematic.

ECG patterns recorded during LV pacing from the coronary venous system

An RBBB pattern in a correctly positioned lead V_1 occurs with few exceptions when the stimulation site is in the posterior or posterolateral vein (Fig. 10) [2–5,7,9,29,30]. Leads V_2 and V_3 may or may not be positive. With apical sites, leads V_4 to V_6 are typically negative. With basal locations, leads V_4 to V_6 are usually positive, as with the concordant positive R waves during overt preexcitation in left-sided accessory pathway conduction in the Wolff-Parkinson-White syndrome [3]. Pacing from the middle cardiac vein or the great (anterior) vein may occasionally produce a LBBB pattern, depending on the site of stimulation [31].

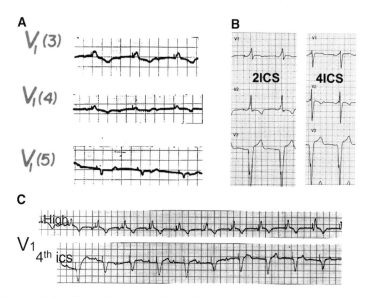

Fig. 8. Dominant R wave in lead V_1 during uncomplicated RV pacing. (*A*) Lead V_1 shows a dominant R wave in the third and fourth intercostal spaces (ICS) but a negative QRS complex is recorded one space lower in the fifth ICS. (*B*) Dominant R wave in lead V1 in ECG when leads V_1 and V_2 were recorded in the second ICS. The dominant R wave in V1 disappeared when V_1 and V_2 were recorded in the fourth ICS. (*C*) Tall R wave recorded in lead V_1 placed too high and its disappearance when V_1 was recorded in the correct fourth ICS. (*Reproduced from* Barold SS, Falkoff MD, Ong LS, et al. Electrocardiographic diagnosis of pacemaker malfunction. In: Wellens HJJ, Kulbertus HE, editors. What's new in electrocardiography? The Hague [The Netherlands]: Martinus Nijhoff; 1981, with permission. With permission from Springer Science and Business Media.)

LV pacing from the traditional site for resynchronization produces a RBBB pattern in lead V_1 virtually without exception. When lead V_1 shows a negative QRS complex during LV pacing, one should consider incorrect ECG lead placement (lead V_1 too high as in Fig. 11), location in the middle or great (anterior) cardiac vein, or an undefined mechanism requiring elucidation. The frontal plane axis often points to the right inferior quadrant (right axis deviation) and less commonly to the right superior quadrant. In an occasional patient with uncomplicated LV pacing with a typical RBBB pattern in lead V_1, the axis may point to the left inferior or left superior quadrant. The

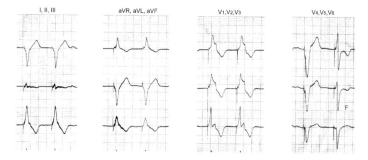

Fig. 9. ECG of a patient who received a dual-chamber pacemaker for sick sinus syndrome. Three years after pacemaker implantation, he presented with several transient ischemic attacks (TIAs). An ECG taken when the pacemaker was programmed to the VVI mode showed ventricular paced beats with a dominant R wave in leads V_1 to V_3 and right axis deviation in the frontal plane. There was a ventricular fusion beat in leads V_4 to V_6. A transesophgeal echocardiogram confirmed the position of the ventricular lead in the LR passing from the right atrium to the left atrium and crossing the mitral valve. The lead was successfully extracted percutaneously without complications using a modified technique to prevent embolization. A new lead in the RV produced ventricular-paced beats with the typical left bundle branch pattern and left superior axis deviation in the frontal plane.

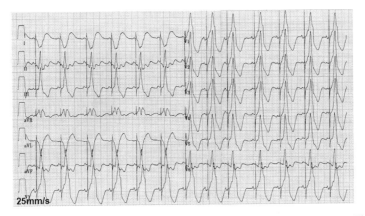

Fig. 10. Twelve-lead ECG showing monochamber LV pacing from the coronary venous system. There is typical right bundle branch pattern and right axis deviation. Note the dominant R wave from V_1 to V_6 consistent with basal LV pacing. LV pacing shown in all the subsequent figures was performed from the coronary venous system. (*Reproduced from* Barold SS, Herweg B, Giudici M. Electrocardiographic follow-up of biventricular pacemakers. Ann Noninvasive Electrocardiol 2005;10:231–55; with permission.)

reasons for these unusual axis locations are unclear.

ECG patterns and follow-up of biventricular pacemakers

So far, evaluation of the overall ECG patterns of biventricular pacing has focused mostly on simultaneous RV and LV stimulation [2,5,7,32–35]. A baseline 12-lead ECG should be recorded at the time of implantation during assessment of the independent capture thresholds of the RV and LV to identify the specific morphology of the paced QRS complexes in a multiplicity of leads [1]. This requires having the patient connected to a multichannel 12-lead ECG during the implantation procedure. A total of four 12-lead ECGs are required. (1) Intrinsic rhythm and QRS complex before any pacing. (2) Paced QRS associated with RV pacing. (3) Paced QRS

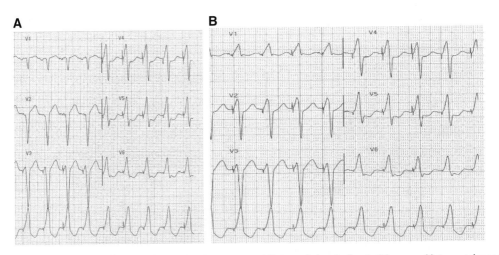

Fig. 11. (*A*) ECG recorded during LV pacing with leads V_1 and V_2 recorded at the level of the second intercostal space in a patient with a thin patient with an elongated chest during LV pacing. There is no dominant R wave in lead V_1. The ECG during biventricular pacing also failed to show a dominant R wave in V_1 at the level of the second intercostals space. (*B*) The dominant R wave in V_1 becomes evident only when lead V_1 is recorded in the fourth ICS. The R wave in V_1 recorded in the fourth ICS during biventricular pacing also became dominant. (*Reproduced from* Barold SS, Herweg B, Giudici M. Electrocardiographic follow-up of biventricular pacemakers. Ann Noninvasive Electrocardiol 2005;10:231–255; with permission.)

Table 1
Change in frontal plane axis of paced QRS when programming from biventricular to monochamber LV and RV pacing

Pacing site	QRS in lead I	QRS in lead III	Axis shift
BiV → RV	Greater positivity	Greater negativity[a]	Clockwise
BiV → LV	Greater negativity	Greater positivity	Counterclockwise

[a] QRS in lead III is more negative than in lead II.
Abbreviations: BiV, biventricular, LV, left ventricle; RV, right ventricle.

associated with LV pacing. (4) Paced QRS associated with biventricular pacing. The four tracings should be examined to identify the lead configuration that best demonstrates a discernible and obvious difference between the four pacing states (inhibited, RV only, LV only, and biventricular). This ECG lead should then be used as the surface monitoring lead for subsequent evaluations. Loss of capture in one ventricle will cause a change in the morphology of ventricular paced beats in the 12-lead ECG similar to that of either single chamber RV pacing or single-chamber LV pacing. A shift in the frontal plane axis may be useful to corroborate loss of capture in one of the ventricles [2,3,6,7]. If both the native QRS and the biventricular paced complex are relatively narrow, then a widening of the paced QRS complex will identify loss of capture in one chamber with effectual capture in the other.

Paced QRS duration and status of mechanical ventricular resynchronization

The paced QRS during biventricular pacing is often narrower than that of monochamber RV or LV pacing. Thus, measurement QRS duration during follow-up is helpful in the analysis of appropriate biventricular capture and fusion with the spontaneous QRS [3,4,7]. If the biventricular ECG is virtually similar to that recorded with RV or LV pacing alone and no cause is found, one should not automatically conclude that one of the leads does not contribute to biventricular depolarization without a detailed evaluation of the pacing system.

Chronic studies have shown that the degree of narrowing of the paced QRS duration is a poor predictor of the mechanical cardiac resynchronization response [7,36,37]. In other words, the degree of QRS narrowing or its absence does not correlate with the long-term hemodynamic benefit of biventricular pacing [7,36,37], because the paced QRS does not reflect the underlying level of mechanical dyssynchrony. In this respect some patients with monochamber LV pacing exhibit an

equal or superior degree of mechanical resynchronization compared with biventricular pacing despite a very wide-paced QRS complex [7,36,38].

Usefulness of the frontal plane axis of the paced QRS complex

Table 1 and Fig. 12 show the importance of the frontal plane axis of the paced QRS complex in determining the arrangement of pacing during testing of biventricular pacemakers [2,5,7]. The shift in the frontal plane QRS axis during programming the ventricular output is helpful in determining the site of ventricular stimulation in patients with first-generation devices without separately programmable RV and LV outputs (see Table 1).

Biventricular pacing with the right ventricular lead located at the apex

The frontal plane QRS axis usually moves superiorly from the left (RV apical pacing) to the right superior quadrant (biventricular pacing) in an anticlockwise fashion if the ventricular mass is predominantly depolarized by the LV pacing lead (Figs. 12 and 13) [2,3,6,7]. The frontal plane axis may occasionally reside in the left superior rather than the right superior quadrant during uncomplicated biventricular pacing.

The QRS is often positive in lead V_1 during biventricular pacing when the RV is paced from the apex (Fig. 13). A negative QRS complex in lead V_1 may occur under the following circumstances: incorrect placement of lead V_1 (too high on the chest), lack of LV capture, LV lead displacement, or marked latency (exit block or delay from the stimulation site, an important but poorly studied phenomenon with LV pacing) associated with LV stimulation, ventricular fusion with the conducted QRS complex, coronary venous pacing via the middle cardiac vein (also the anterior cardiac vein), or even unintended placement of two leads in the RV [39]. A negative QRS complex in lead V_1 during uncomplicated biventricular pacing probably reflects different activation of an heterogeneous biventricular substrate (ischemia, scar, His-Purkinje participation in view of

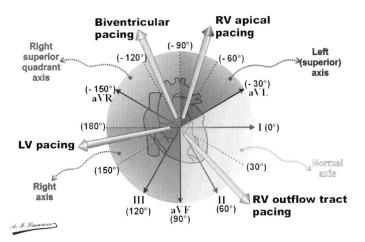

Fig. 12. Diagram showing the usual direction of the mean frontal plane axis during apical RV pacing, RV outflow tract pacing, LV pacing from the coronary venous system, and biventricular pacing with LV from the coronary venous system + RV from the apex. The axis during biventricular pacing from the LV from the coronary sinus + RV outflow tract usually points to the right inferior quadrant (right axis) as with monochamber LV pacing. (*Reproduced from* Barold SS, Stroobandt RX, Sinnaeve AF. Cardiac pacemakers step by step. An illustrated guide. Malden [MA]: Blackwell-Futura; 2004; with permission.)

the varying patterns of LV activation in spontaneous LBBB, and so on), and does not necessarily indicate a poor (electrical or mechanical) contribution from LV stimulation.

Biventricular pacing with the right ventricular lead in the outflow tract

In our limited experience we have found that during biventricular pacing with the RV lead in the outflow tract, the paced QRS in lead V_1 is often negative and the frontal plane paced QRS axis

is often directed to the right inferior quadrant (right axis deviation) (Fig. 14). Further studies are required to confirm these preliminary findings and to determine the significance of these ECG patterns of biventricular pacing according to the RV pacing site.

Q, or q and QS configuration in lead 1

Georger and colleagues [34] observed a q wave in lead I in 17 of 18 patients during biventricular pacing (Fig. 15). As indicated previously, a q wave

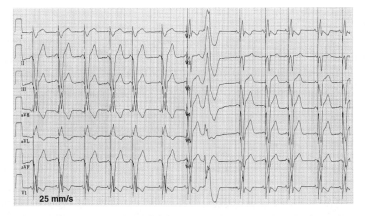

Fig. 13. ECG during biventricular pacing with the RV lead at the apex. There is a dominant R wave is V_1 and a right superior axis in the frontal plane. The QRS complex is relatively more narrow (170 milliseconds) than during single-chamber RV or LV pacing. (*Reproduced from* Barold SS, Herweg B, Giudici M. Electrocardiographic follow-up of biventricular pacemakers. Ann Noninvasive Electrocardiol 2005;10:231–55; with permission.)

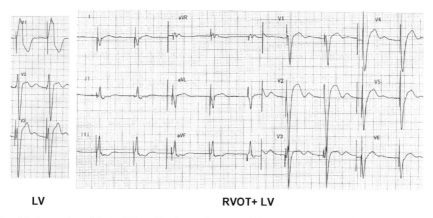

LV   **RVOT+ LV**

Fig. 14. Biventricular pacing with the RV lead in the outflow tract. There was a very prominent R wave in lead V_1 during monochamber LV pacing. Note the typical absence of a dominant R wave in lead V_1, and the presence of right axis deviation, an uncommon finding during biventricular pacing with the RV lead at the apex. The presence of ventricular fusion with the spontaneous conducted QRS complex was ruled out. (*Reproduced from* Barold SS, Herweg B, Giudici M. Electrocardiographic follow-up of biventricular pacemakers. Ann Noninvasive Electrocardiol 2005;10:231–55; with permission.)

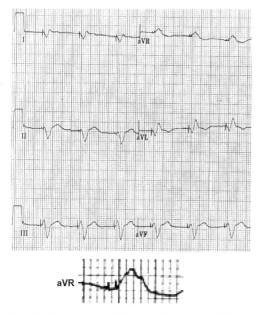

Fig. 15. Uncomplicated biventricular pacing (RV lead at the apex) in a patient with nonischemic cardiomyopathy. The interventricular (V-V) interval is 40 milliseconds with LV activation first. The six-lead ECG shows a Qr complex in lead I and a QR complex in lead aVL. This pattern does not indicate an old myocardial infarction. The frontal plane axis lies in the right superior quadrant as expected with this pacing arrangement. Bottom: magnified lead aVR showing separate RV and LV stimuli.

in lead I during uncomplicated RV apical pacing is rare, and these workers observed it in only one patient. Loss of the q wave in lead I was 100% predictive of loss of LV capture [34]. It therefore appears that analysis of the Q/q wave or a QS complex in lead I may be a reliable way to assess LV capture during biventricular pacing.

Ventricular fusion beats with native conduction

In patients with sinus rhythm and a relatively short PR interval, ventricular fusion with competing native conduction during biventricular pacing may cause misinterpretation of the ECG, and a common pitfall in device follow-up (Fig. 16) [2,7]. QRS shortening mandates exclusion of ventricular fusion with the spontaneous QRS complex, especially in the setting of a relatively short PR interval. The presence of ventricular fusion should be ruled out by observing the paced QRS morphology during progressive shortening of the AS-VP (atrial sensing-ventricular pacing) interval in the VDD mode or the AP-VP (atrial pacing-ventricular pacing) interval in the DDD mode. The AS-VP interval should be programmed to ensure pure biventricular pacing under circumstances that might shorten the PR interval such as increased circulating catecholamines. It is important to remember that a very narrow paced QRS complex may represent ventricular fusion (possibly associated with a suboptimal hemodynamic response) with the conducted QRS complex rather than near-perfect electrical ventricular resynchronization. In this respect, remarkable narrowing of the paced QRS complex occurs with triventricular pacing (two RV sites + LV), advocated by the French group for heart failure patients who have become refractory to conventional biventricular pacing [40].

Long-term ECG changes

Many studies have shown that the paced QRS duration does not vary over time as long as the LV pacing lead does not move from its initial site [7,36,41]. Yet, surface ECGs should be performed periodically because the LV lead may become displaced into a collateral branch of the coronary sinus. Dislodgement of the LV lead may result in loss of LV capture with the ECG showing an RV pacing QRS pattern with an increased QRS duration and superior axis deviation. Ricci and colleagues [41] suggested that variation of the QRS duration over time may play a determinant role if correlated with remodeling of the ventricles by echocardiography. Finally, the underlying spontaneous ECG should be exposed periodically to confirm the presence of a LBBB type of intraventricular conduction abnormality. In this respect, turning off the pacemaker could potentially improve LV function and heart failure in patients who have lost their intraventricular conduction delay or block through ventricular remodeling. In other words, a spontaneous narrow QRS is better than biventricular pacing.

Anodal stimulation in biventricular pacemakers

Although anodal capture may occur with high output traditional bipolar RV pacing, this phenomenon is almost always not discernible electrocardiographically. Biventricular pacing systems may use a unipolar lead for LV pacing via a coronary vein. The tip electrode of the LV lead is the cathode, and the proximal electrode of the bipolar RV lead often provides the anode for LV pacing. This arrangement creates a common anode for RV and LV pacing. A high current density (from two sources) at the common anode during biventricular pacing may cause anodal capture manifested as a paced QRS complex with a somewhat different configuration from that derived from pure biventricular pacing (Fig. 17) [42,43]. Anodal capture during biventricular pacing disappears by reducing the LV output of the pacemaker or when the device (even at high output) is programmed to a true unipolar system with the common anode on the pacemaker can,

a function that may not be available in devices with an ICD. Anodal capture was recognized in first-generation transvenous biventricular pacemakers (without separately programmable RV and LV outputs) when three distinct pacing morphologies were observed exclusive of fusion with the spontaneous QRS complex: Biventricular with anodal capture (at a high output), biventricular (at a lower output), and RV (with loss of LV capture) or rarely LV (with loss of RV capture). This form of anodal stimulation may also occur during biventricular pacing with contemporary devices [44,45] only if there is a common anode on the RV lead.

A different form of anodal capture involving the ring electrode of the bipolar RV lead can also occur with contemporary biventricular pacemakers with *separately programmable ventricular outputs* (Fig. 18). During monochamber LV pacing at a relatively high output, RV anodal capture produces a paced QRS complex identical to that registered with biventricular pacing. Occasionally, this type of anodal capture prevents electrocardiographic documentation of pure LV pacing if the LV pacing threshold is higher than that of RV anodal stimulation. Such anodal stimulation may complicate threshold testing, and should not be misinterpreted as pacemaker malfunction. Furthermore, if the LV threshold is not too high, appropriate programming of the pacemaker output should eliminate anodal stimulation in most cases. The use of true bipolar LV leads eliminates all forms of RV anodal stimulation.

Effect of interventricular V-V timing on the electrocardiogram of biventricular pacemakers

The electrocardiographic consequences of temporally different RV and LV activation with programmable V-V timing in the latest biventricular devices have not yet been studied in detail (Fig. 15). Contemporary biventricular devices permit programming of the interventricular interval usually in steps from +80 milliseconds (LV first) to −80 milliseconds (RV first) to optimize LV hemodynamics. In the absence of anodal stimulation, increasing the V-V interval gradually to 80 milliseconds (LV first) will progressively increase the duration of the paced QRS complex, alter its morphology with a larger R wave in lead V_1, indicating more dominant LV depolarization [46]. The varying QRS configuration in lead V_1 with

482 BAROLD et al

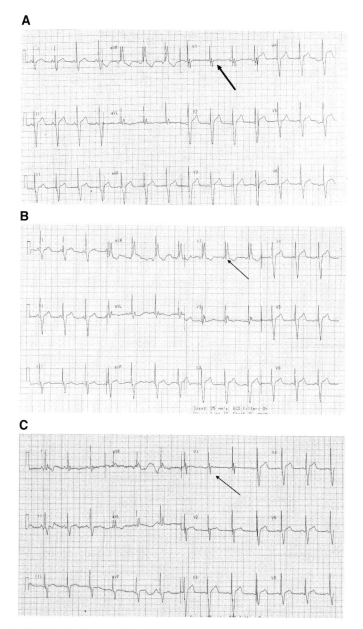

Fig. 16. (*A*) Twelve-lead ECGs showing ventricular fusion. Narrowing of the paced QRS complex (well seen in V$_1$) due to ventricular fusion with the spontaneous conducted QRS complex. This ECG was the initial recording taken upon arrival to the pacemaker follow-up center. AV delay = 100 milliseconds. The marked narrowing of the QRS complex in lead V$_1$ suggests ventricular fusion rather than QRS narrowing from satisfactory biventricular pacing. (*B*) The ECG taken 15 minutes later (same parameters and AV delay) when the patient was more relaxed shows no evidence of ventricular fusion. (*C*) Immediately after the tracing in (B), ventricular fusion was demonstrated only when the AV delay was lengthened to 130 milliseconds. The serial tracings illustrate the dynamic nature of AV conduction (emotion, catecholamines, and so on) and the importance of appropriate programming of the AV delay to prevent ventricular fusion with the spontaneous conducted QRS complex. (*Reproduced from* Barold SS, Herweg B, Giudici M. Electrocardiographic follow-up of biventricular pacemakers. Ann Noninvasive Electrocardiol 2005;10:231–55, with permission.)

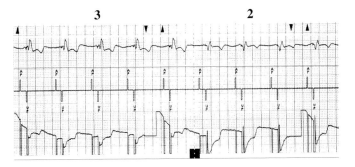

Fig. 17. Anodal capture during first-generation biventricular pacing. There is anodal capture on the left (three pacing sites). It disappears on the right (two pacing sites) with reduction of the common ventricular output revealing pure biventricular pacing. (*Reproduced from* Garrigue S, Barold SS Clémenty J. Electrocardiography of multisite ventricular pacing. In: Barold SS, Mugica J, editors. The fifth decade of cardiac pacing. Elmsford [NY]: Blackwell-Futura; 2004; with permission.)

different V-V intervals has not yet been correlated with the hemodynamic response.

RV anodal stimulation during biventricular pacing interferes with a programmed interventricular (V-V) delay (often programmed with the LV preceding the RV) aimed at optimizing cardiac resynchronization because RV anodal capture causes simultaneous RV and LV activation (The V-V interval becomes zero). In the presence of anodal stimulation, the ECG morphology and its duration will not change if the device is programmed with V-V intervals of 80, 60, and 40

milliseconds (LV before RV). The delayed RV cathodal output (80, 60, and 40 milliseconds) then falls in the myocardial refractory period initiated by the preceding anodal stimulation. At V-V intervals ≤20 milliseconds, the paced QRS may change because the short LV-RV interval prevents propagation of activation from the site of RV anodal capture in time to render the cathodal site refractory. Thus, the cathode also captures the RV and contributes to RV depolarization, which then takes place from two sites: RV anode, and RV cathode [46].

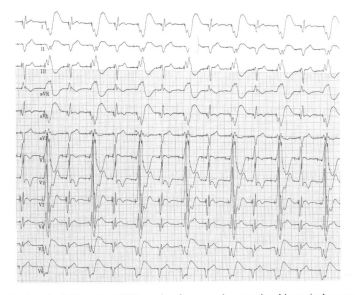

Fig. 18. Anodal pacing (on the left) in the DDD mode of a second-generation biventricular pacemaker seen during monochamber LV pacing with an LV output of 3.5 V and 0.5-millisecond LV. The ECG pattern was identical to that recorded during biventricular pacing. On the right, anodal stimulation alternates with pure LV pacing when the LV output is slightly less than 3.5 V at 0.5 milliseconds. (*Reproduced from* Herweg B, Barold SS. Anodal capture with second-generation biventricular cardioverter-defibrillator. Acta Cardiol 2003;58:435–6; with permission.)

Underlying arrhythmias

The presence of chronic atrial fibrillation is often poorly recognized in a continuously paced rhythm with resultant denial of anticoagulant therapy [47–49]. In a study by Patel and colleagues [47], atrial fibrillation was correctly identified in only 20% of patients with continuous pacing and in 40% with intermittent pacing. A single-lead is clearly unreliable for the diagnosis. A routine 12-lead ECG can provide the diagnosis of underlying atrial fibrillation in most patients, and reprogramming the pacemaker is usually unnecessary in the presence of a continuously paced rhythm.

Hypertrophic obstructive cardiomyopathy

Selection of the longest AV delay that achieves complete ventricular capture by QRS criteria may not be hemodynamically optimal during pacing for obstructive hypertrophic cardiomyopathy. In searching for a shorter more favorable AV delay, a 12-lead ECG is essential to verify the absence of ventricular fusion [50,51]. Lack of improvement may require repositioning of the RV lead with echocardiography to ensure a distal apical position because fluoroscopy and QRS morphology in the 12-lead ECG during pacing are imprecise markers of lead position.

Pacemaker alternans

Pacemaker QRS alternans is characterized by alternate changes in paced QRS morphology [52].

The causes include respiratory fluctuation, pericardial effusion, mechanical pulsus alternans leading to electrical alternans from varying depolarization, and true alternating intraventricular alternans from the pacing site. Alternans can only be diagnosed after ventricular bigeminy or alternate fusion beats (Fig. 19) are ruled out by changing the pacing rate. True alternans represents a form of exit block (persisting over a range of rates) seen only in severe myocardial disease under circumstances that also cause latency and second-degree Wenckebach exit block from the pacing site.

Atrial capture and resynchronization

Evaluation of atrial capture can be difficult in a single-lead ECG. In conventional dual-chamber pacing systems, the configuration, duration, and delay (and degree of atrial latency) of the paced P waves should be carefully evaluated in a 12-lead ECG for evidence of capture, and interatrial conduction delay (where the paced P wave is buried in the QRS complex) [53,54]. The 12-lead ECG taken at double standardization often brings out atrial deflections unclear in a standard tracing. Interatrial conduction delay requires reprogramming of the AV delay or the addition of a second atrial lead for biatrial pacing to provide optimal mechanical AV synchrony on the left side of the heart [55].

Latency

The delay from the pacing stimulus to the onset of ventricular depolarization is called

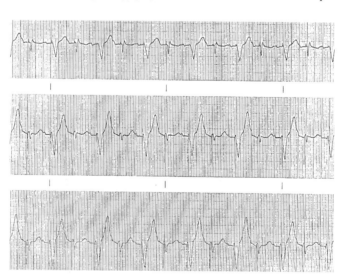

Fig. 19. Three-lead ECG (II, V1, and V5) showing pacemaker alternans in a patient with sinus rhythm, 2:1 AV block, and a DDD pacemaker. Every alternate beat is a ventricular fusion beat (pacing + spontaneous QRS complex).

latency (Fig. 20). An isoelectric onset of QRS complex in one or a few leads can mimic latency. Consequently, latency requires a 12-lead ECG for diagnosis. The normal values measures less than 40 milliseconds. Latency may progress to type I second-degree Wenckebach exit block with gradual prolongation of the spike-to-QRS interval, eventually resulting in an ineffectual stimulus [56,57]. Latency can only be evaluated by looking at a 12-lead ECG to rule out an isoelectric initial part of the QRS complex.

Causes of latency:

Right ventricular infarction
Anterior infarction
Severe myocardial disease
Hyperkalemia
Antiarrhythmic drug toxicity
Variant (Prinzmetal's) angina

These abnormalities usually occur in terminal situations, often with a combination of ischemia, acidosis, hypoxia, antiarrhythmic drugs, and hyperkalemia. Occasionally, latency and second-degree exit block occurs secondary to potentially reversible causes such as hyperkalemia and antiarrhythmic drug toxicity. In biventricular pacing, latency related to LV pacing may produce

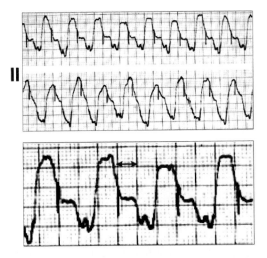

Fig. 20. Latency or first-degree pacemaker ventricular block. (Above) Two pacing rhythm strips, lead II taken at different times, showing a delay of up to 200 milliseconds between the unipolar stimulus artifact and the very broad QRS. (Below) Magnified view of four complexes from the above rhythm strip. The arrow highlights the latency period. (*Reproduced from* Kistler PM, Mond HG, Vohra JK. Pacemaker ventricular block. Pacing Clin Electrophysiol 2003;26:1997–9; with permission.)

suboptimal hemodynamics associated with an ECG showing the pattern of RV pacing because LV depolarization is delayed and overshadowed by RV stimulation. The electrical and hemodynamic problem can often be corrected by advancing LV stimulation by programming the interventricular (V-V) delay, a feature available only in contemporary devices.

Hyperkalemia

The paced QRS complex widens with hyperkalemia. Other common causes of a wide-paced QRS complex include amiodarone therapy and severe myocardial disease. Hyperkalemia can cause pacemaker–myocardial block, which may be reversible with or without a contribution from antiarrhythmic drug toxicity, especially type IA agents [58–65]. This produces first-degree exit block (latency) and second-degree type I (Wenckebach) exit block from the region of the pacemaker stimulus, eventually progressing to complete exit block with total lack of capture. In a dual-chamber device, hyperkalemia may cause failure of atrial capture associated with preservation of ventricular pacing (Fig. 21) [61–63]. This differential effect on atrial and ventricular excitability (pacing) correlates with the well-known clinical and experimental observations that the atrial myocardium is more sensitive to hyperkalemia than the ventricular myocardium. In this situation, the loss of atrial capture should be demonstrated at the maximum programmable AV delay to rule out latency.

Paced QRS duration during conventional right ventricular pacing

Sweeney and colleagues [66] recently found that a long-paced QRS duration was a significant, independent predictor of heart failure hospitalization in patients with sinus node dysfunction (hazard ratio 1.15; 95% confidence interval 1.07,1.23) for each 10-millisecond increase in paced QRS duration ($P = 0.001$). Paced QRS duration was not significant for mortality ($P = 0.41$) or atrial fibrillation ($P = 0.20$) when baseline QRS duration and other predictors were included [66]. The association of a wide paced QRS complex with the increased development of heart failure was confirmed by Miyoshi and colleagues [67], who also found that a prolonged paced QRS duration (≥ 190 milliseconds) was associated with a significant increase in the overall morbidity of heart

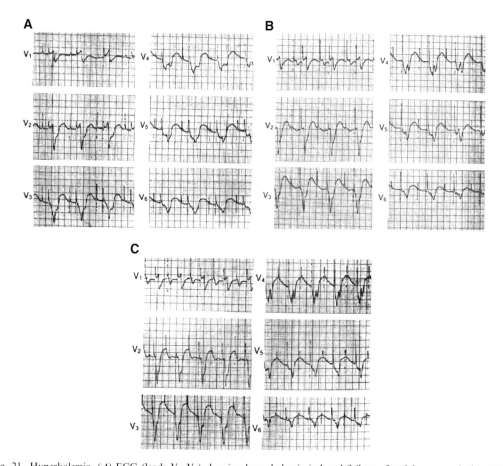

Fig. 21. Hyperkalemia. (*A*) ECG (leads V₁–V₆) showing hyperkalemia-induced failure of atrial capture during DDD pacing in a patient with severe congestive heart failure (K = 6.3 mEq/L). The paced QRS complex is widened to 0.36 seconds. Pacemaker variables: Lower rate = 70 ppm, AV delay = 200 milliseconds, atrial output = 8.1 V at a 1.0-millisecond pulse duration, and ventricular output = 5.4 V at a 0.6-millisecond pulse duration. (*B*) ECG showing restoration of atrial capture a few minutes after initial treatment of hyperkalemia. The pacemaker variables are the same as in (*A*). The duration of the QRS complex has shortened to 0.30 seconds. The interval from the atrial stimulus to the isoelectric segment of the PR interval measures approximately 0.22 seconds, and represents delay in interatrial conduction. (*C*) ECG recorded 24 hours after (*A*). Pacemaker variables: Lower rate = 90 ppm (increased from 70 because of congestive heart failure and ventricular ectopy), AV interval = 300 milliseconds, atrial output = 5.4 V at a 0.6-millisecond pulse duration, ventricular output = 5.4 V at a 0.6-millisecond pulse duration. The QRS complex has further shortened to 0.24 seconds. The interval from the atrial stimulus to the isoelectric segment of the PR interval has shortened to 0.16 seconds. (*Reproduced from* Barold SS, Falkoff MD, Ong LS, et al. Hyperkalemia-induced failure of atrial capture during dual-chamber cardiac pacing. J Am Coll Cardiol 1987;10:467–9; with permission from American College of Cardiology Foundation.)

failure (*P* < 0.05). On this basis, serial determinations of the paced QRS duration may be clinically useful to evaluate LV function and the risk of developing heart failure.

Unusual pacemaker stimuli

The ventricular triggered mode in some biventricular devices automatically attempts to provide ventricular resynchronization in the presence of ventricular sensing (Fig. 22). A ventricular-sensed event initiates an immediate emission of a ventricular or usually a biventricular output (according to the programmed settings) in conformity with the programmed upper rate interval. For example, Medtronic (Minneapolis, Minnesota) devices offer this function in the VVIR mode, but in dual-chamber devices triggering occurs upon sensing only in the programmed AV delay [2]. The ventricular output will be

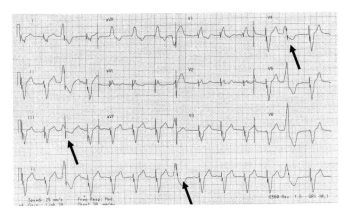

Fig. 22. Ventricular-triggered mode of third-generation Medtronic biventricular ICD (VVIR mode). The device triggers a biventricular output upon sensing the RV electrogram in an attempt to provide resynchronization upon sensing. The pacemaker stimuli (RV and LV) deform the sensed ventricular premature beats. The degree of electrical resynchronization cannot be determined from this tracing. (*Reproduced from* Barold SS, Herweg B, Giudici M. Electrocardiographic follow-up of biventricular pacemakers. Ann Noninvasive Electrocardiol 2005;10:231–55; with permission.)

ineffectual in the chamber where sensing was initiated because the myocardium is physiologically refractory. The stimulus to the other ventricle thus attempts to provide a measure of resynchronization. Ventricular triggering may be helpful in some patients, but its true benefit is difficult to assess as the ventricles may be activated in an order that may not be hemodynamically favorable.

Closely coupled (double) ventricular stimuli occur in two circumstances: (1) Biventricular pacing with V-V programming (Fig. 15) [46]. (2) Biventricular pacing with a conventional DDD pacemaker in patients with persistent atrial fibrillation where the "atrial" channel usually paces the LV and the ventricular channel paces the RV [68]. Two ventricular stimuli are often seen because such devices do not usually permit programming an AV interval of zero.

Artifacts resembling pacemaker stimuli

Artifacts occurring in the ECG of a paced patient create confusion. The term "triboelectric phenomena" is often used to describe high-voltage deflections generated by static electricity. Triboelectric signals are usually wider and more irregular than pacemaker stimuli, and often recognizable as artifacts. Occasionally, the diagnosis depends on finding subtle differences from the pacing stimulus [69–71]. Magnification of the questionable artifact may reveal a relatively prolonged overshoot not present with pacemaker stimuli. Such an overshoot is typical of electrostatic discharges, and should be sought in the evaluation of artifacts mimicking

pacemaker stimuli to avoid the diagnosis of pacemaker malfunction.

Summary

The paced 12-lead ECG is a valuable tool in the assessment of patients with pacemakers, and ideally should be recorded routinely at the time of implantation and during follow-up. It has become particularly important in patients undergoing cardiac resynchronization. The multiplicity of clinical situations described in this review highlight the pitfalls of using a single ECG lead in the overall evaluation of pacemaker patients. The design of programmers capable of registering a 12-lead ECG would obviate the need of an additional electrocardiograph and encourage the routine recording of the paced 12-lead ECG with each patient encounter. Such an arrangement would improve the care of pacemaker patients.

References

[1] Barold SS, Levine PA, Ovsyshcher IE. The paced 12-lead electrocardiogram should no longer be neglected in pacemaker follow-up. PACE 2001;24: 1455–8.

[2] Barold SS, Herweg B, Giudici M. Electrocardiographic follow-up of biventricular pacemakers. Ann Noninvasive Electrocardiol 2005;10:231–55.

[3] Asirvatham SJ. Electrocardiogram interpretation with biventricular pacing devices. In: Hayes DL, Wang PJ, Sackner-Bernstein J, Asirvatham SJ, editors. Resynchronization and defibrillation for heart

failure. A practical approach. Oxford (UK): Black-well-Futura; 2004. p. 73–97.

[4] Kay GN. Troubleshooting and programming of cardiac resynchronization therapy. In: Ellenbogen KA, Kay GN, Wilkoff BL, editors. Device therapy for congestive heart failure. Philadelphia (PA): WB Saunders; 2004. p. 232–93.

[5] Steinberg JS, Maniar PB, Higgins SL, et al. Noninvasive assessment of the biventricular pacing system. Ann Noninvasive Electrocardiol 2004;9:58–70.

[6] Lau CP, Barold S, Tse HF, et al. Advances in devices for cardiac resynchronization in heart failure. J Interv Card Electrophysiol 2003;9:167–81.

[7] Garrigue S, Barold SS, Clémenty J. Electrocardiography of multisite ventricular pacing. In: Barold SS, Mugica J, editors. The fifth decade of cardiac pacing. Elmsford (NY): Blackwell-Futura; 2004. p. 84–100.

[8] Barold SS. Normal and abnormal patterns of ventricular depolarization during cardiac pacing. In: Barold SS, editor. Modern cardiac pacing. Mt. Kisco (NY): Futura; 1985. p. 545–69.

[9] Barold SS, Falkoff MD, Ong LS, et al. Electrocardiographic analysis of normal and abnormal pacemaker function. In: Dreifus LS, editor. Pacemaker therapy, cardiovascular clinics. Philadelphia (PA): F.A.Davis; 1983. p. 97–134.

[10] Barold SS, Falkoff MD, Ong LS, et al. Electrocardiographic diagnosis of myocardial infarction during ventricular pacing. Cardiol Clin 1987;5:403–17.

[11] Klein HO, Becker B, Sareli P, et al. Unusual QRS morphology associated with transvenous pacemakers. The pseudo RBBB pattern. Chest 1985;87:517–21.

[12] Yang YN, Yin WH, Young MS. Safe right bundle branch block pattern during permanent right ventricular pacing. J Electrocardiol 2003;36:67–71.

[13] Coman JA, Trohman RG. Incidence and electrocardiographic localization of safe right bundle branch block configurations during permanent ventricular pacing. Am J Cardiol 1995;76:781–4.

[14] Ciolli A, Trambaiolo P, Lo Sardo G, et al. Asymptomatic malposition of a pacing lead in the left ventricle: the case of a woman untreated with anticoagulant therapy for eight years. Ital Heart J 2003;4:562–4.

[15] Paravolidakis KE, Hamodraka ES, Kolettis TM, et al. Management of inadvertent left ventricular permanent pacing. J Interv Card Electrophysiol 2004;10:237–40.

[16] Ergun K, Tufekcioglu O, Karabal O, et al. An unusual cause of stroke in a patient with permanent transvenous pacemaker. Jpn Heart J 2004;45:873–5.

[17] Arnar DO, Kerber RE. Cerebral embolism resulting from a transvenous pacemaker catheter inadvertently placed in the left ventricle: a report of two cases confirmed by echocardiography. Echocardiography 2001;18:681–4.

[18] Sharafi M, Sorkin R, Sharifi V, et al. Inadvertent malposition of a transvenous inserted pacing lead in the left ventricular chamber. Am J Cardiol 1995;76:92–5.

[19] Burkart TA, Lewis JF, Conti JB, et al. Malpositioned ventricular pacing l lead in the left ventricle. Clin Cardiol 2000;23:123–4.

[20] Agnelli D, Ferrari A, Saltafossi D, et al. A cardiac embolic stroke due to malposition of the pacemaker lead in the left ventricle. A case report. Ital Heart J 2000;1(1 Suppl):122–5.

[21] Van Gelder BM, Bracke FA, Oto A, et al. Diagnosis and management of inadvertently placed pacing and ICD leads in the left ventricle: a multicenter experience and review of the literature. PACE 2000;23:877–83.

[22] Agarwal A, Kapoor A, Garg N. Inadvertent transvenous left ventricular pacing. A case report. Indian Heart J 2000;52:331–4.

[23] Blommaert D, Mucumbitsi J, de Roy L. Images in cardiology. Ventricular pacing and right bundle branch block morphology: diagnosis and management. Heart 2000;83:666.

[24] Trigano JA, Paganelli F, Fekhar S, et al. Pocket infection complicating inadvertent transarterial permanent pacing. Successful percutaneous explantation. Clin Cardiol 1999;22:492–3.

[25] Chun JK, Bode F, Wiegand UK. Left ventricular malposition of pacemaker lead in Chagas' disease. Pacing Clin Electrophysiol 2004;27:1682–5.

[26] Orlov MV, Messenger JC, Tobias S, et al. Transesophageal echocardiographic visualization of left ventricular malpositioned pacemaker electrodes: implications for lead extraction procedures. Pacing Clin Electrophysiol 1999;22:1407–9.

[27] AL-Dashti R, Huynh T, Rosengarten M, et al. Transvenous pacemaker malposition in the systemic circulation and pacemaker infection: a case report and review of the literature. Can J Cardiol 2002;18:887–90.

[28] Firschke C, Zrenner B. Images in clinical medicine. Malposition of dual-chamber pacemaker lead. N Engl J Med 2002;346:e2.

[29] Shettigar UR, Loungani RR, Smith CA. Inadvertent permanent ventricular pacing from the coronary vein: an electrocardiographic, roentgenographic, and echocardiographic assessment. Clin Cardiol 1989;12:267–74.

[30] Altmiks R, Nathan AW. Left ventricular pacing via the great cardiac vein in a patient with tricuspid and pulmonary valve replacement. Heart 2001;85:91.

[31] Barold SS, Banner R. Unusual electrocardiographic pattern during transvenous pacing from the middle cardiac vein. Pacing Clin Electrophysiol 1978;1:31–4.

[32] Ammann P, Sticherling C, Kalusche D, et al. An electrocardiogram-based algorithm to detect loss of left ventricular capture during cardiac resynchronization therapy. Ann Intern Med 2005;142:968–73.

[33] Yong P, Duby C. A new and reliable method of individual ventricular capture identification during

biventricular pacing threshold testing. PACE 2000;
23:1735–7.

[34] Georger F, Scavee C, Collet B, et al. Specific electrocardiographic patterns may assess left ventricular
capture during biventricular pacing [abstract].
PACE 2002;25:56.

[35] Hart D, Luiza P, Arshad R, et al. Assessment of ventricular capture in patients with cardiac resynchronization devices; a simple surface electrocardiographic
algorithm [abstract]. PACE 2003;26:1083.

[36] Leclercq C, Kass DA. Retiming the failing heart:
principles and current clinical status of cardiac
resynchronization. J Am Coll Cardiol 2002;39:
194–201.

[37] Kass DA. Predicting cardiac resynchronization response by QRS duration: the long and short of it.
J Am Coll Cardiol 2003;42:2125–7.

[38] Leclercq C, Faris O, Tunin R, et al. Systolic improvement and mechanical resynchronization does
not require electrical synchrony in the dilated failing
heart with left bundle-branch block. Circulation
2002;106:1760–3.

[39] Kistler PM, Mond HG, Corcoran SJ. Biventricular
pacing: it isn't always as it seems. PACE 2003;26:
2185–7.

[40] Alonso C, Goscinska K, Ritter P, et al. Upgrading to
triple-ventricular pacing guided by clinical outcomes
and echo assessment; a pilot study [abstract]. Europace 2004;6(Suppl 1):195.

[41] Ricci R, Pignalberi C, Ansalone G, et al. Early and
late QRS morphology and width in biventricular
pacing: relationship to lead site and electrical
remodeling. J Interv Card Electrophysiol 2002;6:
279–85.

[42] Van Gelder BM, Bracke FA, Pilmeyer A, et al. Triple-site ventricular pacing in a biventricular pacing
system. PACE 2001;24:1165–7.

[43] Bulava A, Ansalone G, Ricci R, et al. Triple-site
pacing with biventricular device. Incidence of the
phenomenon and cardiac resynchronization benefit.
J Interv Card Electrophysiol 2004;10:37–45.

[44] Herweg B, Barold SS. Anodal capture with second-
generation biventricular cardioverter-defibrillator.
Acta Cardiol 2003;58:435–6.

[45] Thibault B, Roy D, Guerra PG, et al. Anodal right
ventricular capture during left ventricular stimulation in CRT-implantable cardioverter defibrillators.
Pacing Clin Electrophysiol 2005;28:613–9.

[46] van Gelder BM, Bracke FA, Meijer A. The effect of
anodal stimulation on V–V timing at varying V–V
intervals. Pacing Clin Electrophysiol 2005;28:771–6.

[47] Patel AM, Westveer DC, Man KC, et al. Treatment
of underlying atrial fibrillation: paced rhythm obscures recognition. J Am Coll Cardiol 2000;36:784–7.

[48] McLellan CS, Abdollah H, Brennan FJ, et al. Atrial
fibrillation in the pacemaker clinic. Can J Cardiol
2003;19:492–4.

[49] Sparks PB, Mond HG, Kalman JM, et al. Atrial
fibrillation and anticoagulation in patients with

permanent pacemakers: implications for stroke
prevention. Pacing Clin Electrophysiol 1998;21:
1258–67.

[50] Fananapazir L, McAreavey D. Therapeutic options
in patients with obstructive hypertrophic cardiomyopathy and severe drug-refractory symptoms.
J Am Coll Cardiol 1998;31:259–64.

[51] Barold SS. New indications for cardiac pacing. In:
Singer I, Barold SS, Camm AJ, editors. Nonpharmacological therapy of arrhythmias for the 21st
century. The state of the art. Armonk (NY): Futura;
1998. p. 775–95.

[52] Kleinfeld M, Barold SS, Rozanski JJ. Pacemaker
alternans. A review. Pacing Clin Electrophysio
1987;10:924–33.

[53] Daubert JC, Pavin D, Jauvert G, et al. Intra- and
interatrial conduction delay: implications for
cardiac pacing. PACE 2004;27:507–25.

[54] Parravicimi U, Mezzani A, Bielli M, et al. DDD pacing and interatrial conduction block:importance of
optimal interval setting. PACE 2000;23:1448–50.

[55] D'Allones GR, Pavin D, Leclercq C, et al. Long-
term effects of biatrial synchronous pacing to prevent drug-refractory atrial tachyarrhythmia:
a nine-year experience. J Cardiovasc Electrophysiol
2000;11:1081–91.

[56] Kistler PM, Mond HG, Vohra JK. Pacemaker ventricular block. Pacing Clin Electrophysiol 2003;26:
1997–9.

[57] Klein HO, Di Segni E, Kaplinsky E, et al. The
Wenckebach phenomenon between electric
pacemaker and ventricle. Br Heart J 1976;38:961–5.

[58] Peter T, Harper R, Hunt D, et al. Wenckebach
phenomenon in the exit area from a transvenous
pacing electrode. Br Heart J 1976;38:201–352.

[59] Mehta J, Khan AH. Pacemaker Wenckebach
phenomenon due to antiarrhythmic drug toxicity.
Cardiology 1976;61(3):189–94.

[60] Varriale P, Manolis A. Pacemaker Wenckebach
secondary to variable latency: an unusual form of
hyperkalemic pacemaker exit block. Am Heart J
1987;114:189–92.

[61] Barold SS. Loss of atrial capture during DDD
pacing: what is the mechanism? Pacing Clin Electrophysiol 1998;21:1988–9.

[62] Barold SS, Falkoff MD, Ong LS, et al. Hyperkalemia-induced failure of atrial capture during dual-
chamber cardiac pacing. J Am Coll Cardiol 1987;
10:467–9.

[63] Ortega-Carnicer J, Benezet J, Benezet-Mazuecos J.
Hyperkalaemia causing loss of atrial capture and
extremely wide QRS complex during DDD pacing.
Resuscitation 2004;62:119–20.

[64] Varriale P, Manolis A. Pacemaker Wenckebach
secondary to variable latency: an unusual form of
hyperkalemic pacemaker exit block. Am Heart J
1987;114:189–92.

[65] Dohrmann ML, Goldschlager NF. Myocardial
stimulation threshold in patients with cardiac

pacemakers: effect of physiologic variables, pharmacologic agents, and lead electrodes. Cardiol Clin 1985;3:527–37.

[66] Sweeney MO, Hellkamp AS, Lee KL, et al and Mode Selection Trial (MOST) Investigators. Association of prolonged QRS duration with death in a clinical trial of pacemaker therapy for sinus node dysfunction. Circulation 2005;111:2418–23.

[67] Miyoshi F, Kobayashi Y, Itou H, et al. Prolonged paced QRS duration as a predictor for congestive heart failure in patients with right ventricular apical pacing. Pacing Clin Electrophysiol 2005;28: 1182–8.

[68] Barold SS, Gallardo I, Sayad D. The DVI mode of cardiac pacing: a second coming? Am J Cardiol 2002;90:521–3.

[69] Kahan S, Miller CW, Hayes DL, et al. Triboelectric simulation of pacemaker malfunction. Europace 2002;4:325–7.

[70] Barold SS. Images is cardiology: initiation of pacemaker endless loop tachycardia by triboelectricity. Heart 2001;85:248.

[71] Barold SS, Falkoff MD, Ong LS, et al. Differential diagnosis of pacemaker pauses. In: Barold SS, editor. Modern cardiac pacing. Mt Kisco (NY): Futura; 1985. p. 587–613.

Status of Computerized Electrocardiography

Richard H. Hongo, MD[a],*, Nora Goldschlager, MD[b]

[a]Division of Cardiology, California Pacific Medical Center, 2100 Webster Street, Suite 516,
San Francisco, CA 94115, USA
[b]Division of Cardiology, San Francisco General Hospital, 1001 Potrero Avenue, Room 5G1,
San Francisco, CA 94110, USA

In the 1950s, the first step toward computerized electrocardiogram (ECG) analysis was taken with the successful development of the analog-to-digital converter. Electrical ECG signals could now be transformed into digital information that could then be processed by computer. The first published reports on computerized ECG analysis emerged in the early 1960s from two separate laboratories [1,2]. Pipberger and colleagues [1] championed the use of the Frank XYZ lead system, and Caceres and colleagues [2] developed the first analysis program for 12-lead ECGs. Initially, the simultaneously obtained three-orthogonal lead system had an advantage over the 12-lead system that was recorded sequentially. Eventually, the 12-lead system became capable of recording groups of three or more leads simultaneously. The familiar lead configuration (I–II–III, aVR–aVL–aVF, V1–V2–V3, V4–V5–V6) was introduced by Bonner and colleagues in 1972 [3]. Clinician preference ultimately led to the predominance of the 12-lead system over the orthogonal Frank XYZ lead system. By the mid-1970s, European and Japanese investigators were actively contributing to this new field.

The development of signal filtering in the 1960–1970s was a crucial step in advancing computerized ECG analysis. It was recognized that by changing the filtering, the same raw data could be manipulated into any number of different ECG signal tracings. The ECG signal was first processed using a 50-Hz low-pass filter (passage of lower frequency component with attenuation of frequencies above the cutoff frequency); this facilitated the blocking of electrical interference by 60-Hz alternating current (AC) power lines. It became apparent, however, that there was important information in the ECG signal in the 100-Hz region, especially in patients with heart disease, making higher cutoff frequencies necessary. AC noise was independently blocked with band-stop, or notch filters. Determination of the ideal cutoff frequency, in turn, influenced other processing parameters such as the sampling rate of the analog-to-digital converters.

Early computer analysis programs used "deterministic" algorithms that processed ECG data though multiple logical decision rules created by expert ECG readers. The algorithms used sharply defined "cutoff points" that determined whether or not a decision rule was fulfilled. With this type of analysis, "long-QT syndrome" could be diagnosed in one person but not another when the respective QT intervals differed by only 1 millisecond. Since the 1980s, probability theories and statistics have been incorporated into computerized ECG analysis. The use of Bayesian analysis better accounts for the complexities of ECG diagnosis, and introduces influences from elements such as pretest probabilities. Multivariate statistics, in turn, are used to analyze demographic parameters that affect pretest probabilities. More recently, artificial neural networks have also been looked at as a way to better mimic how expert ECG readers arrive at a diagnosis; that is, through pattern recognition [4,5].

The lack of standardization of technical parameters, logic systems, and diagnostic

---

There was no funding support in the writing of this article. There are no relationships that would pose a conflict of interest for either coauthor.

  * Corresponding author.
  E-mail address: rhongo@cpcmg.com (R.H. Hongo).

classifications has led to variability in performance among the different computer programs [6]. In 1975, the American Heart Association made comprehensive technical recommendations that were further expounded upon in 1990 [7,8]. In Europe, the "Common Standards for Quantitative Electrocardiography" project was launched in 1980. In collaboration with six North American and one Japanese center, and with follow-up studies performed in 1985 and 1989, this project was an effort to set an international standard for computerized ECGs [9]. An expanding reference database was created from ECGs obtained from actual patients with corresponding clinical data (ie, cardiac catheterizations, echocardiograms, and so on), as well as from computer-generated ECGs. Despite these efforts and the advances resulting from them, an international standard is still unrealized.

Despite the significant limitations of the initial systems, computerized ECG analysis was recognized early on as having the potential to make an important clinical contribution [10], and development gradually shifted from academic centers to industry. With the advent of the microprocessor in the 1970s, ECG analysis moved from mainframes housed in large rooms to portable carts at the bedside. The first commercial 12-lead ECG analysis program was made available in the early 1980s by Marquette Electronics, followed closely by Siemens-Elema. In an important and popular advance, Hewlett Packett and Marquette made computer analysis available on their portable ECG carts. In 1975, it was estimated that a mere 4 million ECGs were being processed by computer in the United States [11]. This estimate had increased to 15 million by 1983 [12]. The last comprehensive survey was performed in 1988 by Drazen and colleagues [11], at which time 52 million ECGs were being processed by computer, with revenues exceeding $70 million. It is estimated today that over 100 million ECGs are analyzed by computer annually in the United States, with a similar number in Europe and in the rest of the world. The ECG is still the most commonly performed cardiac test [13], and in the United States, virtually 100% are analyzed by computer.

Technical aspects of computer analysis

Computerized ECG analysis can be divided into three distinct stages: (1) signal processing,

(2) measurements, and (3) interpretation. In the first stage, electrical data are acquired and converted from analog to digital signals. The fidelity of the signal is better preserved with faster sampling rates. The signal is then filtered to eliminate noise. Data compression, transmission, and archiving are additional important aspects of digital processing. In the second stage, the processed signal undergoes wave recognition. This involves the computer first selecting the signal (or ECG complex) to be measured. The underlying basic rhythm is distinguished from premature complexes. The computer can also make a template from the composite of several complexes as a way to minimize the effects of small beat-to-beat variations. Simultaneous acquisition of ECG leads aids in wave recognition. Once there is appropriate labeling of wave onset and offset, interval and amplitude parameters are measured. In the final stage, the measured parameters are subjected to multiple criteria to arrive at the computer diagnosis.

Acquisition, conversion, and filtering of data

Simultaneous signal acquisition is today's standard. The ability to cross reference multiple signals improves the determination of wave onset and offset, especially of the QRS complex [14], and yields more accurate interval measurements and wave recognition. The conversion of the analog electrical signal to digital data inevitably results in a loss of information. The fidelity of the signal is better preserved when a higher bit resolution and a faster sampling rate are used. These parameters are limited by both microprocessing capability and also by storage capacity. A higher fidelity is required for computer analysis compared with visual reading. For the former, expert opinion recommends a maximum resolution of 10 mV and at least a 500-Hz sampling rate [8,9].

Filtering is performed before wave recognition to eliminate extraneous noise from the signal of interest. An example of high-frequency noise is myopotentials; movement artifact and baseline wander from respiration are common examples of low-frequency noise. Electrical interference from local power circuits, or "60-Hz AC noise," is another important source of unwanted signal that is frequently encountered in medical office and hospital environments. Low-pass filters (passage of lower frequency component, with attenuation of frequencies above the cutoff frequency) are effective in minimizing high-frequency noise.

Initial cutoff frequencies of 50 Hz were designed to also filter out "AC noise." As mentioned above, it has since been recognized that there is clinically significant information in the 100-Hz region, and a cutoff of 150 Hz is now recommended [8]. A band-stop, or notch filter (attenuation of component within a frequency band), is used to blanket 60-Hz noise.

High-pass filters (passage of higher frequency components, with attenuation of frequencies below the cutoff frequency) with a 0.5 Hz cutoff frequency will eliminate most baseline wander and motion artifact while allowing heart rates of more than 30 beats per minute to be detected. This cutoff, however, encroaches on the frequencies of ventricular repolarization (1–3 Hz) and distortion in the ST-segment and T-wave can occur. A lower cutoff of 0.05 Hz was the initial (1975) recommendation by the American Heart Association [7]

that effectively avoided repolarization distortion, but some baseline wander would still be present. As sophisticated filters that specifically target low-frequency distortions have become available, the low-frequency cutoff can be relaxed back up into the 0.5-Hz range.

The type of filtering and the choice of each cutoff frequency can dramatically alter the final processed signal. For instance, higher cutoff frequencies for the low-pass filter can result in uncovering high-frequency notches in the QRS complex that have been suggested by some to have clinical significance [15–17]. Higher cutoff frequencies also allow for more accurate amplitude measurements because less high-frequency signal is filtered out; a difference between 40 Hz and 100 Hz results in significant changes in measured amplitude [18]. Diagnoses that rely heavily on accurate amplitude measurements, such as

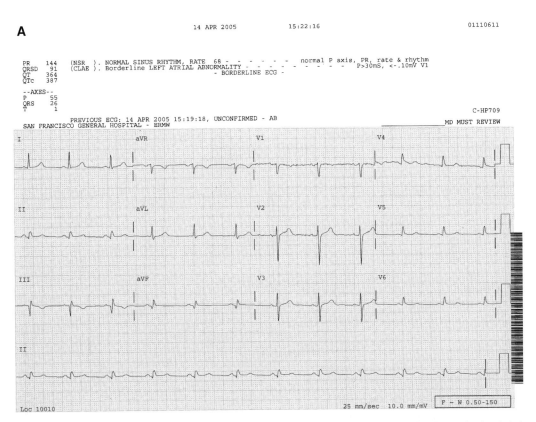

Fig. 1. (*A*) Significant Q waves in the inferior leads are not recognized by the computer, and the diagnosis of an inferior wall myocardial infarction is missed. (*B*) The QRS complex width is grossly undermeasured to be 100 milliseconds (manually measured to be 180 milliseconds), and the diagnosis of right bundle branch block is not made. (*C*) Ventricular preexcitation (delta waves) is not recognized by the computer, and is misinterpreted as Q waves in the lateral leads, leading to a diagnosis of lateral wall infarction. The prominent anterior forces, also due to ventricular preexcitation, lead to a misdiagnosis of right ventricular hypertrophy versus posterior myocardial infarction.

ventricular hypertrophy, are susceptible to these types of parameter changes. Filtering parameters also affects the limits on sampling rate, as the sampling frequency should be several times faster than the "high-frequency cutoff" [8].

Wave recognition and measurements

Before components of the ECG signal can be measured, the waves that make up the ECG signal must be identified. When the signal is taken during normal sinus rhythm, and patterns are regular and predictable, this process is relatively reliable. On the other hand, in the setting of atrial arrhythmias, this step can be challenging. Much of the accuracy of rhythm diagnosis depends on the proper recognition of irregular wave activity. The difficulties in diagnosing premature atrial complexes, atrial flutter, and atrial fibrillation stem from the inadequacies of atrial wave recognition. Techniques such as time-domain analysis of QRST-wave-subtracted electrograms have been used to unmask underlying atrial activity so that

ventricular electrical activity does not drown out the atrial signal. Spectral analysis can be used to detect regularity in the atrial activity, and can help distinguish atrial flutter from atrial fibrillation [19].

Once the waves are properly identified, duration and amplitude measurements are made. Although this step is seemingly straightforward, there are factors that can influence the precision and accuracy of these measurements. Despite significant improvements in the ability to analyze simultaneous ECG leads, identification of wave onset and offset varies among different computer programs. Identical raw digital data have been shown to result in differences in QRS duration and QT interval measurements, with mean differences of up to 18 and 24 milliseconds, respectively [20]. This is partly explained by the different ways various algorithms treat wave components such as isoelectric segments involving the Q or QS waves, or the U waves within the QT interval [9]. Imprecise measurement of the QRS complex and incorrect identification of wave components can lead to

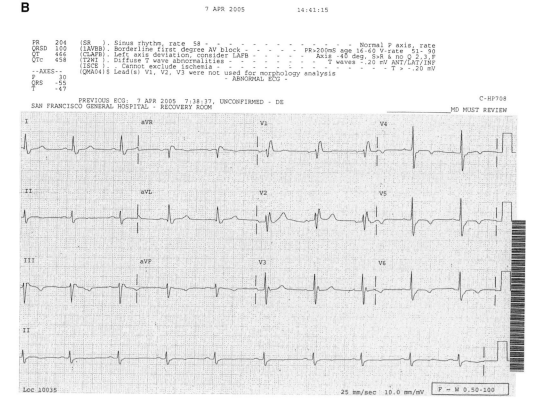

Fig. 1 (*continued*)

misinterpretation of important ECG diagnoses such as myocardial infarctions, bundle branch blocks, and ventricular preexcitation (Fig. 1).

Variability in amplitude measurement has been found to be less than that of interval measurements [20], but there can be day-to-day variability in voltage measurement of up to 20% that can result in reclassification and consequent differences in the computer diagnosis [21]. Some of the known factors that contribute to variability in voltage include fluctuation in metabolic and fluid status, variable lung and torso impedances, and changes in patient position that lead to change in the position of the heart within the chest. There are also procedural and equipment-related factors such as accuracy and consistency of electrode placement, low-pass filter settings, digital sample error, and variable performance among machines [22].

Interpretation and diagnostic classification

The foundation for computerized ECG interpretation has been a "deterministic" approach, or one that uses an algorithm with predictable behavior. This method relies on diagnostic criteria constructed by human experts. These criteria, in turn, are either met or not met, and do not allow for gradations. External factors that influence the likelihood of a diagnosis, such as pretest probability, are ignored. Bayesian probability theory has introduced a "statistical" approach. Considerations such as pretest probability, or clinical suspicion, can now be factored into the computer interpretation. For example, ST-segment elevation is much more likely be a manifestation of acute myocardial infarction if the patient is male, 65 years old, has a history of coronary disease, and is experiencing severe substernal chest pain, as opposed to an asymptomatic 30-year-old woman undergoing a routine screening ECG. Multivariate statistical methods are used to analyze the demographic parameters. The effectiveness of this type of statistical analysis, however, depends on the reliability of available ECG databases that become the basis for determining key determinants such as the prevalence of

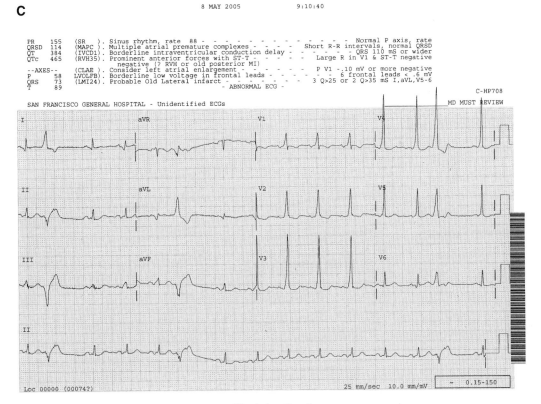

Fig. 1 (*continued*)

a particular diagnosis. Artificial neural networks, which use pattern recognition, have been incorporated into some programs [4,5].

The inability to know the specific details of the computer algorithms is a reality of industry-driven technology development, and the logic systems for ECG interpretation have become proprietary information of manufacturers. To a certain degree, programs are developed by trial and error, or by retesting against ECG databases [23]. These databases are created from real patient data, and from "electronically generated ECG signals" or "electronic test patients" [24,25]. Manufacturers report a high sensitivity and specificity for the major diagnoses when tested in this fashion [23]. A relatively small number of studies have evaluated the performance of computer analysis in the clinical setting. The rate of computer-generated diagnostic errors reported in these studies, however, is much larger than what would

be expected from the performance indices reported by the manufacturers. This suggests that the ECG databases used in testing these computer programs do not yet sufficiently represent the clinical population.

Current status of computerized electrocardiography

Willems and colleagues [26] compared the diagnostic abilities of nine computer programs with that of eight experienced cardiologists, using a database comprised of 1220 ECGs. The database was limited to patients with hypertrophy and infarction, and a control group. The final diagnoses were verified by nonelectrocardiographic clinical data. The combined overall accuracy of the computer programs was 76.3% compared with an accuracy of 79.2% for the cardiologists

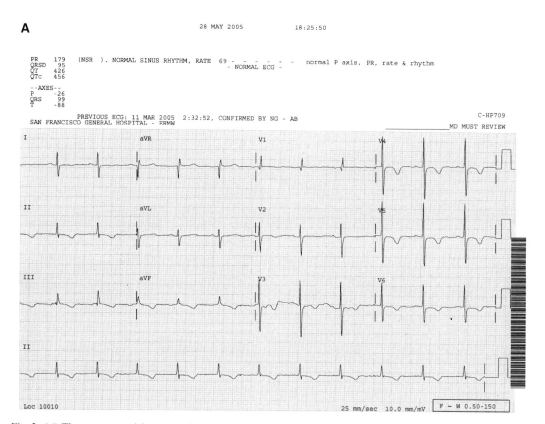

Fig. 2. (*A*) The computer misinterprets the 12-lead ECG to be a "normal ECG." Right axis deviation, qR complex in lead V1, and T-wave inversions in multiple leads are not detected by the computer algorithm. (*B*) The computer misinterprets the presence of "multiple atrial premature complexes" in this 12-lead ECG, missing the diagnosis of normal sinus rhythm. It is not clear from the tracing what is being misidentified as atrial premature complexes.

as a group. When the accuracy of the computer programs and cardiologists were assessed separately within each group, the median accuracy of computer programs was lower (69.7%) than that of the cardiologists (76.3%). Although some computer programs were clearly inferior to the interpretation of cardiologists, others were comparably accurate. In the detection of acute myocardial injury by ST-segment assessment, computer ECG analysis has been found to have lower sensitivity compared with expert readers (52% versus 66%, $P < 0.001$), but higher specificity (98% versus 95%, $P < 0.001$) [23].

Although computer ECG analysis can be comparable to interpretations by expert ECG readers, misinterpretations do occur. Bogan and colleagues [27] reported that out of 2298 computer diagnoses of atrial fibrillation, 19% were in error. Of particular concern was that of the inaccurate interpretations, 24% were not corrected by the ordering physician, and 10% received inappropriate therapy that included initiation of anticoagulation therapy and hospitalization. Misinterpretation of

the ECG, however, is not unique to computerized analysis. In a comprehensive review of the current literature on ECG interpretation, Salero and colleagues [28] found that 4% to 33% of physician interpretations contained errors of major importance, and inappropriate management occurred in up to 11% of patients. Adverse clinical outcomes, however, including preventable death, was observed in only 0.1% to 1.4% of cases.

Perhaps the major reason that computerized misinterpretations lead to clinical mismanagement is an overreliance on the accuracy of the computer algorithms. Primary care physicians have been observed to change up to 45% of their initial ECG interpretations after seeing a computerized interpretation [29], and the computer reading has been shown to mislead clinical decision making [30]. The computerized interpretation was found to not reduce major errors in ECG reading by senior house officers [31]. Many house officers fold over the computer reading at the top of the ECG tracing so it cannot influence their interpretation. Although this is done partly so that they

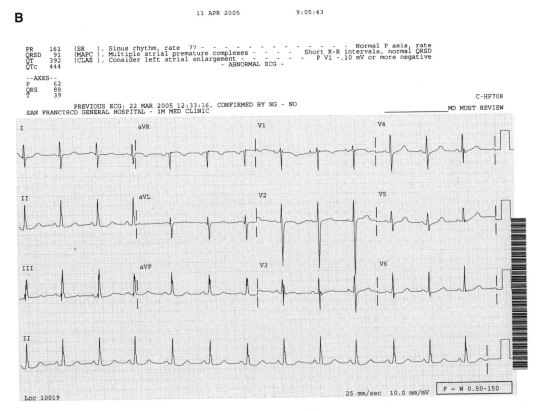

Fig. 2 (*continued*)

can practice their own interpretive skills, there is also a general mistrust of the computer reading. Because computerized ECG analysis is seldom reviewed during medical training, most physicians do not gain a sense of how reliable the computer reading is unless they become ECG readers.

As is true with any diagnostic test, computerized ECG analysis should be an adjunct to, not a substitute for, physician interpretation. When the limitations of the computer program are not known (which is usually the case), there is a real danger of physicians accepting the interpretation either without overreading, or without understanding the findings. A certain level of interpretive skill is needed by physicians overreading the ECG if they are expected to recognize misinterpretations by the computer. A firm understanding of the strengths and limitations of computer analysis is necessary if one is to use this diagnostic tool effectively.

Strengths of computerized ECG analysis

One of the most obvious strengths of computer analysis is the automated measurement of key parameters such as the heart rate, PR interval, QRS duration, and QT interval. Calculation of the corrected QT interval and axes are also performed automatically. This is an important component of ECG reading, but one that is extremely tedious if done manually. One should be aware of potential variability in the measured intervals, however, that stems from variability in inscribing wave onset and offset. The QT interval is the most difficult measurement because of a lack of agreement in the way T-wave offset is determined [32,33]; additional errors are made if TU waves are present. For this reason, when serial QT or QTU intervals are being monitored during antiarrhythmic drug therapy, it is not sufficient to follow the computerized measurement without

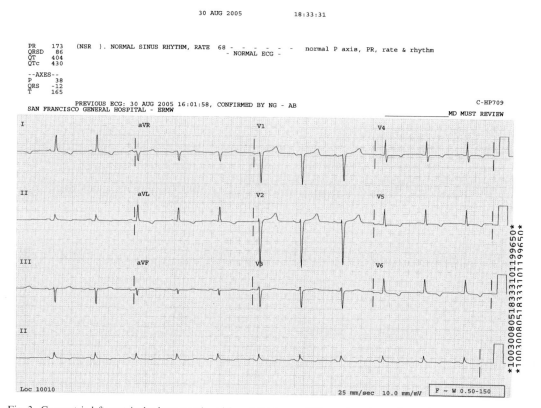

Fig. 3. Concentric left ventricular hypertrophy with wall thickness of 15 mm by echocardiography was not detected by the 12-lead ECG. The QRS complex amplitudes do not reach criteria for an ECG diagnosis. The accompanying repolarization changes with characteristic "strain" are seen, but not read by the computer.

verifying the intervals manually in multiple ECG leads.

Although a rare report can be found [34] that argues that computer interpretation slows readers down, the consensus of multiple studies [30,31,35–37] is that it saves time. Hillson and colleagues [30] performed a study in which 40 primary care physicians (family physicians and general internists) interpreted 10 ECGs with accompanying clinical vignettes. There was an average decrease in the time it took to read each tracing of 15 seconds (24%) when a computer reading was made available to the readers. Brailer and colleagues [35] evaluated 22 cardiologists that as a group read 1760 ECGs. Computerized analysis cut the time spent reading a tracing from an average of 81 seconds to 64 seconds (28%), while improving the accuracy of the readings.

The more straightforward diagnoses appear to be better detected by the computer, and most time is saved when the ECG is simple but tedious (multiple diagnoses) to read [35,38]. The computerized reading also offers a real-time second opinion that may prevent "inadvertent oversight." When the diagnoses are ambiguous or controversial, computerized interpretations can make over reading more time consuming [35].

The anecdotal experience of many ECG readers is that a computer interpretation of "normal ECG" is usually, but not always, correct (Fig. 2). Poon and colleagues [39] found the computer to have high sensitivity of 98.7% (3531/3579), but somewhat lower specificity of 90.1% (338/375) in diagnosing sinus rhythm. The authors cautioned against routinely accepting a computer interpretation of "sinus rhythm" because close to 10% of nonsinus rhythms were erroneously interpreted as sinus rhythm. Because the prevalence of sinus rhythm was high in this study (3579/3954), however, the positive predictive

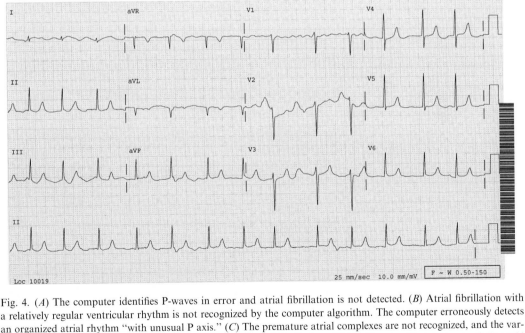

Fig. 4. (A) The computer identifies P-waves in error and atrial fibrillation is not detected. (B) Atrial fibrillation with a relatively regular ventricular rhythm is not recognized by the computer algorithm. The computer erroneously detects an organized atrial rhythm "with unusual P axis." (C) The premature atrial complexes are not recognized, and the variability in the ventricular rate lead to the misdiagnosis of atrial fibrillation. (D) Significant artifact that potentially could lead a reader to misdiagnose atrial fibrillation does not mislead the computer.

value of a computer diagnosis of "sinus rhythm" was 99.0%, supporting the sentiment that a computer statement of "sinus rhythm" is generally reliable.

Limitations of computerized ECG analysis

Limitations of electrocardiography as a diagnostic modality carry over to computerized electrocardiography. One of the most important limitations of electrocardiography is the inability to effectively detect certain anatomic and pathophysiologic conditions. Despite the development of multiple diagnostic ECG criteria, electrocardiography has only around a 50% sensitivity in detecting left ventricular hypertrophy that has been established by echocardiography (Fig. 3) [40–42]. It has been recognized for years that electrocardiography is better at diagnosing arrhythmias and conduction disturbances than structural cardiac or metabolic abnormalities. Ironically, rhythm interpretation is recognized to be one of the most difficult tasks for the computer.

Only a handful of studies have specifically evaluated the accuracy of computerized rhythm diagnosis. Shirataka and colleagues [24] found that although sinus rhythm with first-degree AV block had 100% agreement with the reference standard across five different computer programs, the accuracy of diagnosing second-degree AV block varied between 0% and 100%. In a study that assessed 11,610 consecutive computerized ECG interpretations, Varriale and colleagues [43] reported that multifocal atrial tachycardia was universally misdiagnosed as atrial fibrillation, accounting for 14% of ECGs interpreted as atrial fibrillation. Bogun and colleagues [27] found that of 2298 ECGs interpreted to be atrial fibrillation, 19% were misinterpreted by the computer. The difficulties in diagnosing atrial fibrillation is one of the most commonly encountered problems with computerized rhythm analysis (Fig. 4). More recently, Poon and colleagues [39] examined computerized rhythm interpretation by analyzing 4297 consecutive ECGs using one of the more advanced programs currently available (GE

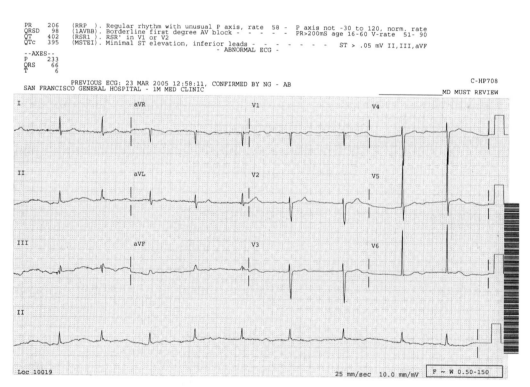

Fig. 4 (*continued*)

Marquette, version 19). The computerized interpretation was assessed against a consensus interpretation by reading cardiologists. Overall, 13.2% of the rhythm interpretations made by the computer were incorrect, and 7.8% if cardiac pacemaker activity misinterpretation was excluded.

The correct identification of pacemaker activity is still a major problem for today's computer software [44]. Poon and colleagues [39] reported that 75.2% of all pacemaker rhythms were misinterpreted. Because pacemaker stimulus outputs are very short in duration (generally 0.4–0.6 milliseconds), high sampling rates (>1000 Hz) are needed for adequate detection. In addition, current bipolar pacemaker systems are able to capture the myocardium with smaller amounts of energy, in turn resulting in progressively smaller pacemaker stimulus outputs that can be undetectable on the surface ECG. This reduction in stimulus output is facilitated by autocapture algorithms that allow the device to deliver its output just above the capture threshold, achieving pacemaker battery conservation while maintaining patient safety. Current algorithms "write in" the pacing output stimulus to make pacing activity apparent. High-frequency components of the ECG, such as pacemaker output stimuli, can sometimes disappear when the tracing is reprinted after data has been compressed for storage; the noncompressed ECG has the best signal fidelity and is the most appropriate for determining pacemaker rhythm. Considerable improvement has been made [45], however, especially in the detection of ventricular pacemaker activity, and newer iterations of the available algorithms are expected to have even further enhanced ability to define ventricular and atrial pacemaker stimuli.

There does appear to be progressive improvement in rhythm analysis software. The Marquette 12SL ECG Analysis software program (GE Health Care Technologies, Waukesha, Wisconsin) has been the single most studied commercial computer algorithm through its many versions [22,23,29,31,38,39]. The most current version 20 has been found to need physician correction of a rhythm interpretation in only 4.1% of cases [44] compared with 7.8% reported with version

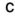

C

7 APR 2005
13:40:17
PR
QRSD 88
QT 310
QTc 419
(AFIB0). Atrial fibrillation, mean V-rate = 110 - - - V-rate varies, ? atrial activity
(T2WI). Diffuse T wave abnormalities - - - - - - - - T waves -.20 mV ANT/LAT/INF
(ISCE) . Cannot exclude ischemia - - - - - - - - - - - - - - T > -.20 mV
- ABNORMAL ECG -
--AXES--
P
QRS 70
T. 251
C-HP708
PREVIOUS ECG: 7 APR 2005 9:28:07, UNCONFIRMED - AB
SAN FRANCISCO GENERAL HOSPITAL - 5E ICU
MD MUST REVIEW
I
aVR
V1
V4
II
aVL
V2
V5
III
aVF
V3
V6
II
Loc 10055
25 mm/sec 10.0 mm/mV
F ~ W 0.50-100

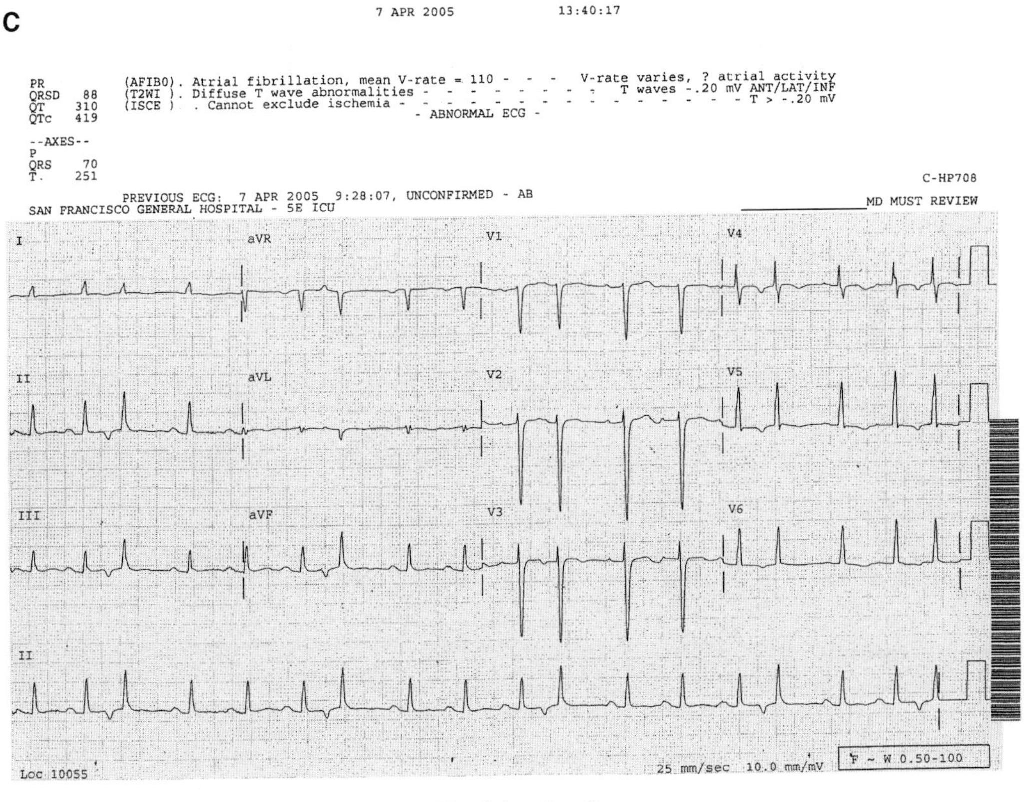

Fig. 4 (*continued*)

19 [39]. Although interpretive software from major manufacturers, such as GE Marquette and HP Phillips, include more sophisticated programming that specifically address difficult aspects of rhythm analysis, such as pacemaker activity recognition and analysis of pediatric ECGs, continued development is still needed [38].

Future directions

There are many challenges if current computerized ECG analysis programs are to be used to their fullest capabilities. On an individual physician level, there needs to be a fuller understanding of the strengths and limitations of the programs, so that overreliance on the computer reading is avoided. Continued improvement in the physician's own ECG interpretative skills will aid in recognition of computer misinterpretations, and will help steer clear of inappropriate management of patients. Teaching institutions are needed in this process, not only by encouraging higher standards

in ECG reading skills, but also by incorporating into their curricula instruction on the current status of computerized electrocardiography.

On the level of institutions and industry, medical centers are faced with the need to better integrate computer ECG analysis with expert physician overreading. Not only should computerized interpretations be verified in a timely manner that actually impacts clinical decision making, but also expert ECG readers should be made readily available for physicians at the point of patient care, both in the inpatient and outpatient setting [46]. Finally, developers are faced with the continued challenge of improving the accuracy of computer algorithms. ECG databases, used to test newer programs, should be sufficiently large, diverse, and contain all clinical diagnoses. True standardization within the industry should help facilitate this process, and efforts should continue toward this goal.

The reliability of computerized ECG analysis programs will only continue to improve, and the degree to which expert readers will continue to be

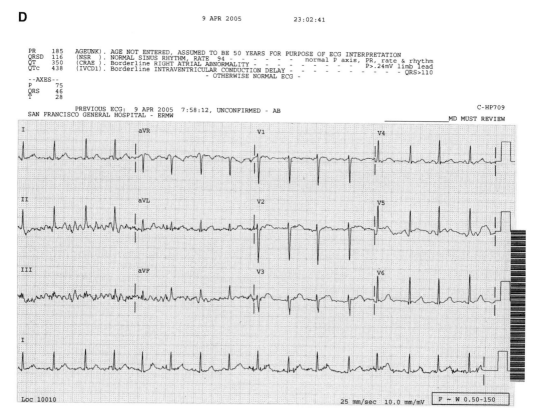

Fig. 4 (*continued*)

needed remains to be seen. The importance of understanding the technical aspects of computerized electrocardiography may, therefore, wane as computers become more accurate and physicians find that computerized interpretations can be trusted. In the meantime, until there is true automated ECG analysis, computerized interpretations should be viewed as an adjunct to, not a substitute for, interpretation by a competent and experienced physician.

Acknowledgments

The authors thank Dr. E. William Hancock, Professor of Medicine at Stanford University, and Dr. Paul D. Kligfield, Professor of Medicine at Cornell University, for their expert insights during the preparation of this manuscript.

References

[1] Pipberger HV, Arms RJ, Stallman FW. Automatic screening of normal and abnormal electrocardiograms by means of a digital electronic computer. Proc Soc Exp Biol Med 1961;106:130–2.

[2] Caceres CA, Steinberg CA, Abraham S, et al. Computer extraction of electrocardiographic parameters. Circulation 1962;25(2):356–62.

[3] Bonner RE, Crevasse L, Ferrer MI, et al. A new computer program for analysis of scalar electrocardiograms. Comput Biomed Res 1972;5(6):629–53.

[4] Holst H, Ohlsson M, Peterson C, et al. A confident decision support system for interpreting electrocardiograms. Clin Physiol 1999;19(5):410–8.

[5] Kaiser W, Faber TS, Findeis M. Automatic learning of rules: a practical example of using artificial intelligence to improve computer-based detection of myocardial infarction and left ventricular hypertrophy in the 12-lead ECG. J Electrocardiol 1996; 29(Suppl):17–20.

[6] Willems JL, Abreu-Lima C, Arnaud P, et al. Evaluation of ECG interpretation results obtained by computer and cardiologists. Methods Inf Med 1990;29(4):308–16.

[7] Pipberger HV, Arzbaecher RC, Berson AS, et al. Recommendations for standardization of leads and of specifications for instruments in electrocardiography and vectorcardiography: report of the Committee on Electrocardiography. Circulation 1975;52: 11–31.

[8] Bailey JJ, Berson AS, Garson A Jr, et al. Recommendations for standardization and specifications in automated electrocardiography: bandwidth and digital signal processing. A report for health professionals by an ad hoc writing group of the Committee on Electrocardiography and Cardiac Electrophysiology of the Council on Clinical Cardiology, American Heart Association. Circulation 1990;81(2):730–9.

[9] Willems JL, Arnaud P, van Bemmel JH, et al. Common standards for quantitative electrocardiography: goals and main results. Methods Inf Med 1990;29(4): 263–71.

[10] Burchell HB, Reed J. A test experience with a machine-processed electrocardiography diagnosis: the recognition of "normal" and some specific patterns. Am Heart J 1976;92(6):773–80.

[11] Drazen E, Mann N, Borun R, et al. Survey of computer-assisted electrocardiography in the United States. J Electrocardiol 1988;21(Suppl):S98–104.

[12] Grauer K, Kravitz L, Curry R Jr, et al. Computerized electrocardiogram interpretations: are they useful for the family physician? J Fam Pract 1987;24(1): 39–43.

[13] Kadish AH, Buxton AE, Kennedy HL, et al. ACC/ AHA clinical competence statement on electrophysiology and ambulatory electrocardiography. Circulation 2001;104(25):3169–78.

[14] Willems JL, Arnaud P, van Bemmel JH, et al. A reference database for multilead electrocardiographic computer measurement programs. J Am Coll Cardiol 1987;10(6):1313–21.

[15] Goldberger AL, Bhargava V, Froelicher V, et al. Effect of myocardial infarction on high-frequency QRS potentials. Circulation 1981;64(1):34–42.

[16] Pettersson J, Warren S, Mehta N, et al. Changes in high-frequency QRS components during prolonged coronary artery occlusion in humans. J Electrocardiol 1995;28(Suppl):225–7.

[17] Pettersson J, Carro E, Edenbrandt L, et al. Spatial, individual, and temporal variation of the high-frequency QRS amplitudes in the 12 standard electrocardiographic leads. Am Heart J 2000;139(2 Pt 1): 352–8.

[18] Garson A Jr. Clinically significant differences between the "old" analog and the "new" digital electrocardiograms. Am Heart J 1987;114(1 Pt 1):194–7.

[19] Taha B, Reddy S, Xue Q, et al. Automated discrimination between atrial fibrillation and atrial flutter in the resting 12-lead electrocardiogram. J Electrocardiol 2000;33(Suppl):123–5.

[20] Willems JL. A plea for common standards in computer aided ECG analysis. Comput Biomed Res 1980;13(2):120–31.

[21] McLaughlin SC, Aitchison TC, Macfarlane PW. The value of the coefficient of variation in assessing repeat variation in ECG measurements. Eur Heart J 1998;19(2):342–51.

[22] Farb A, Devereux RB, Kligfield P. Day-to-day variability of voltage measurement used in electrocardiographic criteria for left ventricular hypertrophy. J Am Coll Cardiol 1990;15(3):618–23.

[23] Kudenchuk PJ, Ho MT, Weaver WD, et al. Accuracy of computer-interpreted electrocardiography in selecting patients for thrombolytic therapy. J Am Coll Cardiol 1991;17(7):1486–91.

[24] Shirataka M, Miyahara H, Ikeda N, et al. Evaluation of five computer programs in the diagnosis of second-degree AV block. J Electrocardiol 1992; 25(3):185–95.

[25] Teppner U, Lobodzinski S, Neuberg D, et al. A technique to evaluate the performance of computerized ECG analysis systems. J Electrocardiol 1987; 20(Suppl):S68–72.

[26] Willems JL, Abreu-Lima C, Arnaud P, et al. The diagnostic performance of computer programs for the interpretation of electrocardiograms. N Engl J Med 1991;325(25):1767–73.

[27] Bogun F, Anh D, Kalahasty G, et al. Misdiagnosis of atrial fibrillation and its consequences. Am J Med 2004;117(9):636–42.

[28] Salerno SM, Alguire PC, Waxman HS. Competency in interpretation of 12-lead electrocardiograms: a summary and appraisal of published evidence. Ann Intern Med 2003;138(9):751–60.

[29] Grauer K, Kravitz L, Ariet M, et al. Potential benefits of a computer ECG interpretation system for primary care physicians in a community hospital. J Am Board Fam Pract 1989;2(1):17–24.

[30] Hillson SD, Connelly DP, Liu Y. The effects of computer-assisted electrocardiographic interpretation on physicians' diagnostic decisions. Med Decis Making 1995;15(2):107–12.

[31] Goodacre S, Webster A, Morris F. Do computer generated ECG reports improve interpretation by accident and emergency senior house officers? Postgrad Med J 2001;77(909):455–7.

[32] Xue Q, Reddy S. Algorithms for computerized QT analysis. J Electrocardiol 1998;30(Suppl):181–6.

[33] Azie NE, Adams G, Darpo B, et al. Comparing methods of measurements for detecting drug-induced changes in the QT interval: implications for thoroughly conducted ECG studies. Ann Noninvasive Electrocardiol 2004;9(4):166–74.

[34] Phibbs BP, Marriott HJL. Computer ECG programs: a critical evaluation. Primary Cardiol 1981; 7:49–60.

[35] Brailer DJ, Kroch E, Pauly MV. The impact of computer assisted test interpretation on physician decision making: the case of electrocardiograms. Med Decis Making 1997;17(1):80–6.

[36] Salerno SM, Alguire PC, Waxman HS. Training and competency evaluation for interpretation of 12-lead electrocardiograms: recommendation from the American College of Physicians. Ann Intern Med 2003;138(9):747–50.

[37] Sridharan MRL, Flowers NC. Computerized electrocardiographic analysis. Mod Concepts Cardiovasc Dis 1984;53:37–41.

[38] Snyder CS, Fenrich AL, Friedman RA, et al. The emergency department versus the computer: which is the better electrocardiographer? Pediatr Cardiol 2003;24(4):364–8.

[39] Poon K, Okin PM, Kligfield P. Diagnostic performance of a computer-based ECG rhythm algorithm. J Electrocardiol 2005;38(3):235–8.

[40] Romhilt DW, Bove KE, Norris RJ, et al. A critical appraisal of the electrocardiographic criteria for the diagnosis of left ventricular hypertrophy. Circulation 1969;40(2):185–95.

[41] Devereux RB, Casale PN, Eisenberg RR, et al. Electrocardiographic detection of left ventricular hypertrophy using echocardiographic determination of left ventricular mass as the reference standard. Comparison of standard criteria, computer diagnosis and physician interpretation. J Am Coll Cardiol 1984; 3(1):82–7.

[42] Casale PN, Devereux RB, Alonso DR, et al. Improved sex-specific criteria of left ventricular hypertrophy for clinical and computer interpretation of electrocardiograms: validation with autopsy findings. Circulation 1987;75(3):565–72.

[43] Varriale P, David W, Chryssos BE. Multifocal atrial arrhythmia—a frequent misdiagnosis? A correlative study using the computerized ECG. Clin Cardiol 1992;15(5):343–6.

[44] Farrell RM, Xue JQ, Young BJ. Enhanced rhythm analysis for resting ECG using spectral and time-domain techniques. Comput Cardiol 2003;30:733–6.

[45] Helfenbein ED, Lindauer JM, Zhou SH, et al. A software-based pacemaker pulse detection and paced rhythm classification algorithm. J Electrocardiol 2002;35(Suppl):95–103.

[46] Hongo RH, Goldschlager N. Overreliance on computerized algorithms to interpret electrocardiograms. Am J Med 2004;117(9):706–8.

ELSEVIER SAUNDERS

CARDIOLOGY CLINICS

Cardiol Clin 24 (2006) 505–513

Index

Note: Page numbers of article titles are in **boldface** type.

Moving?

Make sure your subscription moves with you!

To notify us of your new address, find your **Clinics Account Number** (located on your mailing label above your name), and contact customer service at:

E-mail: elspcs@elsevier.com

800-654-2452 (subscribers in the U.S. & Canada)
407-345-4000 (subscribers outside of the U.S. & Canada)

Fax number: 407-363-9661

Elsevier Periodicals Customer Service
6277 Sea Harbor Drive
Orlando, FL 32887-4800

*To ensure uninterrupted delivery of your subscription, please notify us at least 4 weeks in advance of move.